Artificial Vision

Veit Peter Gabel
Editor

Artificial Vision

A Clinical Guide

Springer

Editor
Veit Peter Gabel
Munich
Germany

ISBN 978-3-319-41874-2 ISBN 978-3-319-41876-6 (eBook)
DOI 10.1007/978-3-319-41876-6

Library of Congress Control Number: 2016958299

Printed on acid-free paper

This Springer imprint is published by Springer Nature
The registered company is Springer International Publishing AG Switzerland
The registered company address is Gewerbestrasse 11, 6330 Cham, Switzerland

Foreword

These are fascinating times for efforts toward restoring vision in individuals who are severely impaired or blind from retinal disease or injury. There is a long history of efforts to create prostheses for the sensory system. Hearing was the first to receive concerted attention. Of course, many hearing impaired individuals benefit from hearing aids which amplify sound and assist millions who are hearing impaired, particularly from presbycusis of hearing loss with age. But for individuals with essentially total absence of hearing, often on a congenital basis from genetic disease, simply amplifying the sound is insufficient, and one must stimulate the cochlea directly with electrodes. Efforts to design a cochlear implant were underway by the 1950s. The auditory system has the advantage that the sensory organ of the ear is readily accessible and that hair cells are laid out in linear one-dimensional order in the cochlea, from low to progressively higher tones. Simply snaking a continuous thread of many electrodes alongside the hair cells allows for stimulating residual cellular function in an orderly and tonally topographic fashion, and this was being done by 1964.

Work on developing a visual prosthesis was being considered in the 1980s. The task for vision is more complex, as stimulating the visual system requires transmitting two-dimensional spatial information, beginning with the retina. The retina is encased within the back of the eye, and access is possible but difficult. I recall that in 1984, during my ophthalmology fellowship at UCSF, vision scientists in the San Francisco Bay area gathered to review lessons learned from the auditory prosthesis and to consider the feasibility of developing a prosthesis for the visual system. Vision requires viewing a scene in two-dimensions, and the density of information is far greater than required for one-dimensional sound. The consensus at the time was a visual prosthesis based on stimulating the retina was too difficult to envision proceeding. Thus, it is gratifying now in 2016, that two visual retinal-based prostheses devices have actually been developed and are available commercially.

The technical challenges for a visual prosthesis are daunting. The majority of blinding conditions involve death of the photoreceptor cells that normally respond directly to light. These photoreceptors are the first stage of the visual process, and they send the visual signals progressively through the retina beginning with the bipolar cells, and then on to the ganglion cells which send their output through the optic nerve to visual centers in the brain. The death of photoreceptor cells obviously limits vision, as losing all photoreceptor cells consigns one to blindness. Hence, the early quest in the retina was to provide a substitute system to transduce light into electrical impulses and communicate this to the remaining bipolar cells. Such work was underway in the 1990s but proceeded slowly.

Two cellular targets were considered in the retina by different groups. One was the obvious replacement of the missing photoreceptor cells, to stimulate the retinal bipolar cells. Conceptually this could be accomplished by untethered photovoltaic photocells, but ultimately these were found to generate electrical impulses insufficient to activate bipolar cells. The solution required a passive electrode array, energized through a wire harness connected outside the eye. The second target was the ganglion cells which lie at the surface of the retina in orderly fashion in a two-dimensional topography of vision. Stimulating ganglion cells at the far periphery of the retina gives a visual sensation in one's peripheral vision, whereas stimulating ganglion cells in the macula near the center of the retina will generate a visual percept directly ahead in the line of sight.

However, technical challenges are immediately evident from considering the biology of neural visual processing in the retina. The millions of photoreceptor cells each correspond to individual discreet pixels of vision that recapitulate the visual scene. Signal processing through the successive layers of retinal neurons progressively extract visual information, and the initial, discreet pixilated vision of photoreceptors is systematically analyzed by an elaborate neural network in the retina, beginning with the bipolar cells. By the time the visual scene is communicated to ganglion cells at the retinal surface, the information has been recoded into abstract features of intensity, contrast and movement across the visual space from right to left, or top to bottom.

With these neural challenges, it is nothing short of remarkable that two visual prosthesis devices have passed through US and European regulatory approvals and have reached the marketplace and are available for patients. These devices are colloquially termed "retinal implants for artificial vision." Both consist of a two-dimensional array of electrodes to stimulate the remaining retinal cells electrically. One group produced the Tübingen MPDA Project Alpha IMS device that is implanted underneath the retina at the retinal location of the original photoreceptor cells that are lost from disease. This sub-retinal implant has 1500 microelectrodes that contact the retinal bipolar cells, to replace the photoreceptors lost in macular degeneration. Alpha-IMS obtained CE marking in 2013. A second device, the Argus II implant, is a two-dimensional array of 64 electrodes that sits on the surface of the retina, adjacent to the ganglion cells. This was approved for commercial use in Europe in 2012 and in the United States in 2013.

This book explores a range of topics pertinent to moving the field forward. Among these is a consideration of extra-retinal locations to stimulate the visual system, such as at the visual cortex or the optic nerve. The history of stimulating the visual cortex goes back to the 1980's with the first cortical implant based on work of William Dobelle. There has been modest success with this approach, including work by

Richard Norman, and his reflections on this approach are quite useful. This approach uses a matrix of spike electrodes positioned on the brain surface to penetrate into the visual cortex and stimulate cells to generate a complex visual percept. Alternately, stimulating more proximally in the visual pathway is possible by a cuff electrode around the optic nerve which is the ensemble of axons projecting from the retinal ganglion cell to the lateral geniculate nucleus. An optic nerve-based stimulating prosthesis must deal with the unique spatial arrangement of the axons to engage the topography of vision. If successful, one might expect this to yield an abstract visual percept resembling that from stimulating ganglion cells directly at the retinal surface.

For patients a very practical question remains as to what degree of spatial resolution can be obtained by these approaches. Reading vision requires high spatial resolution to achieve the 6/6 acuity that is the hallmark of excellent natural vision enjoyed by the majority of people. There is general agreement that restoring 6/6 acuity is beyond what can be obtained by an electrical visual prosthesis. Other approaches to stimulating the neurons chemically are being developed. In theory this may give tighter spatial localization and higher resolution. But even then, ultimately the spatial resolution at the level of the retina will be limited by retinal disorganization consequent to disease pathology, as collateral cellular damage from disease compromises the visual neural processing network. It has been known for some time that for retinitis pigmentosa, end-stage disease causes disarray even of retinal neurons not directly involved, and the remaining cells sustain damage that ultimately limits the quality of "vision" that could be obtained. Consequently, the topic of assessing the vision of individuals after receiving these prosthetic vision devices is important to consider.

In sum, the technical and biological context to developing retinal and visual neural prostheses is presents a complex challenge. And the topic is critically important to assist individuals with advanced and even end-stage vision loss. One readily finds that the topics are interconnected in complex ways and warrant dedicated study by a variety of disciplines, including scientists, engineers, physicians and sensory psychologists, to envision how best to proceed. That puts us back to the opening statement - that these are fascinating times to work in the arena of restoring sight to vision-limited individuals.

National Eye Institute, NIH Paul A. Sieving, MD, PhD,
April 14, 2016 Bethesda, MD, USA

Preface

The socioeconomic impact of blindness is an increasing worldwide problem and every attempt to reduce it is to be welcomed. During the last decades the scientific approaches to restore lost vision in blind patients either by gene and stem cell therapy or by technology development are continuously growing.

Artificial Vision is an exciting and rapidly developing field in both ophthalmology and basic science. The technology has been published in highly specialised scientific journals as well as in the lay press. The latter, however, has often overemphasised single experimental results which can mislead the non-specialist.

My goal as editor was therefore to put together a comprehensive collection of all the leading groups worldwide working on Artificial Vision, by authoring their own work in single chapters. This should give an updated overview on the different approaches currently discussed. The book begins with four introductory contributions on the difficulties in comparing and interpreting functional results in the area of very low vision and the principal prospects and limitations of spatial resolution with artificial tools. This is followed by eight chapters by workers who stimulate the surface or the pigment epithelial side of the retina and five further chapters by experts who work on stimulating the optic nerve, the lateral geniculate body and the superficial layers of the visual cortex.

I do hope this book will be helpful for our colleagues who are working in the wider field of ophthalmology so that they may knowledgeably inform their patients who are often desperate to hear of these exciting medical breakthroughs.

Munich, Bavaria, Germany
April, 2nd 2016

Veit Peter Gabel

Contents

Contributors

Editor

Veit Peter Gabel, MD, FARVO University of Regensburg, Germany, Munich, Bavaria, Germany

Contributors

Mark Armstrong, DIP, ART, RMIT Department of Design, Monash Art Design and Architecture, Caulfield, VIC, Australia

Lauren N. Ayton, PhD, B.Optom, FAAO, FACO Centre for Eye Research Australia, The University of Melbourne, Royal Victorian Eye and Ear Hospital, East Melbourne, VIC, Australia

Karl Ulrich Bartz-Schmidt, MD Center for Ophthalmology, University of Tübingen Medical Centre, Tübingen, Germany

Ryad Benosman INSERM, Sorbonne Universités, UPMC Univ Paris 06, UMR_S968, CNRS UMR7210, Institut de la Vision, Paris, France

Dorothea Besch, PhD Center for Ophthalmology, University of Tuebingen Medical Centre, Tuebingen, Germany

Tamara-Leigh E. Brawn, BA, BBSc, PostGradDip Ed, MBA Bionic Vision Australia, University of Melbourne, Parkville, VIC, Australia

Emma Brunton, PhD Department of Electrical and Computer Systems Engineering, Monash University, Clayton, VIC, Australia

Anthony N. Burkitt, PhD, BSc (Hon), BSc Department of Electrical and Electronic Engineering, The University of Melbourne, Melbourne, VIC, Australia

Pengjia Cao, PhD School of Biomedical Engineering, Shanghai Jiao Tong University, Shanghai, People's Republic of China

Xinyu Chai, PhD School of Biomedical Engineering, Shanghai Jiao Tong University, Shanghai, People's Republic of China

Yao Chen, PhD School of Biomedical Engineering, Shanghai Jiao Tong University, Shanghai, People's Republic of China

Gislin Dagnelie, PhD Department of Ophthalmology, Johns Hopkins University School of Medicine, Baltimore, MD, USA

Marcus Dapper Pixium Vision, Paris, France

Paulo Falabella, MD Department of Ophthalmology, University of Southern California, Los Angeles, CA, USA

Eduardo Fernández, MD, PhD Department of Neural Engineering, Miguel Hernández University, CIBER BBNElche, Alicante, Spain

Angélica Pérez Fornos, PhD Western Switzerland Cochlear Implants Center, Geneva University Hospitals, Geneva, Switzerland

Takashi Fujikado, MD, PhD Department of Applied Visual Science, Osaka University Graduate School of Medicine, Suita, Osaka, Japan

Florian Gekeler, MD Center for Ophthalmology, University of Tübingen and Klinikum Stuttgart, Stuttgart, Germany

Robert Hill Pixium Vision, Paris, France

Ralf Hornig Pixium Vision SA, Paris, France

Mark S. Humayun, MD, PhD Department of Ophthalmology, University of Southern California, Los Angeles, CA, USA

Khalid Ishaque Pixium Vision, Paris, France

Eric Le Joliff Pixium Vision, Paris, France

Horace Josh, BEng (Hons), PhD Department of Electrical and Computer Systems Engineering, Monash Vision Group, Clayton, VIC, Australia

Steven Katz, MD Department of Ophthalmology & Visual Science, Havener Eye Institute, Ohio State University, Columbus, OH, USA

Shawn K. Kelly, PhD Institute for Complex Engineered Systems, VA Pittsburgh Healthcare System, Carnegie Mellon University, Pittsburgh, PA, USA

Nathaniel J. Killian, PhD Department of Neurosurgery, Massachusetts General Hospital, Harvard Medical School, Boston, MA, USA

Lindsay Kleeman, BE, BMath, PhD Department of Electrical and Computer Systems Engineering, Monash Vision Group, Clayton, VIC, Australia

Assen Koitschev, MD Department of Otorhinolaryngology, Klinikum Stuttgart, Stuttgart, Germany

Margee J. Kyada Department of Behavioral Neuroscience, Northeastern University, Boston, MA, USA

Yannick LeMer Fondation Ophtalmologique Adolphe de Rothschild, Paris, France

Liming Li, PhD School of Biomedical Engineering, Shanghai Jiao Tong University, Shanghai, People's Republic of China

Menghui Li, PhD Department of Biomedical Engineering, College of Engineering, Peking University, Beijing, People's Republic of China

Wai Ho Li, BE (HONS I), PhD Department of Electrical and Computer Systems Engineering, Monash Vision Group, Clayton, VIC, Australia

Henri Lorach, PhD Department of Ophthalmology, Stanford University, Stanford, CA, USA

Nigel H. Lovell, BE (Hons), PhD Graduate School of Biomedical Engineering, University of New South Wales, Sydney, NSW, Australia

Arthur James Lowery, BSc Dunelm, PhD Department of Electrical and Computer Systems Engineering, Monash University, Clayton, VIC, Australia

Yiliang Lu, PhD School of Biomedical Engineering, Shanghai Jiao Tong University, Shanghai, People's Republic of China

Zengguang Ma, PhD School of Biomedical Engineering, Shanghai Jiao Tong University, Shanghai, People's Republic of China

Collette Mann, PhD Department of Electrical and Computer Systems Engineering, Monash University, Clayton, VIC, Australia

Anand Mohan, BE (FCD), ME, PhD Department of Electrical and Computer Systems Engineering, Monash University, Clayton, VIC, Australia

David A.X. Nayagam, BSc/BE(ElecEng)(Hons), PhD Bionics Institute, The University of Melbourne, East Melbourne, VIC, Australia

Hossein Nazari, MD Department of Ophthalmology, University of Texas Medical Branch (UTMB), Galveston, TX, USA

Richard A. Normann, PhD Department of Bioengineering, University of Utah, Salt Lake City, UT, USA

Daniel Palanker, PhD Department of Ophtalmology, Stanford University, Stanford, CA, USA

Matthew A. Petoe, BSc, BEng (Hons), PhD Department of Medical Bionics, Bionics Institute of Australia, Melbourne, VIC, Australia

John S. Pezaris, PhD Department of Neurosurgery, Massachusetts General Hospital, Harvard Medical School, Boston, MA, USA

Serge Picaud, PhD INSERM, Sorbonne Universités, UPMC Univ Paris 06, UMR_S968, CNRS UMR7210, Institut de la Vision, Paris, France

Christoph Posch INSERM, Sorbonne Universités, UPMC Univ Paris 06, UMR_S968, CNRS UMR7210, Institut de la Vision, Paris, France

Jeanette Pritchard, BSc (Hons), MPhil, PhD Department of Electrical and Computer Systems Engineering, Monash Vision Group, Clayton, VIC, USA

Ramesh Rajan, BSc(Hons), PhD Department of Physiology, Monash University, Neuroscience Program, Biomedicine Discovery Institute, Clayton, VIC, USA

Qiushi Ren, PhD Department of Biomedical Engineering, College of Engineering, Peking University, Beijing, People's Republic of China

Joseph Rizzo, MD Director of the Neuro-Ophthalmology Service, Harvard Medical School and the Massachusetts Eye and Ear Infirmary, Boston, MA, USA

Marcello G.P. Rosa, BSc, MSc, PhD Department of Physiology, Monash Vision Group, Australian Research Council Centre of Excellence for Integrative Brain Function, Clayton, VIC, Australia

Jeffrey V. Rosenfeld, MD, MS, FRACS, FRCS, FACS Monash Institute of Medical Engineering, Alfred Hospital, Clayton, VIC, Australia

Gary S. Rubin, PhD Department of Visual Neuroscience, UCL Institute of Ophthalmology, London, UK

Helmut G. Sachs, PhD, MD Eye Clinic, Klinikum Dresden Friedrichstadt, Dresden, Germany

José-Alain Sahel INSERM, Sorbonne Universités, UPMC Univ Paris 06, UMR_S968, CNRS UMR7210, Institut de la Vision, Fondation Ophtalmologique Adolphe de Rothschild, Paris, CHNO des Quinze-Vingts, Paris, Academie des Sciences, Paris, Paris, France

Paulo Schor, MD, PhD Department of Ophthalmology and Visual Sciences, São Paulo Hospital, Federal University of São Paulo, São Paulo, SP, Brazil

Jörg Sommerhalder, PhD Department of Ophthalmology, Geneva University Hospitals, Geneva, Switzerland

Katarina Stingl, MD Center for Ophthalmology, University of Tübingen Medical Centre, Tübingen, Germany

Gregg J. Suaning, BSc, MSc, PhD Graduate School of Biomedical Engineering, University of New South Wales, Sydney, NSW, Australia

Jingjing Sun, PhD School of Biomedical Engineering, Shanghai Jiao Tong University, Shanghai, People's Republic of China

Pengcheng Sun, PhD School of Biomedical Engineering, Shanghai Jiao Tong University, Shanghai, People's Republic of China

Philip R. Troyk, PhD Department of Biomedical Engineering, Illinois Institute of Technology, Chicago, IL, USA

Peter Walter, MD Department of Ophthalmology, University Hospital RWTH Aachen, Aachen, NRW, Germany

James D. Weiland, PhD Department of Ophthalmology, University of Southern California, Los Angeles, CA, USA

Kaijie Wu, PhD School of Biomedical Engineering, Shanghai Jiao Tong University, Shanghai, People's Republic of China

Yan Yan, PhD School of Biomedical Engineering, Shanghai Jiao Tong University, Shanghai, People's Republic of China

Eberhart Zrenner, PhD, MD Werner Reichardt Center for Integrative Neuroscience (CIN), Eberhard Karls Universität Tübingen, Institute for Ophthalmic Research, Tübingen, Germany

Part I
Introduction or Principles of Functional Assessment

Chapter 1
Assessing Patient Suitability and Outcome Measures in Vision Restoration Trials

Lauren N. Ayton and Joseph Rizzo

Abstract One of the challenging aspects of visual prosthesis clinical trials is the assessment and reporting of efficacy. In this relatively early phase of development, visual prosthesis devices are not able to provide high-resolution visual acuity, and hence standard vision tests such as logMAR acuity charts are not sufficient to measure post-intervention improvements in vision. This has led to the development of a number of functional vision assessments, such as tests of orientation and mobility and activities of daily living, which aim to show the "real-world" benefit of the devices. These challenges face all research groups and companies who are developing vision restoration interventions (including stem cells, gene therapy and optogenetics), and sharing of techniques and knowledge between the groups can only further our quest to provide patient benefit. As such, an International Taskforce was developed in 2014 to generate consensus on the methods of testing and reporting outcomes in vision restoration trials, and has become known as the Harmonization of Outcomes and Vision Endpoints in Vision Restoration Trials (HOVER) Taskforce. This chapter outlines the structure and aims of the Taskforce, and provides an update of the progress to date. In addition, a summary of the patient characteristics that are desirable for a visual prosthesis candidate are provided for the practicing ophthalmologist.

Keywords HOVER Taskforce • Consensus • Outcome measures • Clinical trials

L.N. Ayton, PhD, B.Optom, FAAO, FACO (✉)
Centre for Eye Research Australia, The University of Melbourne, Royal Victorian Eye and Ear Hospital, East Melbourne, VIC, Australia
e-mail: lnayton@unimelb.edu.au

J. Rizzo, MD
Harvard Medical School and the Massachusetts Eye and Ear Infirmary, Boston, MA, USA

V.P. Gabel (ed.), *Artificial Vision*, DOI 10.1007/978-3-319-41876-6_1

Key Points

- At the present time, there are no internationally-accepted gold standards for the assessment and reporting of patient outcomes in vision restoration clinical trials.
- An international group, the Harmonization of Outcomes and Vision Endpoints in Vision Restoration Trials (HOVER) Taskforce, is currently working to generate consensus in this area.
- There are a number of clinical characteristics that practicing ophthalmologists should assess for when considering referral of a patient for vision restoration clinical trials or treatments.

Developing an International Consensus on the Measurement and Reporting of Patient Outcomes: The Harmonization of Outcomes and Vision Endpoints in Vision Restoration Trials (HOVER) Taskforce

As is evident from the contributions to this book, the field of vision restoration is rapidly progressing. Treatment options such as stem cells, gene therapy and optogenetics, which were once considered science fiction, are now becoming real options for the future treatment of people with blindness. But of all the vision restoration techniques, visual prosthetic devices (or "bionic eyes") are the most advanced and have yielded the best visual outcomes to date for people with profound vision loss. There have been over ten chronic human clinical trials of these devices, with implants placed in various locations in the brain, the optic nerve and retina. These trials have shown that the devices are generally safe to implant and can, in the better cases, produce improvements in visual function for patients who are otherwise severely vision impaired [1–6]. However, to date these devices have provided vision with relatively low spatial resolution, which confounds attempts to convincingly demonstrate improvements in vision and functional vision.

Assessment of low vision has historically been recognized as demanding, with variability in test results and patient fatigue increasing with lower levels of vision [7]. These factors conspire with other confounding factors, like improved motivation and performance that can occur when patients know an assistive device is being used, given their heightened expectations of benefit. For these and other reasons, it can be challenging to convincingly prove the benefits of vision restoration interventions.

These challenges have long been recognized by the field, both in publications [8–11] and through conference discussions [12]. Guidelines for the measurement of patient outcomes were published by the Food and Drugs Administration (FDA) in 2009, and updated in 2013 [13], and outlined a number of considerations, including methodological standards. This FDA document also detailed the two main areas of outcome assessment that it considered necessary for the report of visual prosthesis outcomes; visual function (acuity, spatial mapping of phosphenes and form vision assessments) and functional vision (orientation and mobility, activities of daily living and patient reported outcomes).

In more recent years, there has been a call for international cooperation and a higher level of discussion from the researchers themselves, which ultimately led to the formation of the Harmonization of Outcomes and Vision Endpoints in Vision Restoration Trials (HOVER) International Taskforce, founded by Joseph Rizzo (Boston, USA) and Lauren Ayton (Melbourne, Australia) in 2014 [14]. This Taskforce was formed to engage a wide swathe of experts in the fields of vision restoration, low vision, and clinical trial outcomes to work toward developing an international consensus on preferred methods to measure and to report patient outcomes in vision restoration clinical trials, whether of prosthetic devices or any other form of intervention. For several reasons, improving consistency in methodology and reporting will become even more important as the number of vision restoration treatments increases.

To date, over 100 eminent researchers and clinicians have joined the HOVER Taskforce and have been cooperating to develop consensus on areas ranging from visual acuity testing to methods of performing electrical stimulation studies. The Taskforce is overseen by a guidance committee formed of representatives of research groups who have completed clinical trials, experts in each of the fields of stem cells, gene therapy and optogenetics, and a representative of the Food and Drug Administration (FDA) who is an expert on regulatory issues. This guidance committee provides counsel and support to the working groups with the aim of producing a set of consensus documents that will be relevant to all forms of vision restoration technologies. The Taskforce is supported by Detroit Institute of Ophthalmology, with the director, Dr Philip Hessburg, providing executive oversight for the work.

The most important aspect of the HOVER Taskforce is its philosophy of inclusiveness and openness. The committee is aware and sensitive to the fact that there are notable differences among the various approaches to prosthetic intervention. As such, there was no intent to seek detailed specification of methods that would be appropriate for all groups. Rather, this Taskforce was motivated by the goal of improving transparency by developing guidelines to obtain more consistent measures of visual function and more consistent means of reporting results. The guidelines generated by the HOVER Taskforce will reflect the knowledge and experience of a broad, international cohort of researchers, which should provide benefit for all emerging forms of visual restoration trials for decades to come. The Taskforce intends to continuously seek input from its constituency, which will likely lead to modifications to its recommendations as new information and experience is acquired. The Taskforce seeks to distribute the collective wisdom of many experts, not to control but rather to guide future work in this field. Draft guidelines from each of the working groups are being collated and will be published in the near future.

Another aim of the HOVER Taskforce is to provide patients, the low vision community and clinicians with accurate and up-to-date information about the status of vision restoration research. To this end, we have designed a website to provide this interface between the medical researchers and the patient community, at www.artificialvision.org.

The progress of the HOVER Taskforce has been inspirational, with international experts from all backgrounds working together for a common good. This work will only serve to strengthen the field and advance the development of treatment options for our visually-impaired patients whom we are proud to serve.

Advice to the Practicing Ophthalmologist: How to Test and Advise Patients Interested in Restoration Therapies at Present

With the significant general public interest in vision restoration therapies, it is inevitable that many ophthalmologists will be approached by potential candidates. As evident above, there is still controversy on the most appropriate outcome measures for defining efficacy in vision restoration trials, but it is easier to define a candidate's suitability based on three main aspects:

1. Level of residual vision

   At the present time, vision restoration interventions are only suitable for people with extremely poor levels of vision. Most trials of visual prostheses have included participants with vision of bare light perception or less, with a few including those who are able to identify hand movements. Candidates for a vision prosthesis must have this low vision in both eyes. At present, candidates must also have a history of prior useful form vision, as this is indicative of posterior visual pathway integrity (which may be compromised in cases of congenital blindness).
2. Cause of vision loss

   As detailed in this book, the type of vision loss is a key factor when deciding on which visual prosthesis is the most suitable for a patient. Retinal prostheses, which are the only commercially available prosthesis at this time, are suitable for people with retinal degenerative diseases such as retinitis pigmentosa or choroideremia. In 2015, the first clinical trials were commenced in patients with complete vision loss from geographic atrophy from age-related macular degeneration, but at this time this is not a regulatory- approved indication for the devices. There are no approved cortical prostheses on the market, but clinical trials are anticipated to commence in the coming years. It is believed that a cortical prosthesis could be an option for people who have lost their sight from other diseases, including glaucoma, diabetic retinopathy and trauma.
3. Patient motivation and expectations

   Possibly one of the most important factors to consider when deciding if a patient would be a good candidate for a visual prosthesis is their own expectations and motivations. At the present time, the improvements in vision that such

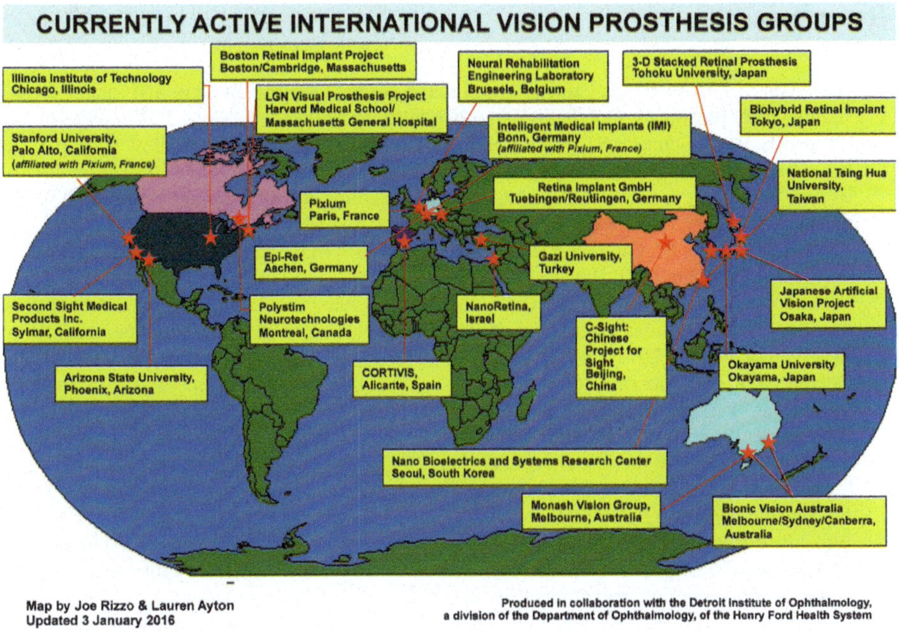

Fig. 1.1 Currently active visual prosthesis groups, January 2016 (Map by Joe Rizzo & Lauren Ayton Updated 3 January 2016. Produced in collaboration with the Detroit Institute of Ophthalmology, a division of the Department of Ophthalmology, of the Henry Ford Health System)

devices afford is still modest, and so it is vital that patients are aware of the limitations of the technology. In most trials to date, there have been significant variations in patient performance with prostheses, and hence it is not possible to guarantee an improvement in vision to someone who undergoes the treatment. The best candidates for visual prostheses are those who understand these limitations, and who have reasonable and fair expectations.

The best way to be sure of a patient's suitability for a visual prosthesis is to contact the research group or medical device supplier directly. They can then provide practitioners with up-to-date information and advice. A map showing the active visual prosthesis groups in 2015 is shown below (Fig. 1.1), and up to date information can be located online. To date, the three regulatory approved and commercially available retinal prostheses are:

(a) The Argus II retinal implant by Second Sight Medical Products, USA (CE mark and FDA approval); http://www.secondsight.com/
(b) The Alpha IMS retinal implant by Retina Implant AG, Germany (CE mark approval); http://www.retina-implant.de/en
(c) The Iris 150 retinal implant by Pixium Vision, France (CE mark approval); http://www.pixium-vision.com/en

References

1. Humayun MS, Dorn JD, da Cruz L, et al. Interim results from the international trial of second sight's visual prosthesis. Ophthalmology. 2012;119(4):779–88.
2. Zrenner E, Bartz-Schmidt KU, Benav H, et al. Subretinal electronic chips allow blind patients to read letters and combine them to words. Proc Biol Sci. 2011;278(1711):1489–97.
3. Brelen ME, Duret F, Gerard B, et al. Creating a meaningful visual perception in blind volunteers by optic nerve stimulation. J Neural Eng. 2005;2(1):S22–8.
4. Ayton LN, Blamey PJ, Guymer RH, et al. First-in-human trial of a novel suprachoroidal retinal prosthesis. PLoS One. 2014;9(12):e115239.
5. Fujikado T, Kamei M, Sakaguchi H, et al. Testing of semichronically implanted retinal prosthesis by suprachoroidal-transretinal stimulation in patients with retinitis pigmentosa. Invest Ophthalmol Vis Sci. 2011;52(7):4726–33.
6. Dobelle WH. Artificial mac for the blind by connecting a television camera to the visual cortex. ASAIO J. 2000;46(1):3–9.
7. Bittner AK, Ibrahim MA, Haythornthwaite JA, et al. Vision test variability in retinitis pigmentosa and psychosocial factors. Optom Vis Sci. 2011;88(12):1496–506.
8. Lepri BP. Is acuity enough? Other considerations in clinical investigations of visual prostheses. J Neural Eng. 2009;6(3):035003.
9. Wilke R, Bach M, Wilhelm B, et al. Testing visual functions in patients with visual prostheses. In: Humayun M, Weiland J, Chader GJ, Greenbaum E, editors. Artificial sight: basic research, biomedical engineering, and clinical advances. Oak Ridge: Springer Science; 2007. p. 91–110.
10. Geruschat DR, Bittner AK, Dagnelie G. Orientation and mobility assessment in retinal prosthetic clinical trials. Optom Vis Sci. 2012;89(9):1308–15.
11. Dagnelie G. Psychophysical evaluation for visual prosthesis. Annu Rev Biomed Eng. 2008;10:339–68.
12. Ayton LN, Rizzo JF. The challenges of measuring extremely low vision in vision restoration trials. Detroit: The Eye and the Chip World Congress; 2012.
13. US Food and Drug Administration. Investigational device exemption (IDE) guidance for retinal prostheses. USA; 2013.
14. Rizzo 3rd JF, Ayton LN. Psychophysical testing of visual prosthetic devices: a call to establish a multi-national joint task force. J Neural Eng. 2014;11(2):020301.

Chapter 2
Functional Assessment of Artificial Vision

Gary S. Rubin

Abstract "Functional Assessment" refers to tests that capture a person's ability to use vision to perform everyday tasks. These include assessments ranging from basic psychophysical tests of light perception and discrimination to performance-based tests such as reading a newspaper or navigating through an obstacle course. Like all types of clinical tests, functional assessments must use methods that are adequately standardised, but not so rigorously standardised that they lose their relevance to everyday life. Functional assessment can be time-consuming and much effort has gone into making these assessments efficient through the use of intelligent, adaptive testing and scoring algorithms. As for other types of clinical tests, functional assessments must be shown to be reliable, valid, and responsive. The chapter concludes with an overview of currently available functional tests and evaluates their standardisation, reliability and validity, where such data are available.

Keywords Visual function • Reading • Mobility • Navigation • Reliability • Validity • Bayesian adaptive algorithms

Key Points

- Functional assessment must strike a balance between standardisation, to insure that the tests are reproducible across sites, and natural conditions, to insure that the tests reflect performance in real-world conditions.
- Functional assessment typically does not inform us about the mechanisms or aetiology of disease, but it does tell us about the impact of disease and the safety and effectiveness of its treatment
- Forced-choice testing procedures should be used whenever possible to reduce the influence of criterion effects
- Adaptive test procedures significantly reduce test time

G.S. Rubin
Department of Visual Neuroscience, UCL Institute of Ophthalmology, London, UK
e-mail: g.rubin@ucl.ac.uk

V.P. Gabel (ed.), *Artificial Vision*, DOI 10.1007/978-3-319-41876-6_2

Introduction

In the field of artificial or prosthetic vision, “functional assessment” refers to any of a variety of tests that capture a person’s ability to use vision to perform everyday tasks. Functional assessment stands in contrast to structural assessment, such as measurements of retinal thickness made with the OCT. Functional assessment also differs from tests designed to assess eye health such as intraocular pressure. But what about such common tests as visual acuity which are used to predict reading performance, to assess photoreceptor density, and to monitor refractive error? Indeed, many eye tests can have functional, structural, and eye health uses, but in this chapter we will focus our attention on the functional application. Functional assessment is important for the evaluation of treatments applied across the entire range of visual abilities, from patients looking to achieve “super-normal” vision with wavefront LASIK to blind participants hoping for restoration of visual function through gene or stem cell therapies. But as most of the candidates for visual prostheses must have vision worse than counting fingers upon entry into the study, we will limit our discussion to what has been termed “ultra-low vision” (ULV)

Patient reported outcome measures (questionnaires) play an important role in functional assessment, but we will not be discussing them in this chapter. We will also limit our discussion to applications within the field of artificial or prosthetic vision, bypassing much interesting work with sensory substitution such as vibriotactile displays and text-to-speech.

Functional assessment runs the gamut from basic psychophysical tests of light perception and discrimination to performance based tests such as reading a newspaper or navigating through an obstacle course. Functional assessment is used as an outcome measure to assess safety and efficacy of prosthetic devices, and to develop training or rehabilitation plans to improve the use of such devices.

Standardisation

To be useful, especially for multi-centre investigations, functional vision tests need to be carefully standardized. That much is obvious. But it is less obvious that functional tests can be over standardized. Take reading tests. There are many types of tests that are designed to measure reading speed. These include tests based on random words that are matched only for length and word frequency, to sentence based tests that have carefully controlled syntax word length word frequency and syntax [1].

It is argued that the random word reading tests are linked more closely to purely visual factors whereas the controlled sentence tests are strongly influenced by cognitive factors. But which is better related to every day reading? That question has not been addressed for most reading tests, but in our study of the impact of visual impairment on function and quality of life in the elderly [2], we compared a standardized laboratory reading test to reading under natural conditions in the home. The laboratory reading test used short paragraphs of meaningful, continuous text that was constrained only by grade level and presented on a computer monitor at a fixed luminance and contrast. The home reading test used a selection of text from the local newspaper, read directly from the newsprint and illuminated however the participant wished. Nevertheless, the correlation between the two tests was high ($\rho = 0.86$) indicating that the laboratory test predicted everyday reading performance. We will return to this issue later when discussing some of the specific tests used in recent clinical trials.

Forced Choice Testing

Tests of visual function are often faulted for being "subjective", compared to "objective" tests like ERGs. Without delving into the complex philosophical issue of how to distinguish between the objective and subjective, there is one principle of psychophysical testing that can reduce the subjectivity of visual assessment – forced-choice testing [3]. A forced-choice test requires the participant to choose among two or more alternatives, only one of which is the correct answer. A forced-choice letter acuity test requires the participant to name each letter on the chart until he reaches a pre-determined stopping criterion, such as 4 errors in a row of 5 letters. To understand the importance of forced-choice testing, consider the following example: Two people are taking a visual acuity test that does not use forced-choice. Instead, each individual reads down the chart until they don't think they can see any more letters, then stops. Participant 1 is doesn't like to make mistakes so they don't venture a response unless they are sure it's correct. Participant 2 is bold and carefree and will happily guess as long as they can see something. Participant 1 stops responding after letter 45 (end of line 9 having made no mistakes up to this point. Participant 2 starts making occasional errors on line 8 but still gets most of the letters right on the next 3 lines. Not until line 12 do they reach the limit and miss all 5 letters. Participant 1 has a score of 45 letters; participant 2's score is 63, a difference of 18 letters or .36 logMAR (more than 3½ lines). But if forced-choice testing had been used, participant 1 would have had to continue responding until they made enough errors on a line to reach the stopping rule. Participant 1 would have undoubtedly gotten a few more letters correct (our experience suggests a minimum of 5 letters or 1 line, but possibly 2 or 3 lines more). The large difference in acuity turns out to be a difference in criterion, at least in part. Criterion shifts occur with age, onset of disease, and with treatment. One can well imagine that a patient receiving a new experimental therapy, such as a retinal implant, may try harder, guess more willingly, in other words, shift their criterion. Without forced-choice testing it is difficult to distinguish changes in visual function from changes in motivation.

Forced-choice testing should not be confused with "yes-no" procedures where the participant is shown a test target and responds, "yes, I saw it" or "no, I didn't see it". Although the participant may be forced to make a choice, these procedures are not criterion free. Our timid Participant 1 above will still score lower than bold Participant 2 because of differences in criteria, instead of, or in addition to differences in vision.

Efficient Testing Algorithms and Scoring Methods

Clinical trials often require a large number of tests. Therefore it is extremely important that the psychophysical measurements use an efficient algorithm for stimulus selection and scoring. There has been a great deal of work on efficient algorithms that go by names such as QUEST, PEST, and BEST PEST [4]. All of these algorithms are adaptive. This means that the choice of stimulus intensity is based on the results of previous trials. If the participant responds incorrectly on a given trial, then the next trial is likely to present a stimulus at higher intensity, or one that is easier to see. These procedures use maximum likelihood estimating techniques to determine the stimulus intensity that will yield the most information. The efficiency of the algorithm is determined by how much information we have about the subject's current threshold estimate and by how well we model the underlying psychometric function. Whereas traditional methods of psychophysical testing frequently required 100 or more trials per estimate, modern algorithms usually need only 25 or 30 trials per point.

It has been elegantly shown [5] that scoring methods with small step sizes produce more reliable measurements than methods that use large steps. For example, when grading cataract severity, grading scales that allow the use of decimal number are more reliable than methods based on integer grades only. Similarly, tests that give partial credit for partially correct answers are more reliable than those that do not. Letter charts are a good example. If partial credit is given for each correctly named letter then the results are more reliable than if the test were scored line by line. The greatest waste of information occurs when a well-designed test with a nearly continuous scale is converted to pass/fail.

Psychometric Properties of Functional Vision Tests

Functional vision tests, like all clinical assessments, need to be reliable and valid. Validity is typically based on measures of association between the test in question and other indicators of functional ability. But in addition to the usual construct, content, and criterion-related validity, these tests must have ecological validity. This term, popularised by Gibson, refers to the link between the laboratory measurement and the participant's performance of similar real-world tasks. A well-constructed mobility task may be administered under carefully standardised lighting conditions on a clean, dry, level surface, but to be ecologically valid it should predict performance in the real world.

Bland and Altman have written popular and easy to understand guides for assessing test reliability [6]. They eschew methods based on correlation coefficients preferring instead methods based on the analysis of differences between scores at test and retest.

Less well understood, but equally important, functional vision tests need to be responsive, that is, they need to be sensitive to change and indicate improvement when it really occurs. Closely linked to responsiveness is the concept of a "Minimally

Important Difference" (MID), the MID specifies the smallest change in a test score that is still sufficient to make a difference to the participant. For example, if a clinical trial is testing a new drug therapy for advanced AMD and the primary outcome measure is a change in ETDRS visual acuity, how large a change should be required? Investigators frequently focus on the effect size needed to demonstrate statistical significance, which depends on the size of the sample. With a very large sample, statistically significant results may be obtained with a tiny change in outcome measure, such as a 1-letter improvement in our acuity example. But is a 1-letter change in acuity noticeable to the patient; does it really make a difference? Probably not.

How do we determine an MID? This topic has been extensively studied and there are excellent reviews of the alternative methods [7, 8]. In brief, there are two types of methods for determining MID, "distributional" and "anchor-based." The former are based on the distribution of results obtained in a study, the most common being ½ the standard deviation of the scores. The latter are anchored to an external measurement, frequently the patients' responses to a questionnaire. For example, to determine the MID for a visual acuity test, patients' acuities are measured at baseline and follow up. At follow up they are also asked whether their vision has got a little better, a lot better, stayed the same, got a little worse or a lot worse since the baseline exam. The visual acuity change associated with those reporting minimal improvement or decline is the MID. Interestingly, MIDs based on the ½ SD rule are often similar to anchor-based MIDs.

Basic Visual Function Tests

Light Perception

A popular strategy for designing a functional assessment is to take a hierarchical approach, beginning with the simplest and most basic visual abilities – light detection and localisation – and moving up through more complex vision tasks – motion detection, and resolution (acuity) before moving on to everyday visual activities such as navigation and object recognition. Several simple test batteries have been developed to monitor basic visual ability. The Basic Assessment of Light and Motion (BaLM) is a group of four tests that assess light perception, localisation, motion, and resolution [9]. All of the tests are presented with a light projector at very high luminance (5100 cd/m^2) and contrast (>99 %). The use of such high luminance raises the issue of whether the tests are valid; whether they predict performance under natural conditions. In addition, all of the components of the BaLM battery are described as "forced choice" However the light perception test uses a standard yes/no procedure that is not forced-choice and not independent of the participant's criterion.

One might ask how such a basic task as light perception could be related to functional vision. Geruschat explains how localisation of a single light source can be used by a person with ULV to orient and navigate more efficiently than if totally blind, and how this rudimentary visual information can be used during rehabilitation for other types of visually-guided behaviour [10].

Spatial Resolution

The BaLM test battery was used to evaluate efficacy of the Alpha IMS subretinal implant, and a similar group of tests (localisation, motion, and orientation) was used to evaluate the Second Sight Argus II epiretinal implant. Following these very basic tests of visual function, we proceed to tests of resolution ability (grating or letter acuity). Conventional wisdom suggests that acuity cannot be measured reliably for vision of count fingers or worse. However Bach has demonstrated with the FRaCT letter acuity test that by simply increasing letter size and decreasing viewing distance it is possible to reliably assess visual acuity down to the level of count fingers and hand motion.

Grating acuity is an alternative to letter acuity that can easily be modified for ULV. Grating acuity should be closely related to letter acuity, however this relationship does break down with certain eye disorders, such as amblyopia and macular degeneration where letter acuity is generally worse than grating acuity for appropriately matched sizes (especially when there are multiple letters shown on a single trial). The Basic Grating Acuity test (BaGA) [11] which can test grating sizes ranging from 0.1 to 3.3 cpd (corresponding to Snellen equivalents of 6/1800–6/50) was used in the alpha-IMS trial and a similar test was used by Second Sight.

Bailey et al. [12] takes a different approach to the assessment of low level visual function. His Berkeley Rudimentary Vision Test (BRVT) uses a combination of tumbling E, gratings, and white and black patches to arrive at a single measure of visual function when acuity is too poor to be measured with conventional eye charts. Although he describes an algorithm for combining these disparate types of data into a single measure, he provides no evidence that the algorithm is valid or reliable.

Activities of Daily Living

Object Recognition

Once it has been established that a retinal implant can support basic visual processing, such as light perception and localisation, the assessment of functional vision turns to everyday visual tasks like reading and recognising faces and objects. While there are several validated, reliable tests for such activities, these are not suitable for people with ULV and correspondingly poor spatial and temporal resolution. New tests have been designed for this purpose, but, disappointingly, each group of investigators has developed their own tests rather than agreeing on a set of common tasks and shared methodology. Beginning with object recognition, the Alpha-IMS group used a black table surface as a backdrop for geometric shapes, dining objects (such as cups and cutlery), individual large letters, and clock hands to test object localisation and identification [13]. All of the objects are uniformly white. That feature severely limits the validity of the test. It is questionable whether the object recognition test is generalizable to objects in the real world; whether it is ecologically valid. Moreover, the letter recognition test allows patients up to 2 min of viewing time. In some of the videos of patients performing the letter recognition task, they appear to be tracing out the letters with head movements, which converts letter recognition into a proprioceptive rather than visual task.

Picture Recognition

We took a different approach when we developed a picture recognition test for Intelligent Medical Implants [14] 100 images of everyday urban scenes were photographed with a digital camera. Each scene had an object of interest (e.g. doorway, staircase, obstacle on the walking path) on the left or right side. 60 subjects with normal vision viewed the pictures through a virtual reality headset. The pictures were rendered on a 7 × 7 grid of Gaussian shaped pixels to simulate vision as it might be experienced with a retinal implant. Subjects indicated whether the object of interest was on the left or right side. All 100 pictures were shown twice in random order. The median score was 85 % correct. We found that a practice session with trial-by-trial feedback was necessary to prevent subjects from adopting a strategy that lead to worse than chance performance. Rasch analysis [15] was used to select 50 pictures that ranged in difficulty along a single underlying dimension. Although the simulation experiment was useful, the results will need to be compared to those who would be eligible or are enrolled in a retinal prosthesis study.

Dagnelie's group [16] took a similar approach to face recognition, using simulated phosphene vision to test whether subjects could match a partially averted face to one of four reference faces viewed straight on. Subjects achieved high accuracy for high contrast images and learned to recognise low contrast faces. Accuracy was heavily influenced by details of the simulation, such as pixel density, separation, and dropout rate.

Navigation Ability

Good vision is not required to navigate safely, and efficiently. With the help of experienced orientation and mobility instructor, people with ultra low or no vision can learn to travel independently. Nevertheless, most travellers do rely on vision and navigation ability is a widely used outcome measure for judging the efficacy retinal prostheses. Geruschat and colleagues [17] created a mobility course for the artificial silicon retina (ASR) that included an 18-m long straight hallway seeded with foam obstacles. Eight subjects with RP were tested before and after implantation of the ASR device. Four of the subjects had reduced navigational ability after implantation (either reduced walking speed or increased number of contacts) and the other four showed no difference. This study showed that navigation ability did not necessarily improve with artificial vision.

Two navigation tasks have been used for evaluation of the Argus II [18]. One required patients to find a white door embedded in a black wall (or the opposite polarity) from across the room. The other requires patients to follow a white line on the black floor. Both tests were scored as a pass if the patient was touching the door or white line at the end of the trial; and as a fail otherwise. After implantation, patients were more likely to succeed with the system on for both tasks.

As mentioned previously, the pass – fail scoring method produces less reliable scores and discards valuable information that could have been retained by using a continuous measure such as distance from the door or deviation from the white line. More importantly, as was the case for the Alpha-IMS object recognition task, the exclusive use of black and white stimuli severely reduces the ecological validity of the navigation task.

An example of another navigational task that tried to balance standardization with ecological validity is the maze used in the clinical trial of gene therapy for Leber's congenital amaurosis [19]. The maze was constructed at the UCL Pedestrian Accessibility and Movement Environment Laboratory (PAMELA). PAMELA is a simulated outdoor sidewalk environment with a paved surface and street lamps overhead. The platform was configured as three mobility tasks: 10 m straight walk through an open doorway; 13 m serpentine course through a simple maze with eight barriers; and 10 m straight walk along a path with simulated curb stones. Light levels were chosen to replicate a range of illumination levels from indoor office light (240 lux) to nighttime residential street lighting (4 lux), and the colour of the barriers was matched to common clothing materials. Barriers in the maze were randomly positioned for each trial. Time to traverse the maze and the numbers of mobility errors (contacts with the walls or barriers and lapses in orientation) were recorded. Mobility errors appear to be the more sensitive measure and were used for the main analysis. The data indicated that half the subjects (6 of 12) showed improved mobility at night 6 months after treatment, but that the benefits diminished by 12 months.

This example demonstrates that a real world task can be standardized while preserving important features that contribute to ecological validity. The problem with the PAMELA maze is that the facilities and equipment required to create the test are expensive and not portable, making them less suitable for multi-centre clinical trials. A paper by Nau et al. [20] describes an obstacle course designed for patients with ULV that is described as "portable" and relatively inexpensive to build. The materials cost about $5000, but that doesn't include labour and the course requires installation of lights and painting walls, so it would hardly be considered portable.

Multimodal Sensory Integration

Working our way up the hierarchy from very basic visual processing to complex everyday visual tasks, we can go a step further and consider the integration of vision with other sensory modalities. Reports of individuals who have vision restored late in life after many years of blindness do not paint an optimistic picture. After the initial fascination with visual sensations, some report that visual stimulation acts as a source of noise; not information. It is as if the visual precepts are never integrated with sensory information from hearing, proprioception, etc. There are some very simple tests of hand eye coordination that address the integration of vision with proprioception and tactile sense. These include a square localization task used with Argus II [21]. A white square, 6 cm on a side, is displayed in a random location on a computer touch screen. The participant is instructed to locate and touch the centre of the screen with their finger. The vast majority of implanted patients touch closer to the centre when the device is on. In the Alpha-IMS version of the test [22], the patient is instructed to touch handheld chess piece to the centre of a box outlined by a large white square. No data are provided.

It is also possible to test for more complex forms of sensory integration using techniques that were designed primarily for studying visual development in children. Garcia and colleagues [23] tested five patients implanted with the Argus II on a vision – touch task, (judging the size of a ball) a vision – hearing task (judging latency of a beep and flash), and a vision – self motion task (navigation). None of the participants showed any improvement with addition visual information on the size or navigation tasks; two showed a gain in speed judgements.

Looking at the navigation task more closely, the participants were asked to perform two tasks. The first was path reproduction. The participant was led along a path that begins at about the 10 o'clock point on an imaginary circle and ended at about 2:30, after taking one turn. The participant was then led back to the beginning and asked to reproduce the two-leg path. A single floor lamp acted as a visual landmark for the task. The second task was path completion. From the 10 o'clock point, the participant was led to the 2:30 point and told to walk back to the beginning (10 o'clock). Performance was compared with the system on and off. It was also compared to performance of controls with normal vision who viewed the path through goggles that simulated vision with the Argus II.

Patients complete the tasks as accurately without the floor lamp as with it. Two patients showed as much improvement with the system on as did controls when using the simulated Argus II the remaining patients were less accurate with the system on than with it off. The authors conclude that prosthetic vision "may not provide sufficiently reliable visual information to improve the precision of patients on tasks for they have learnt to rely on non-visual senses."

Conclusions

Functional assessment is an integral part of the evaluation of new and improved artificial vision devices. It is not sufficient to demonstrate that patients see phosphenes or that they enjoy the visual phenomena that these devices provide. We need reliable, quantifiable evidence that the devices improve visual function enough to make a difference to patients' lives. Each prosthetic vision company uses slightly different functional outcome measures, which is unfortunate, as it increases the burden to demonstrate that the assessment tools are valid, reliable, and responsive.

Functional outcomes are generally considered in a hierarchical fashion, beginning with simple light detection and localisation and ascending through acuity, contrast, and motion to performance-based tasks of everyday living. Basic tests of visual function have generally undergone more testing and evaluation than higher-level tasks. However, more work is needed on reliability and especially MID, the smallest difference that makes a difference, even for basic tasks. Many of the higher order functional tasks suffer from a lack of ecological validity – the laboratory functional assessment is not likely to predict performance in the real world. This problem arises primarily because the tests use illumination levels that are too high or are composed of uniform black and white components. Presumably they are not designed to incorporate features of the world outside the lab but so that they can be passed by patient who have implants

Performance-based functional outcomes, such as those reviewed here, should be considered in conjunction with patient-reported outcomes (PROs, or questionnaire), Not only are the methods for developing reliable and valid PROs more mature, they provide important information from the patients' perspective. We have found the PROs and performance-based measures often agree but even when they don't, the discrepancy can be informative as well [24].

Acknowledgements The research was supported by the National Institute for Health Research (NIHR) Biomedical Research Centre based at Moorfields Eye Hospital NHS Foundation Trust and UCL Institute of Ophthalmology. The views expressed are those of the author(s) and not necessarily those of the NHS, the NIHR or the Department of Health.

References

1. Radner W, Willinger U, Obermayer W, Mudrich C, Velikay-Parel M, Eisenwort B. A new German reading chart for the simultaneous evaluation of reading acuity and reading speed. Klin Monatsbl Augenheilkd. 1998;213:174–81.
2. West SK, Rubin GS, Munoz B, Abraham D, Fried LP. Assessing functional status: correlation between performance on tasks conducted in a clinic setting and performance on the same task conducted at home. The Salisbury Eye Evaluation Project Team. J Gerontol A Biol Sci Med Sci. 1997;52(4):M209–17.
3. Vaegan, Halliday BL. A forced-choice test improves clinical contrast sensitivity testing. Br J Ophthalmol. 1982;66:477–91.
4. Watson AB, Pelli DG. QUEST: a Bayesian adaptive psychometric method. Percept Psychophys. 1983;33:113–20.
5. Bailey IL, Bullimore MA, Raasch TW, Taylor HR. Clinical grading and the effects of scaling. Invest Ophthalmol Vis Sci. 1991;32:422–32.
6. Bland JM, Altman DG. Measuring agreement in method comparison studies. Stat Methods Med Res. 1999;8(2):135–60.
7. Beaton DE, Boers M, Wells GA. Many faces of the minimal clinically important difference (MCID): a literature review and directions for future research. Curr Opin Rheumatol. 2002;14(2):109–14.
8. Copay AG, Subach BR, Glassman SD, Polly DW, Schuler TC. Understanding the minimum clinically important difference: a review of concepts and methods. Spine J. 2007;7(5):541–6.

9. Bach M, Wilke M, Wilhelm B, Zrenner E, Wilke R. Basic quantitative assessment of visual performance in patients with very low vision. Invest Ophthalmol Vis Sci. 2010;51(2): 1255–60.
10. Geruschat DR, Deremeik J. Activities of daily living and rehabilitation with prosthetic vision. In: Dagnelie G, editor. Visual prosthetics: physiology, bioengineering, rehabilitation. New York: Springer Science & Business Media; 2011. p. 413–25.
11. Stingl K, Bartz-Schmidt KU, Besch D, Braun A, Bruckmann A, Gekeler F, et al. Artificial vision with wirelessly powered subretinal electronic implant alpha-IMS. Proc Biol Sci. 2013;280(1757):20130077.
12. Bailey IL, Jackson AJ, Minto H, Greer RB, Chu MA. The Berkeley rudimentary vision test. Optom Vis Sci. 2012;89(9):1257–64.
13. Stingl K, Bartz-Schmidt KU, Besch D, Chee CK, Cottriall CL, Gekeler F, et al. Subretinal visual implant alpha IMS – clinical trial interim report. Vision Res. 2015;111(Pt B):149–60.
14. Gulati R, Roche H, Thayaparan K, Hornig R, Rubin GS. The development of a picture discrimination test for people with very poor vision. Invest Ophthalmol Vis Sci. 2011;52(14):1197.
15. Bond TG, Fox CM. Applying the rasch model: fundamental measurement in the human sciences. Hove: Psychology Press; 2013.
16. Thompson Jr RW, Barnett GD, Humayun MS, Dagnelie G. Facial recognition using simulated prosthetic pixelized vision. Invest Ophthalmol Vis Sci. 2003;44(11):5035–42.
17. Geruschat DR, Bittner AK, Dagnelie G. Orientation and mobility assessment in retinal prosthetic clinical trials. Optom Vis Sci. 2012;89(9):1308–15.
18. Humayun MS, Dorn JD, da Cruz L, Dagnelie G, Sahel JA, Stanga PE, et al. Interim results from the international trial of second sight's visual prosthesis. Ophthalmology. 2012;119(4): 779–88.
19. Bainbridge JW, Smith AJ, Barker SS, Robbie S, Henderson R, Balaggan K, et al. Effect of gene therapy on visual function in Leber's congenital amaurosis. N Engl J Med. 2008; 358(21):2231–9.
20. Nau AC, Pintar C, Fisher C, Jeong J-H, Jeong K. A standardized obstacle course for assessment of visual function in ultra low vision and artificial vision. J Vis Exp. 2014;(84):e51205.
21. Ahuja AK, Dorn JD, Caspi A, McMahon MJ, Dagnelie G, Dacruz L, et al. Blind subjects implanted with the Argus II retinal prosthesis are able to improve performance in a spatial-motor task. Br J Ophthalmol. 2011;95(4):539–43.
22. Stingl K, Bach M, Bartz-Schmidt KU, Braun A, Bruckmann A, Gekeler F, et al. Safety and efficacy of subretinal visual implants in humans: methodological aspects. Clin Exp Optom. 2013;96(1):4–13.
23. Garcia S, Petrini K, da Cruz L, Rubin G, Nardini M. Cue combination with a new sensory signal: multisensory processing in blind patients with a retinal prosthesis. J Vis. 2014; 14(10):1132.
24. Friedman SM, Munoz B, Rubin GS, West SK, Bandeen-Roche K, Fried LP, et al. Characteristics of discrepancies between self-reported visual function and measured reading speed. Invest Ophth Vis Sci. 1999;40(5):858–64.

Chapter 3
Patient-Reported Outcomes (PRO) for Prosthetic Vision

Gislin Dagnelie

Abstract Patient-reported outcome measures have gained an important role in clinical trials, especially for novel treatments where the patient's opinion on quality of life and functional outcomes is valued highly. This chapter discusses the development and calibration of such instruments and emphasizes the need to further develop instruments that are sensitive to measurement and changes of very limited vision levels, such as those afforded by today's visual prostheses.

Keywords Patient reported outcome • Self-report • Questionnaire • Visual prosthesis • Rasch analysis

Key Points
- Visual Functioning Questionnaires can play an important role in understanding how patients are using their prosthetic vision
- Rasch analysis allows systematic and quantitative interpretation of VFQ data
- Most VFQs are not designed to assess low vision levels provided by current retinal implants, and none have been validated for use in prosthesis patients
- The IVI-VLV and ULV-VFQ have the potential to provide quantitative measures of prosthetic visual performance

Introduction

Patient-Reported Outcomes (PRO) are used with increasing regularity as an important outcome measure of clinical trials, especially those where objective outcomes show limited impact, and where the patient's quality of life and ability to function independently are important criteria for success, and even for regulatory decisions.

G. Dagnelie, PhD
Department of Ophthalmology, Johns Hopkins University School of Medicine, Baltimore, MD, USA
e-mail: gdagnelie@jhmi.edu

V.P. Gabel (ed.), *Artificial Vision*, DOI 10.1007/978-3-319-41876-6_3

Originally the term PRO encompassed all reports by the patient regarding effects of a clinical intervention, but more recently it has been applied primarily to data collected with standardized questionnaires, typically using rating scales to capture the impact of vision loss or a change in well-being or vision use. This chapter provides a brief overview of the different types of questionnaires (also called instruments) currently in use, their suitability for retinal prosthesis wearers as a target population, and the need for further developments in this area.

Vision-related PRO instruments typically explore one or both of the following aspects of vision loss: quality of life (QoL) or visual ability. In the former type, patients are asked to rate how severely certain aspects of their life – e.g., work, shopping, social life – have been affected by visual impairment, on a scale that may read: "not at all, a little, moderately, severely, completely." The latter type, usually referred to as a visual function questionnaire (VFQ) asks respondents to rate the difficulty of visual activities, on a scale such as "easy, somewhat difficult, very difficult, impossible;" since not all activities are relevant to every respondent, there usually is an option "don't do this for reasons unrelated to vision." Such items are left out of the analysis, and an average or total score can be computed by assigning numerical values or "raw scores" to the categories; in the examples above, the QoL instrument would be scored as "0" to "4," and the VFQ as "0" to "3."

In both types of survey, although the categories used by all respondents are the same, their meaning may differ. Some respondents will qualify activities as "impossible" even though they could perform them with effort, whereas others would just qualify such effort as "moderately difficult." This limits our ability to compare responses from different patients, a problem that does not arise when comparing responses from the same patient over time: Judgments such as "moderately difficult" by a particular individual are likely to retain their meaning, even if the person's vision status has changed: The internal metric used by the person in answering the question is still the effort it takes to perform the activity.

PRO instruments are used in different ways: to assess the respondent against a norm – e.g., the inclusion criterion for a clinical trial –, against others – e.g., to determine who has the greatest need for treatment –, or against the same person at a different time – e.g., to assess the effect of treatment. For a treatment effect, responses by the same person before and after treatment are compared, so comparing raw scores may tell us whether the treatment was effective. Even this is questionable, though, since we do not know how variable the person's answers are, unless we've determined this by administering the instrument more than once prior to treatment. For this reason, even within the same person, we should use a quantitative (or "psychometric") approach to analyzing PRO data. When comparing one person's responses against those of others, or against a norm, a psychometric approach is the only valid one.

Basic Psychometric Concepts; Rasch Analysis

Scales such as "easy, somewhat difficult, very difficult, impossible" are ordinal, since they rank a quality (in this case effort), whereas a scale from 0 to 3 is cardinal: it not only ranks the categories, but assigns values to them. When administering a test or a questionnaire we are ranking the ability of the persons against the difficulty of the items. The purpose of a psychometric analysis is to transform ranking data into (cardinal) measures, but this requires certain assumptions about the underlying structure of the data, the so-called latent trait we are measuring. In the case of a VFQ the latent trait would be visual ability (from the person's perspective) or visual difficulty (from the item's perspective).

One generally accepted framework for such a transformation is called Item Response Theory, which has found widespread application in test development. A more general approach, formulated by the Danish mathematician Georg Rasch, has led the development of what is now broadly referred to as Rasch analysis [1]. Conceptually, it is based on the assumption that an item rated as more difficult than another by one respondent will also be rated more difficult by other respondents, and that conversely a person more able than another in performing one item (i.e., rating that item as less difficult than the other person) will also be more able in performing all other items. Thus the persons can be ranked in ability, and the items in difficulty, on the basis of the complete set of judgments.

In reality, judgments will not be perfectly consistent: Questionnaire items may be interpreted somewhat differently by different persons. Also, certain assumptions about the variability of the persons and items (which can be thought of as "noise" in the measurement) are required to create a mathematical set of equations that provides the best fitting estimates. The most commonly used Rasch model, formulated by Andrich, has been implemented in a computer program called Winsteps. This software not only provides estimates of the person and item measures, but also confidence intervals on the estimates and information on the quality of the fit, i.e., the extent to which each item fits the model. Winsteps also provides information about the score distributions, and whether there is a meaningful distinction between response categories such as "very difficult" and "extremely difficult." This information is especially helpful during the development of a new questionnaire.

Precision of Item and Person Measure Estimates

The precision of estimates obtained through Rasch analysis depends on the number of responses contributing to them: The more questions a respondent answers, the more precise will be the estimate of the person measure; and the more respondents answer any given question, the more precise will be the estimate of the item measure. However, this is true only if the person abilities and item difficulties contributing to the estimates are broadly distributed: If every item has the same difficulty, they will all elicit the same response, from any respondent, and the estimates of their person measures will remain imprecise. Thus, a well-designed instrument will span a broad range of item difficulties, and to calibrate its items a large set of respondents with a broad range of abilities will be required. It is also important that the ranges of the person and item measures match: An item that is scored "easy" or "impossible" by every respondent has no discriminating power and thus does not contribute to the estimates. Similarly we can't obtain a precise person measure for someone whose vision is too good (every item is rated "easy") or too poor (every item is rated "impossible").

Winsteps software is easily available and well documented, allowing any researcher to analyze questionnaire rating data. Thus it is no wonder that Rasch analysis has become the standard for the analysis of questionnaire data in the scientific literature. Another advantage of such a generally accepted framework is that data from most currently used QoL and VFQ instruments have been analyzed retroactively, and that the properties of those instruments are now well known. Moreover, once the items of these existing questionnaires have been calibrated, the item measures and the weight of each response category can be considered fixed, and calculating the person measure for any new patient answering the questionnaire becomes as simple as entering the responses into a spreadsheet that will instantly calculate the person measure.

Subscales, Visual Domains, Visual Aspects

The items in traditional PRO instruments are often grouped into subscales thought to be informative about the respondent's ability in different areas of daily life. As an example, the NEI-VFQ [2, 3] combines the responses to groups of items to calculate separate scores for general, near, and distance vision; day and night driving; and glare; but also for ocular pain, vision expectations, general health, mental health, and social function. The ratings for most items contribute to more than one subscale, so it is not surprising that subscale scores are highly correlated for most respondents. Note also that the NEI-VFQ, and therefore its subscales, cover both QoL and visual ability. The use of subscales can certainly be informative for clinical application of PRO instruments, but the interdependence of subscales limits their use for research purposes, as it would be inappropriate to use more than one subscale as an outcome measure. Well-designed PRO instruments therefore tend to avoid the use of subscales.

While the use of subscales has been limited to clinical studies, research in the area of visual impairment and low vision rehabilitation has widely accepted the assignment of activities to four separate visual domains: reading (more broadly defined as detail vision), visual information gathering, visually guided mobility, and visually guided activities (often called eye-hand coordination). The advantage of using these domains in rehabilitation is that they are easily translated into training activities and assessments; moreover, it is relatively straightforward to create questionnaire items assessing the patient's ability in these four domains. This use of visual domains can be found in more recent questionnaires developed using psychometric tools, such as the VALVVFQ-48 [4] and the three impact of visual impairment (IVI) [5–7] instruments.

A third approach to classifying human vision is in terms of subjectively experienced visual aspects of the scene such as contrast, illumination (natural and manmade), familiarity, size/distance, movement, color, depth, etc. These visual aspects may not be of particular importance to normally sighted individuals, but as vision becomes more severely compromised and individuals can no longer appreciate complex visual scenes, they report that their visual perception relies on the presence of these elementary visual qualities. This was one of the principal findings in a focus group study involving patients with profound vision loss who were asked to report in which daily activities they still had benefit from their minimal remaining vision; the focus group study was the first phase in the development of the prosthetic low vision rehabilitation (PLoVR) curriculum funded by a grant from the National Eye Institute. Surprisingly some 750 different activities were reported by the 46 members of 7 groups, and for every single activity a specific visual aspect, most often contrast or illumination, was reported to be the determining factor allowing these individuals to perform that activity [8].

None of the classifications above results in independent vision measures (or factors) when analyzing the properties of PRO instruments, but they are useful as conceptual frameworks when thinking about prosthetic vision, and how to analyze patients' self-reports.

Application to Prosthetic Vision

Over the last 25 years the number of PRO instruments developed for vision assessment has reached several dozen, and that just covers those available in English. Some instruments were developed for specific disorders, such as cataract [9] or hemianopia [10], while others were designed for specific populations such as children [6, 10–13] or military veterans [4, 14, 15].

Prosthetic vision is still in its infancy and can best be described as "moving shadows," according to the descriptions provided by recipients of the Argus II [16], Alpha IMS [17], and suprachoroidal retinal implants in Australia [18] and Japan [19]. This poses a particular challenge in the context of PRO instruments, since most items in existing VFQs are aimed at vision that includes shape recognition, i.e., vision that is no worse than "count fingers." Prosthetic vision, in its present form, allows most users to recognize crude shapes [20, 21], but they only do so with great effort, and most of their visual activities fall in the range of movement detection, light localization, of light detection. This imposes a new requirement on PRO instruments used in this population: Most or all of the items in such an instrument should address very basic visual perceptions, such as seeing a person walk past, locating crosswalk lines or a building across the street, or noticing whether room lights are on.

As it turns out, retinal implant users are not the only individuals with extremely poor vision. As mentioned above we gathered 46 individuals with "ultra-low vision" (ULV), defined as vision insufficient to recognize shapes other than through extensive scanning. Most of them had enjoyed better vision earlier in life, but had lost most of that vision due to a variety of disorders. Most of them also reported still using their remaining vision, and had benefited from low vision rehabilitation. Thus, we concluded that individuals with ULV, not just those with visual prostheses, could benefit from the existence of a dedicated PRO instrument. Another potential target group is formed by those with ULV (or completely blind) who may soon become participants in early clinical trials of stem cell and gene therapy approaches, as well as prosthetic devices stimulating higher visual pathways, especially the visual cortex.

One validated and calibrated PRO instrument, the IVI-VLV [7], contains items that can capture vision at the level of movement detection and light localization, although most of its items require shape recognition. This instrument is also geared towards exploring the impact of vision loss, i.e., a combination of QoL and visual ability. To our knowledge, the only VFQ specifically designed for, and calibrated in, individuals with ULV is the ULV-VFQ [22]. It currently exists in 150-, 50-, and 23-item versions; there also is an interactive version, using a Bayesian adaptive approach to estimate a ULV person's visual ability, which can obtain a reliable estimate with fewer than 20 items [23]. The ULV-VFQ will require continued calibration studies in target populations with prosthetic and other types of restored vision, and it is only available in English at this time. Nonetheless, it is an important step forward in the use of PRO instruments for the assessment of visual ability among visual prosthesis recipients.

References

1. Massof RW. Application of stochastic measurement models to visual function rating scale questionnaires. Ophthalmic Epidemiol. 2005;12(2):103–24.
2. Mangione CM, Lee PP, Pitts J, Gutierrez P, Berry S, Hays RD. Psychometric properties of the National Eye Institute Visual Function Questionnaire (NEI-VFQ). NEI-VFQ field test investigators. Arch Ophthalmol. 1998;116(11):1496–504.
3. Mangione CM, Lee PP, Gutierrez PR, Spritzer K, Berry S, Hays RD. Development of the 25-item National Eye Institute Visual Function Questionnaire. Arch Ophthalmol. 2001;119(7):1050–8.
4. Stelmack JA, Massof RW. Using the VA LV VFQ-48 and LV VFQ-20 in low vision rehabilitation. Optom Vis Sci. 2007;84(8):705–9.
5. Lamoureux EL, Pallant JF, Pesudovs K, Rees G, Hassell JB, Keeffe JE. The impact of vision impairment questionnaire: an assessment of its domain structure using confirmatory factor analysis and rasch analysis. Invest Ophthalmol Vis Sci. 2007;48(3):1001–6.
6. Cochrane GM, Marella M, Keeffe JE, Lamoureux EL. The Impact of Vision Impairment for Children (IVI_C): validation of a vision-specific pediatric quality-of-life questionnaire using Rasch analysis. Invest Ophthalmol Vis Sci. 2011;52(3):1632–40.
7. Finger RP, Tellis B, Crewe J, Keeffe JE, Ayton LN, Guymer RH. Developing the impact of Vision Impairment-Very Low Vision (IVI-VLV) questionnaire as part of the LoVADA protocol. Invest Ophthalmol Vis Sci. 2014;55(10):6150–8.
8. Dagnelie G, Jeter PE, Dalvin L, Arnold E. An inventory of visually guided activities self-reported by individuals with profound visual impairment. Invest Ophthalmol Vis Sci. 2013;54(ARVO Abstr):2784.
9. Mangione CM, Phillips RS, Seddon JM, Lawrence MG, Cook EF, Dailey R, et al. Development of the 'Activities of Daily Vision Scale'. A measure of visual functional status. Med Care. 1992;30(12):1111–26.
10. Mennem TA, Warren M, Yuen HK. Preliminary validation of a vision-dependent activities of daily living instrument on adults with homonymous hemianopia. Am J Occ Ther Off Pub Am Occ Ther Asso. 2012;66(4):478–82.

11. Gothwal VK, Sumalini R, Bharani S, Reddy SP, Bagga DK. The second version of the L. V. Prasad-functional vision questionnaire. Optom Vis Sci. 2012;89(11):1601–10.
12. Felius J, Stager Sr DR, Berry PM, Fawcett SL, Stager Jr DR, Salomao SR, et al. Development of an instrument to assess vision-related quality of life in young children. Am J Ophthalmol. 2004;138(3):362–72.
13. Cochrane G, Lamoureux E, Keeffe J. Defining the content for a new quality of life questionnaire for students with low vision (the Impact of Vision Impairment on Children: IVI_C). Ophthalmic Epidemiol. 2008;15(2):114–20.
14. Becker SW, Lambert RW, Schulz EM, Wright BD, Burnet DL. An instrument to measure the activity level of the blind. Int J Rehab Res Int Zeitschrift fur Rehabilitationsforschung Revue internationale de recherches de readaptation. 1985;8(4):415–24.
15. Stelmack JA, Szlyk JP, Stelmack TR, Demers-Turco P, Williams RT, Moran D, et al. Psychometric properties of the veterans affairs low-vision visual functioning questionnaire. Invest Ophthalmol Vis Sci. 2004;45(11):3919–28.
16. Dorn JD, Ahuja AK, Caspi A, da Cruz L, Dagnelie G, Sahel JA, et al. The detection of motion by blind subjects with the epiretinal 60-electrode (Argus II) retinal prosthesis. JAMA Ophthalmol. 2013;131(2):183–9.
17. Stingl K, Bartz-Schmidt KU, Besch D, Braun A, Bruckmann A, Gekeler F, et al. Artificial vision with wirelessly powered subretinal electronic implant alpha-IMS. Proc Biol Sci. 2013;280(1757):20130077.
18. Ayton LN, Blamey PJ, Guymer RH, Luu CD, Nayagam DA, Sinclair NC, et al. First-in-human trial of a novel suprachoroidal retinal prosthesis. PLoS One. 2014;9(12):e115239.
19. Lohmann TK, Kanda H, Morimoto T, Endo T, Miyoshi T, Nishida K, et al. Surgical feasibility and biocompatibility of wide-field dual-array suprachoroidal-transretinal stimulation prosthesis in middle-sized animals. Graefes Arch Clin Exp Ophthalmol. 2016;254(4):661–73.
20. da Cruz L, Coley BF, Dorn J, Merlini F, Filley E, Christopher P, et al. The Argus II epiretinal prosthesis system allows letter and word reading and long-term function in patients with profound vision loss. Br J Ophthalmol. 2013;97(5):632–6.
21. Zrenner E, Bartz-Schmidt KU, Benav H, Besch D, Bruckmann A, Gabel VP, et al. Subretinal electronic chips allow blind patients to read letters and combine them to words. Proc Biol Sci. 2011;278(1711):1489–97.
22. Dagnelie G, Jeter PE, Adeyemo K, Rozanski C, Nkodo AF, Massof RW. Psychometric properties of the PLoVR ultra-low vision (ULV) questionnaire. Invest Ophthalmol Vis Sci. 2014;55(ARVO E-abstr):2150.
23. Dagnelie G, Barry MP, Adeyemo K, Jeter PE, Massof RW. Twenty questions: an adaptive version of the PLoVR ultra-low vision (ULV) questionnaire. Invest Ophthalmol Vis Sci. 2015;56(ARVO E-abstr):497.

Chapter 4
Prospects and Limitations of Spatial Resolution

Jörg Sommerhalder and Angélica Pérez Fornos

Abstract Our sense of vision permanently captures, transmits and interprets enormous amounts of visual information. The amount of visual information that can be transmitted to the brain by the means of visual prosthesis will be severely limited and thus also limit the rehabilitation prospects of such devices. While several parameters contribute to the information content of visual stimuli, this chapter concentrates essentially on *spatial resolution*.

The first part of the chapter is dedicated to discuss the results of simulation studies of prosthetic vision on normal subjects. These studies aimed to respond to the question of how much visual information should be transmitted to the brain to rehabilitate patients. The amount of visual information, necessary to accomplish daily living tasks (such as reading, eye-hand coordination or whole body mobility) is task-dependent and not only image resolution itself, but also other parameters such as the size of the effective visual field seem to be important.

In the second part of the chapter we tried to discuss to which extent the information made available by the stimulation device is lost or degraded before reaching the brain. The experience with actual retinal implants shows us that only part of the information provided by the device finds its way to the central nervous system and that this information loss can be highly variable from patient to patient: the spatial resolution provided by the devices corresponds rarely to the spatial resolution perceived by the patients.

Keywords Visual prosthesis • Artificial vision • Simulation studies • Spatial resolution • Visual psychophysics • Retinal stimulation • Clinical trials

---

J. Sommerhalder (✉)
Department of Ophthalmology, Geneva University Hospitals, Geneva, Switzerland
e-mail: jorg.r.sommerhalder@hcuge.ch

A. Pérez Fornos
Western Switzerland Cochlear Implants Center, Geneva University Hospitals, Geneva, Switzerland

V.P. Gabel (ed.), *Artificial Vision*, DOI 10.1007/978-3-319-41876-6_4

Key Points

- Spatial resolution is clearly an important issue in the context of visual prostheses; it describes the amount of information that can be transmitted by the device.
- Simulation studies are a useful tool to determine what spatial resolution should be targeted by such devices: about 500 retinotopically distributed phospenes would be enough in many everyday situations.
- Only part of the information, made available by the stimulation device, reaches the brain; this information loss at the electrode-nerve interface is highly variable from patient to patient.
- At present, commercially available visual prostheses should be considered as vision aids for blind patients, complementary to traditional vision aids.

Visual prostheses are devices that aim to replace a non-functioning part in the visual pathway by directly stimulating the remaining and still functioning neural tissue mostly using electrical currents (for a review see e.g., [1–6]). Other devices designed to rehabilitate blindness use alternative sensory modalities like hearing or touch to transmit visual information [7, 8]. A common aspect of all these devices is that certain technical constraints can severely limit the quantity of visual information that can be captured and transmitted. Obviously, the final amount of visual information that can be transmitted to the brain will fundamentally limit the rehabilitation prospects of the device.

From a technical point of view, the information content of a visual stimulus can be characterized by several parameters: spatial resolution (number of pixels/dots in an image), hue and brightness information (number of hue and brightness levels that can be represented by each of these pixels), and visual field (size of the visual scene covered by the image). This chapter essentially focuses on how spatial resolution, commonly expressed by visual acuity in daily ophthalmologic practice, impacts on performance with visual prosthesis.

The first part of the chapter is dedicated to discuss the results of simulations of prosthetic (artificial) vision on normal subjects. This strategy has been used by several research groups to explore potential benefits of neural prostheses, in particular cochlear implants (see e.g., [9]) and visual prostheses (see e.g., [10] for a review). The advantages of this strategy are that the effect of a single parameter can be measured without confounding its influence with that of others and that it is easy to repeat experiments on a single subject [11]. Furthermore, it is non-invasive and independent of the availability of patients with visual prostheses.

The second part of the chapter discusses the effect of information loss at the electrode-nerve interface. In other words, we will try to discuss to which extent the information made available by the stimulation device is lost or degraded before reaching the brain. The experience with actual retinal implant wearers shows us that only part of the information provided by the device finds its way to the central nervous system and that this information loss can be highly variable from patient to patient: the spatial resolution provided by the devices corresponds rarely to the spatial resolution perceived by the patients (perceived dots or phosphenes).

Please note that this chapter does not aim to give a global and complete review on the subject of spatial resolution. It is essentially based on our own research work and our experience with patients of the Argus II feasibility study (http://clinicaltrials.gov/show/NCT00407602).

Which Spatial Resolution Should Be Targeted by Visual Prosthesis?

Simulations that mimic the artificial vision provided by visual prostheses have to take into account the main technical constraints of these devices, namely that they would only stimulate a fixed and spatially limited location of the visual field and that the number of stimulation contacts (or stimulating electrodes) is limited (resulting in reduced spatial resolution).

We simulated such viewing conditions by projecting a low resolution (pixelized) image within a limited-size viewing window presented either on a computer screen for reading (Fig. 4.1a) or on a smaller screen attached in front of a portable simulator for tasks involving eye-hand coordination and whole body mobility (Fig. 4.1b). A fast video based eye-tracking system was used to stabilize these (dynamic) stimuli on a fixed area of the retina.

Our psychophysical experiments were designed to determine a "cut-off" or threshold value for performance below which a given task becomes difficult and finally impossible to be executed. It is precisely this "cut-off" value that determines the minimum information (e.g., in terms of spatial resolution) required to achieve important daily living tasks.

Reading

Our experiments on full-page text reading [12] demonstrated that about 500 distinct phosphenes[1], retinotopically distributed[2] on a 10°×7° central visual field could restore significant reading abilities to blind patients (i.e., reading accuracy >95 % and reading rates of 60–71 words/min that improved to 72–122 words/min after some training). In such viewing conditions, displaying at a glance approximately four to six letters and two lines of text [12, 13], a single lower case letter of the visualized text would have to cover about 2° of the entire 10° × 7° visual field. This

[1] Distinct percepts of light produced by stimulating the visual system by other means than light.

[2] Perceived phosphenes are distributed in a way that they can be easily interpreted by the visual system – they spatially represent the original image.

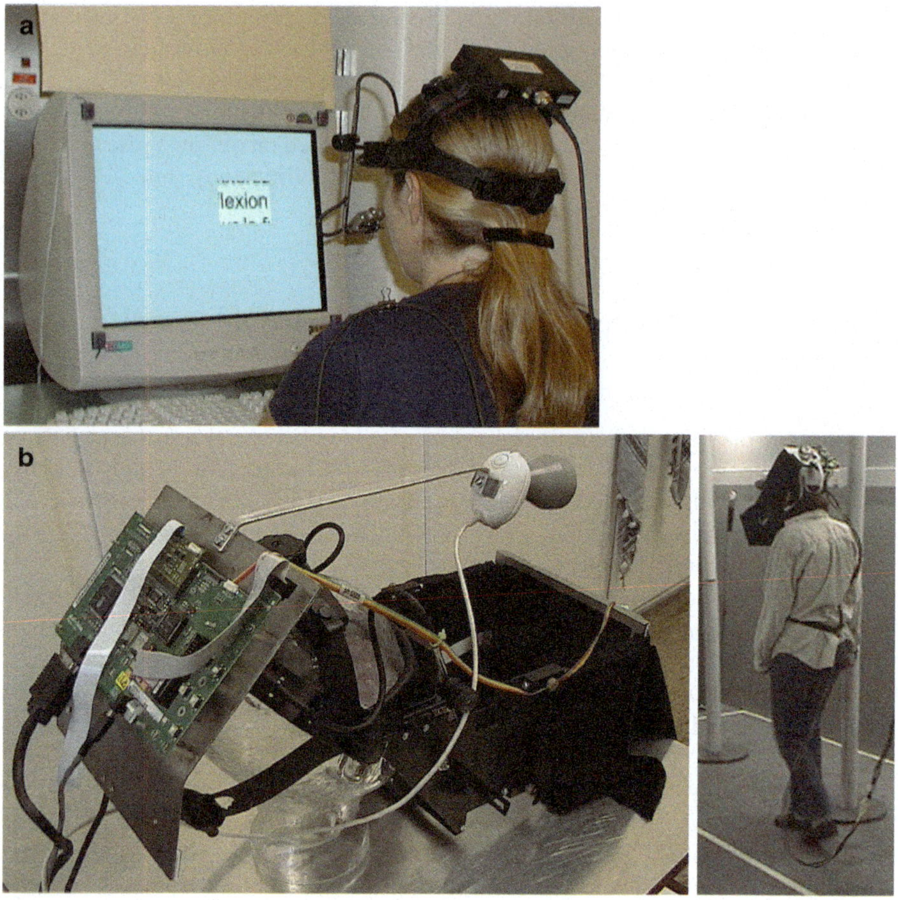

Fig. 4.1 The experimental setup used to simulate the artificial vision provided by an "ideal" retinal implant. (**a**) The stationary setup: the subject was asked to read aloud pixelized text pages. Only a portion of the text was visible inside a restricted low resolution viewing window. The subject had to use her own eye movements to navigate through the page of text on the computer screen. (**b**) The mobile setup: a camera and a screen were attached to the headband of the eye-tracking system for capturing and presenting the stimuli. A bite-bar was used to stabilize the whole mobile setup on the subject's head. A piece of black cloth covered the entire head-mounted setup so that the subject was only able to view the environment through the small, low-resolution viewing window presented on the screen. All experiments were conducted in monocular viewing

corresponds to an effective resolution of 4 pix/char (or about 300 pix/deg^2 for common news-paper text reading).

Cha et al. [14] found similar reading rates when using perphorated masks with a head-mounted display and head-scanning (100 word/min with a 25×25 dot mask). Dagnelie et al. [15] showed that accurate paragraph text reading (>90 % reading accuracy) could be achieved with a 16×16 dot matrix with 30 % phosphene dropout, at reading rates of about 30 words/min.

Reading rates of 50–100 words/min are certainly lower than normal (about 250 words/min [13]) and quite similar to those achieved with Braille reading [16]. Nevertheless, it would be of high interest for visual prosthesis patients to be able to read commonly available printed material, even if this takes four times longer than for normally sighted people.

Visuo-motor Coordination

Our experiments on eye-hand coordination included two simple pointing and manipulation tasks [17]. For the LED pointing task, subjects were facing a panel composed of an array of 6 × 4 light-emitting diodes (LEDs). Subjects had to point as precisely as possible on each one of the LEDs that lighted up randomly on the panel. For the chips manipulating task, subjects were facing a 5 × 4 random template of square chips, each representing one of 20 different black figures drawn on white background (Fig. 4.2a). Scores (pointing precision and correct placements) as well as rapidity were recorded for both tasks. Various effective field of view sizes and image resolutions were tested (Fig. 4.2b). Small effective fields of view increased visual search times, while large effective fields of view limited pointing precision or form recognition. A good compromise between effective field of view and image resolution was found at an effective field of view of 17° × 12° and an image resolution of about 500 pixels which corresponds to a spatial resolution of about 2.5 pixels/deg^2 (Fig. 4.2c).

It is difficult to compare this result with those of other studies, because experimental conditions were not identical. Humayun et al. [18] and Hayes et al. [19] used a head-mounted display and pixelizing software to simulate artificial vision (without stabilized retinal projection). Almost all of their subjects were able to pour candies from one cup to another using a grid of 16 × 16 pixels. Under the same conditions, subjects were able to cut a black square drawn on a white paper sheet with approximately 50 % accuracy. Another study [20] attempted to evaluate the issue of retinal stabilization on a checker placing task using a 10 × 6 array of Gaussian shaped pixels. However, the parameter of spatial resolution was not considered in this study. More recently, Srivastava et al. [21] reported that their eye-hand coordination task (placing black checkers on the white fields of a checker board) could be done using a viewing condition with 325 phosphene dots.

Whole Body Mobility

Whole body mobility is important in daily living. We explored this category of tasks in various environments, representative of different every-day situations.

First, a well-known indoor environment, a laboratory course with six known but randomly placed obstacles was used (Fig. 4.3a, [22]). Performance was measured as

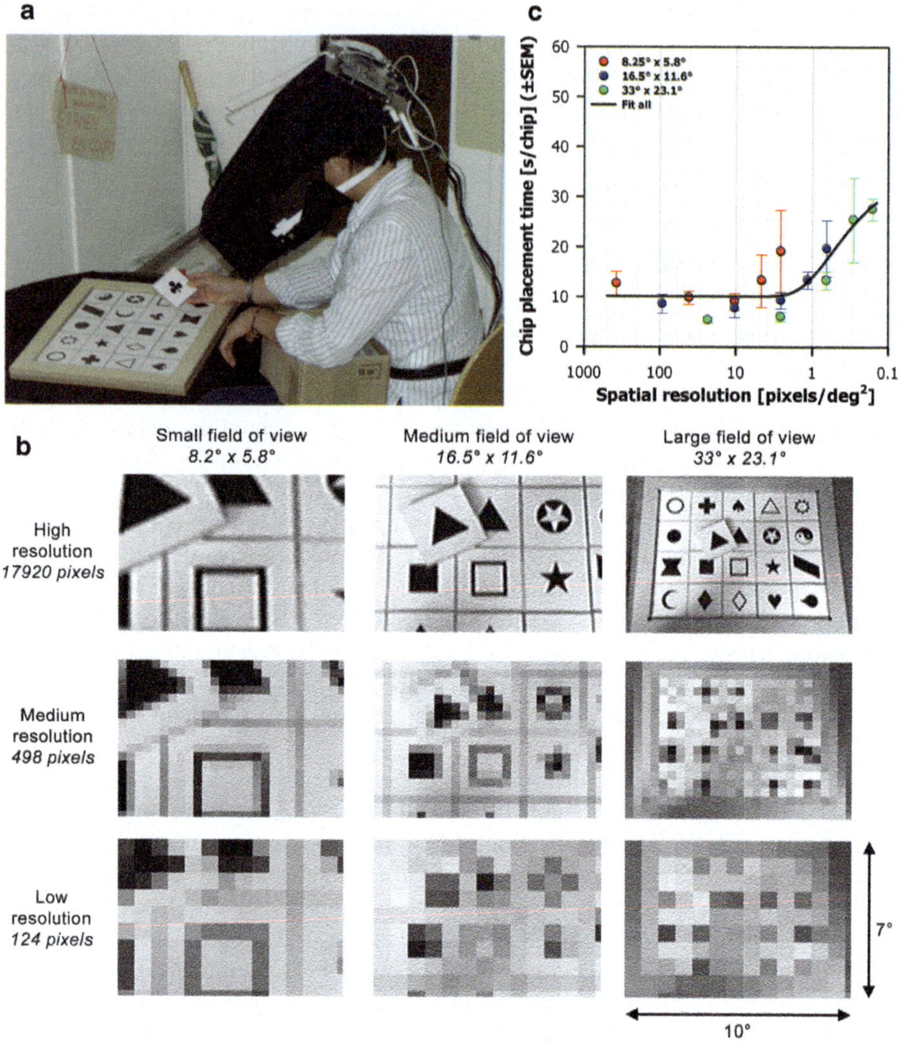

Fig. 4.2 The chips manipulating task covering object recognition and eye hand coordination. (**a**) Subject wearing the artificial vision simulator and placing a chip on the 5 × 4 template board. (**b**) Stimuli presented in the 10° × 7° viewing window to the subject. Illustration of three image resolutions at three different effective fields of view (part of the visual field projected into the viewing window). (**c**) Placement time (per chip) versus spatial resolution expressed in pixels/deg^2 (Modified from Perez Fornos et al. [17])

the total time to complete the course and the number of errors per course. For this task, a good compromise between effective field of view and image resolution was found at 33° × 23° and a relatively low image resolution of about 200 pixels, which corresponds to a spatial resolution of about 0.25 pixels/deg^2 (Fig. 4.3b).

Second, an indoor maze with 52 randomly placed poles ('random forest') on a 16 × 8 m^2 surface was used as a model of a much less predictable environment (Fig. 4.4a, [23]).

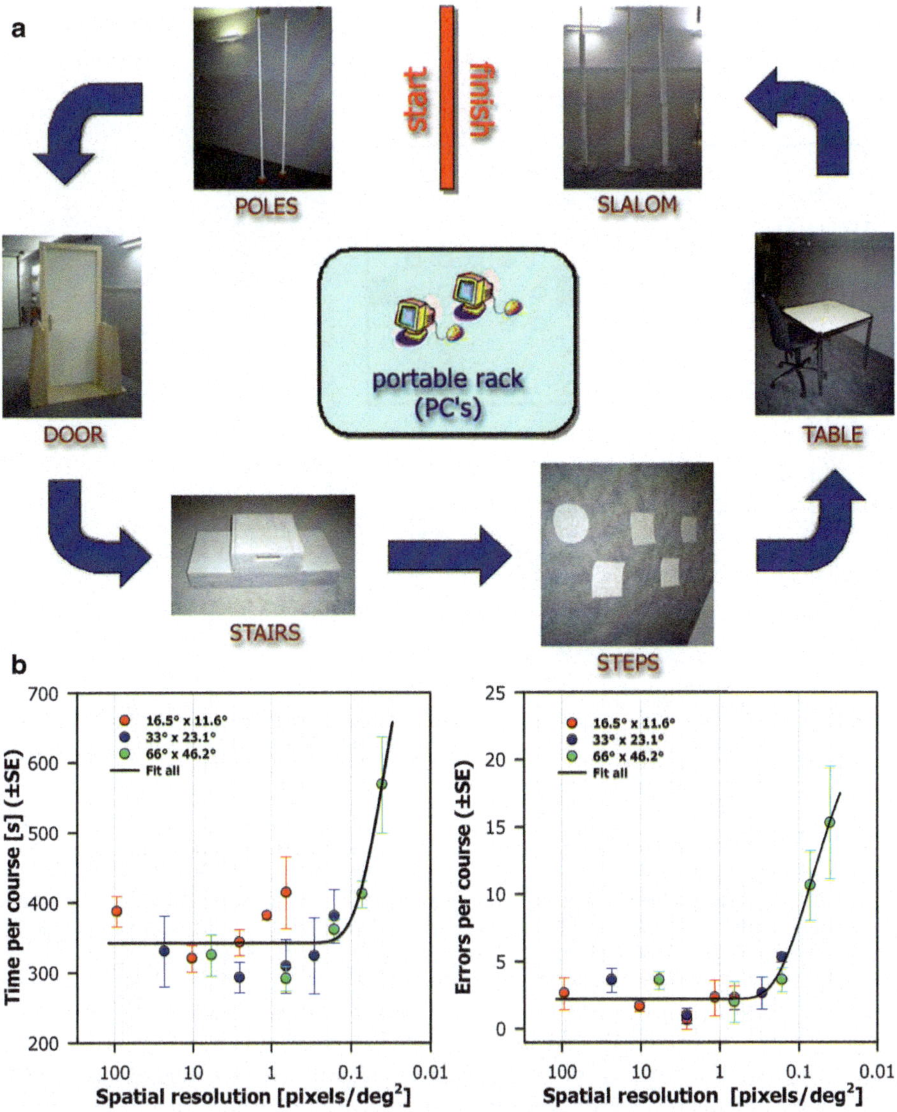

Fig. 4.3 The indoor course mobility task. (**a**) Scheme of a random configuration with six obstacles: the subject had to pass between two poles, open and pass through the door, climb over the stairs, walk on the spots placed on the floor, sit on the chair in front of the table and put a pencil inside the plastic cup, and slalom around three poles. (**b**) Mean performance as a function of spatial resolution in pix/deg^2

Performance was measured as the total time required to complete the course and the number of errors per course. Error counts remained quite stable even for low image resolutions (for the conditions where the effective field of view was not too large). However, time per run began to increase at image resolutions of 500 pixels.

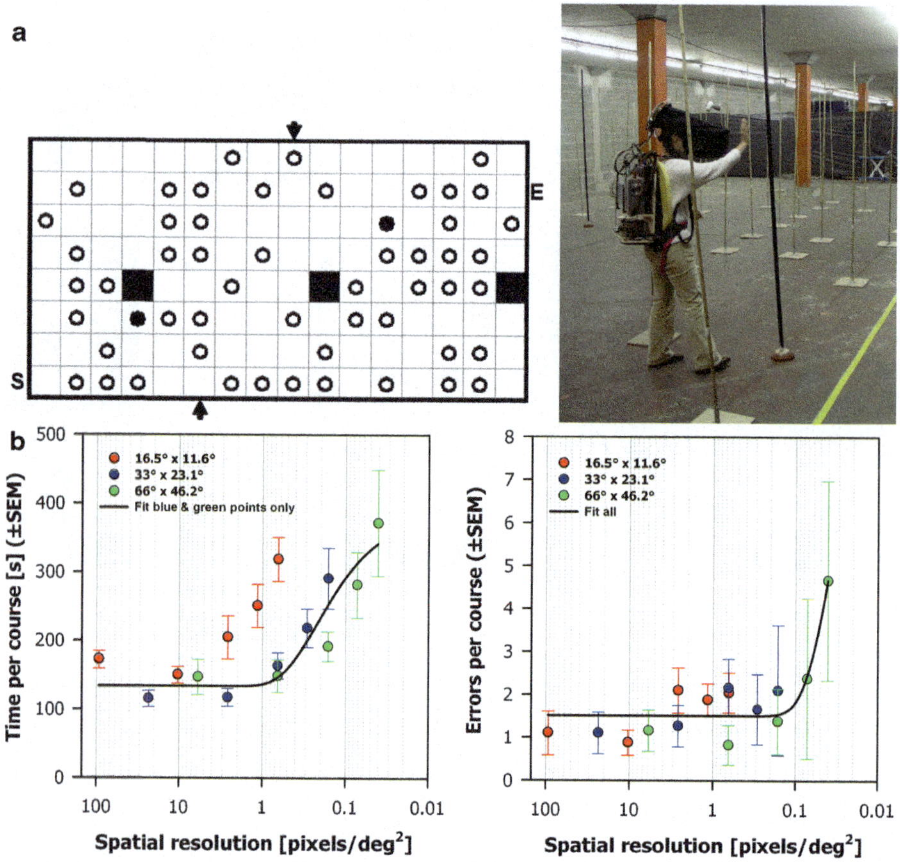

Fig. 4.4 The 'random forest' task. (**a**) Example of a test configuration: empty dots represent 'white trees' to be avoided, filled dots represent 'black trees' to be localized and touched, starting point S, end point E. *Arrows* represent the starting point of dynamic obstacles (0–2 persons could cross the 'forest' at any time and had to be avoided). (**b**) Performance as a function of spatial resolution in pix/deg²

A viewing window with 500 pixels and representing an effective field of view of 33° × 23° appeared to be the best compromise for this task. This corresponds to a spatial resolution of about 0.7 pixels/deg² (Fig. 4.4b).

Finally, a completely unpredictable and visually complex environment was tested in the 'road crossing' task [23]. Subjects were confronted to the real situation of a medium traffic one way road and had to estimate at which moment they could cross the street (without actually crossing it for obvious safety reasons). Subjective danger was evaluated using a questionnaire. Subjects had to indicate the 'difficulty' of the task, the 'safety' of their crossing and the 'reliance on hearing' to accomplish the task. The traffic situation at the moment of the crossing decision was taken in account as a more objective parameter. Both, the 'difficulty' and the 'security' estimates for the task got steadily worse when reducing stimulus resolution (for all tested effective fields of view). Subjects mainly relayed on hearing to complement insufficient visual information. Only a few dangerous situations were detected among several hundreds of attempts. Surprisingly, these were observed at relatively high stimulus resolutions when subjects inappropriately trusted their vision.

The results for these three mobility tasks show that mobility in unpredictable complex (and dynamic) environments needs more visual information than mobility in highly predicable static environments. About 500 distinct phosphenes, retinotopically distributed on a $10° \times 7°$ central retinal area seem to transmit enough visual information to accomplish most mobility tasks that do not include hazardous situations. Much higher stimulus resolutions are needed to rely on vision for avoiding danger in complex visual environments.

The results of other studies on mobility using simulated artificial vision are again difficult to compare because of differences in experimental conditions and scopes/issues. Cha et al. [24] found with their simplified simulation that a 25×25 array of pixels distributed within the foveal visual area could provide useful visually guided mobility in environments not requiring a high degree of pattern recognition.[3] Dagnelie et al. [25] explored simulated artificial vision in a real indoor maze (suite of offices) and found that inexperienced subjects required 16×16 dots for adequate performance, while experienced subjects reached similar levels with 10×6 dots.[4] Wang et al. [26] explored mobility with simulated prosthetic vision in a virtual ten room maze using a gaze-locked 10×6 matrix of Gaussian shaped pixels and found a 40 % performance decrease for a 30 % phosopene dropout.

Synthesis

The simulation studies reported above can be summarized as follows: A visual prosthesis being able to produce about 500 distinct and retinotopically distributed phosphenes could be useful in many daily life situations. The effective visual field that would have to be covered by these devices is task dependent (very small for reading and large for mobility). Such variation of the effective field of view could be realized by using optical or digital zooms for the image capturing devices of the prosthesis. Table 4.1 summarizes corresponding numbers.

It is interesting to mention that other parameters than image or spatial resolution limited performance in our simulation experiments. Due to the particular viewing conditions (using a small viewing window and monocular viewing), fastest speed performances in simulated prosthetic vision were three to seven times lower than those for normal viewing conditions. This was probably due to the limited visual span and difficult page navigation for reading and to the missing peripheral and stereoscopic vision for visuo-motor coordination and mobility tasks.

---

[3] Their experimental setup is closest to our 'random forest' setup (Fig. 4.4).

[4] These authors use a highly simplified (predictable) environment probably closest to our 'indoor course' (Fig. 4.3).

Table 4.1 Approximate (minimal) spatial resolution proposed to reach 'useful' vision for several daily living tasks

Task	Image resolution [n° of phosophenes]	Effective field of view	Spatial resolution
Reading of standard news-papers and small object recognition	~500	1.6° × 1.1°	~300 pixels/deg^2
Visuo-motor coordination (eye-hand coordination)	~500	17° × 12°	~2.5 pixels/deg^2
Mobility in well-known predictable environments (e.g., at home)	~200	33° × 23°	~0.25 pixels/deg^2
Mobility in relatively simple but unpredictable environment (e.g., unknown flat, park, etc.)	≥500	33° × 23°	~0.7 pixels/deg^2
Mobility in complex unpredictable and potentially dangerous environments (e.g., traffic roads, airport hall, mall, etc.)	>2000 (even with high resolution stimuli, these tasks are difficult to perform)		

Our experiments [12, 17, 22] as well as the studies by other authors (e.g., [21, 25]) demonstrate that subjects generally improve their performance with time, thus training is an important factor in simulated prosthetic vision and the experience with retinal implant patients confirms the importance of rehabilitation training.

From Theory to Reality

The above suggested spatial resolutions for 'useful' prosthetic vision indicate which effective image resolutions should be targeted by visual prostheses. Retinal implants that use incorporated photodiodes to transform light directly in-situ into electric stimuli already reach high electrode densities (e.g., the 1500 electrode Alpha IMS sub-retinal implant from Retina Implant AG). This is not yet the case for prostheses that receive the visual information from an external camera (e.g., the 60 electrode Argus II epi-retinal implant from Second Sight Medical Products Inc.) because these are technically more challenging to realize. Devices with external stimulus processing present, however, other advantages, such as the much larger possibilities to vary stimulus parameters.

It is thus also interesting to study the best possible performances that could be reached with existing low resolution devices. Several of the above mentioned simulation studies were conducted with 10 × 6 dot stimuli to simulate the commercially available Argus II system [20, 25, 26]. Our group also explored reading with a simulated 60 channel implant using the simulation techniques described above [27]. Reading performances (reading accuracies and reading rates) were recorded as a function of spatial resolution in pixels/character (Fig. 4.5a). Best reading rates were achieved at about 4.5 pix/char (confirming the results of

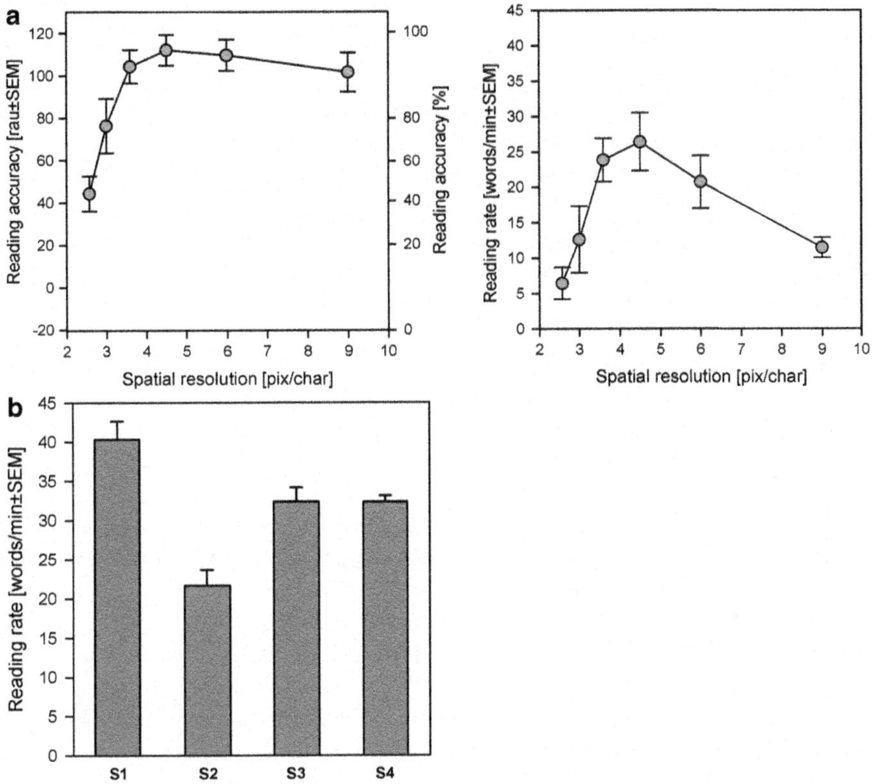

Fig. 4.5 Reading performance with a simulated 60 channel implant (gaze stabilized horizontal 10 × 6 pixel viewing window) on four subjects. (**a**) Mean performance as a function of spatial resolution in pixels/character. (**b**) Individual mean performances at the end of the experiment using the "optimum" spatial resolution (4.5 pix/char) (Modified from Perez Fornos et al. [27])

previous studies in terms of spatial resolution [12, 15]). At the end of the study and under such 'optimum' viewing conditions (4.5 pix/char), subjects achieved almost perfect reading accuracy and mean reading rates of 21–40 words/min (Fig. 4.5b). These reading rates were considerably lower than those obtained with 500 dot stimuli, because of the much lower information content of the viewing window (covering a visual span of 1–2 characters instead of 4–6 characters and just one line instead of two). This resulted in more difficulties for page navigation and a lesser ability to use context information.

It is important to mention that the above reported simulation studies establish ***a theoretical upper limit of performance, assuming that all information provided by the device effectively reaches the brain***. Unfortunately, this is rarely the case. Some autors (such as [14] or [26]) have tried to incorporate information loss at the electrode-nerve interface (e.g., phosphene dropout or reduced contrast discrimination) into their studies, but it is extremely difficult to simulate such information loss realistically.

Effectively, many of the patients participating in the Argus II feasibility study were able to recognize single letters, some of them short words [28], and the best two patients were even able to read short 4-word sentences with maximum reading rates of 5 and 2 words/min [29]. These reading rates are, however, far below the above cited theoretical limit of about 30 words/min. The same would certainly also apply for most of the other tests conducted during the clinical trial, if they would have been compared to theoretical upper limits experienced by simulating the same tasks. This means that a considerable part of the visual information provided by the stimulating device did not reach the brain.

This finding is further supported by the observation that increased spatial resolution (i.e., a higher number of electrodes) provided by the stimulating device does not seem to fundamentally improve the performances of the implanted patients. The high density Alpha IMS device seems to have quite similar outcomes [30–32] than the Argus II system [28, 29, 33, 34].[5] This means that, at the present state of the art, it is probably not useful to target visual performance improvements by simply increasing the number of stimulation electrodes in a visual prosthesis. First the electrode nerve interface has to be extensively studied and new and better stimulation strategies have to be developed to optimize information transfer from the prosthesis to the upper visual centers and limit information loss at this site.[6].

Besides relatively low performance compared to the expectations based on simulation studies, the clinical trials with retinal prostheses also revealed big individual performance differences between subjects [28, 30–34]. Visual performances with these devices go from bare light detection to the capability to read words. One of the reasons for such high inter-subject variability is that for some subjects, only a limited number of electrodes effectively evoked visual sensations at electrical current levels within security limits.[7] This could be due to a sub-optimal contact between the stimulation electrodes and the retina. Another reason can probably be found in the variability of the pathophysiology of retinal degenerations amongst patients (see e.g., [41]).

Some research groups propose to compensate the lack of information content in low resolution stimuli by using real-time image treatment/enhancement (see e.g., [42–46]). Such image processing algorithms can be useful in certain circumstances, they can however not really compensate for missing image information (spatial resolution).

Not only loss of spatial resolution deteriorates prosthetic vision. The temporal properties of the visual perception are also of high importance. Percepts should not only be sharp and well localized, they should also last long enough for the brain to reconstruct meaningful images. Ideally phosphenes should appear as soon as

---

[5] A recent paper [35] tried to compare functional performance of the two devices.

[6] Several research groups work on the question of highly localized retinal stimulation using in vitro or vivo setups or computer models [e.g., 36–40].

[7] High stimulation currents risk damaging either the retinal tissue, or the electrode material, or both. The smaller the stimulating electrode surface (and consequently the higher the spatial resolution of the device), the lower are the currents that can be used to stimulate while respecting such security limits. The latter also depend on electrode material.

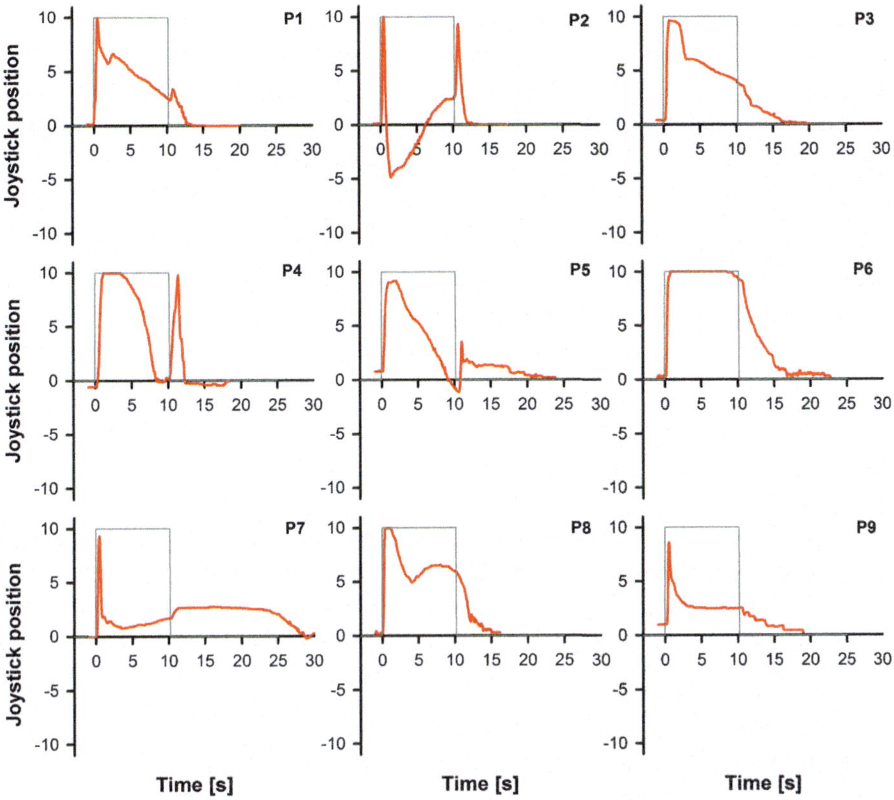

Fig. 4.6 Dynamics of visual perception upon electric stimulation of the retina. Average self-reported responses (*red*) versus time to a 10s duration stimulus (at 20 Hz – grey) for nine patients (Modified from Perez Fornos et al. [47])

stimulation is activated, evoke a stable percept as long as the stimulation lasts, and then disappear instantly when the stimulation is turned off. A recent study on nine patients participating at the Argus II clinical trial revealed important inter-subject variability for the temporal properties of electrically evoked phosphenes [47]. Figure 4.6 illustrates the time course of visual perception evoked by a 10s constant amplitude stimulus. The patient for whom the time course of the percept resembled most to the time course of stimulation (P6 in Fig. 4.6) is also the one who performed best in the clinical trial.

It has been suggested that the dynamic or "fading" behavior of percepts might be due to the stabilization of the stimulation pattern on the retina [30]. In other words, the lack of eye movements allowing to constantly "refresh" the electrical image provided to the retina by the implant would result in neural adaptation leading to some kind of Troxler's "filling-in" [48, 49]. Our results do not allow confirming or rejecting this hypothesis. The observed differences across subjects are, however, difficult to explain in the sole perspective of central neural adaptation.

Conclusion and Final Thoughts

Spatial resolution is definitely a big issue in the context of visual prostheses. Simulation studies can determine what 'ideal' spatial resolution these devices should be able to provide to the patient to achieve a certain level of performance. Being able to fabricate visual prosthesis that can effectively evoke about 500 retinotopically distributed phospenes would be a major step forward towards a visual prosthesis that would be useful in the majority of everyday situations and that would thus significantly improve quality of life. For complete autonomy, a spatial resolution of several 1000 spots distributed over a large visual field would be necessary. Commercially available retinal implants are not yet able to satisfy such high expectations: Performance of implanted patients remains relatively low and there is extremely high variability between patients.

Are state of the art, commercially available devices are really useful for their wearers? In a functional low-vision observer rated assessment, 65 % of the participating Argus II patients (N=23) reported a positive or mild positive effect 3 years after implantation [34]. This does not really tell much about the utility of the device in daily living which can probably best be estimated by analyzing the effective time the devices are used by the patients (on their own). For the Argus II retinal implant, the patients of the clinical trial can be distributed in three groups: one third used the device less than 90 min/week, another third up to 4.8 h/week and the last third up to 18.9 h/week (weekly mean values – personal communication from Second Sight Medical Products Inc.). This suggests that about one third of these users really benefit from the device.

We believe that actually commercially available visual prostheses should be considered as vision aids for blind patients, complementary to traditional vision aids such as the guiding dog, the white cane, Braille reading, technological aids such as voice-over programs in computers or mobile phones, etc. A particular attention has to be given to the screening methods, so that candidates having the best rehabilitation prospects can be appropriately identified. Once implanted, an adapted training with low vision specialists seems mandatory to maximize benefits for the users. It would be contra-productive to raise unrealistic expectations among blind patients.

It is imperative to increase research efforts in the field. Interesting work is done to better understand why the communication of high resolution stimuli to the visual system is so difficult, and how to improve the electrode-nerve interface of visual prostheses. Hopefully, next generation devices will benefit from these efforts and will be able to communicate more effectively with the brain.

References

1. Fernandes RA, Diniz B, Ribeiro R, Humayun M. Artificial vision through neuronal stimulation. Neurosci Lett. 2012;519(2):122–8.
2. Lorach H, Marre O, Sahel JA, Benosman R, Picaud S. Neural stimulation for visual rehabilitation: advances and challenges. J Physiol Paris. 2013;107(5):421–31.

3. Zrenner E. Fighting blindness with microelectronics. Sci Transl Med. 2013;5(210):210 ps16.
4. Luo YH, da Cruz L. A review and update on the current status of retinal prostheses (bionic eye). Br Med Bull. 2014;109:31–44.
5. Weiland JD, Humayun MS. Retinal prosthesis. IEEE Trans Biomed Eng. 2014;61(5):1412–24.
6. Lewis PM, Ackland HM, Lowery AJ, Rosenfeld JV. Restoration of vision in blind individuals using bionic devices: a review with a focus on cortical visual prostheses. Brain Res. 2015;1595: 51–73.
7. Yu X, Ganz A. Audible vision for the blind and visually impaired in indoor open spaces. Conf Proc IEEE Eng Med Biol Soc. 2012;2012:5110–3.
8. Lee VK, Nau AC, Laymon C, Chan KC, Rosario BL, Fisher C. Successful tactile based visual sensory substitution use functions independently of visual pathway integrity. Front Hum Neurosci. 2014;8:291.
9. Shannon RV, Zeng FG, Kamath V, Wygonski J, Ekelid M. Speech recognition with primarily temporal cues. Science. 1995;270(5234):303–4.
10. Chen SC, Suaning GJ, Morley JW, Lovell NH. Simulating prosthetic vision: II. Measuring functional capacity. Vision Res. 2009;49(19):2329–43.
11. Pelli DG. The visual requirements of mobility. In: Woo GC, editor. Low vision: principles and applications. New York: Springer; 1987. p. 134–46.
12. Sommerhalder J, Rappaz B, de Haller R, Perez Fornos A, Safran AB, Pelizzone M. Simulation of artificial vision: II. Eccentric reading of full-page text and the learning of this task. Vision Res. 2004;44(14):1693–706.
13. Legge GE, Pelli DG, Rubin GS, Schleske MM. Psychophysics of reading. I Normal Vis Res. 1985;25(2):239–52.
14. Cha K, Horch KW, Normann RA, Boman DK. Reading speed with a pixelized vision system. J Opt Soc Am A. 1992;9(5):673–7.
15. Dagnelie G, Barnett D, Humayun MS, Thompson Jr RW. Paragraph text reading using a pixelized prosthetic vision simulator: parameter dependence and task learning in free-viewing conditions. Invest Ophthalmol Vis Sci. 2006;47(3):1241–50.
16. Mousty P, Bertelson P. A study of braille reading: 1. Reading speed as a function of hand usage and context. Q J Exp Psychol A. 1985;37(2):217–33.
17. Perez Fornos A, Sommerhalder J, Pittard A, Safran AB, Pelizzone M. Simulation of artificial vision: IV. Visual information required to achieve simple pointing and manipulation tasks. Vision Res. 2008;48(16):1705–18.
18. Humayun MS. Intraocular retinal prosthesis. Trans Am Ophthalmol Soc. 2001;99:271–300.
19. Hayes JS, Yin VT, Piyathaisere D, Weiland JD, Humayun MS, Dagnelie G. Visually guided performance of simple tasks using simulated prosthetic vision. Artif Organs. 2003;27(11): 1016–28.
20. Dagnelie G, Walter M, Liancheng Y. Playing checkers: detection and eye-hand coordination in simulated prosthetic vision. J Mod Opt. 2006;53(9):1325–42.
21. Srivastava NR, Troyk PR, Dagnelie G. Detection, eye-hand coordination and virtual mobility performance in simulated vision for a cortical visual prosthesis device. J Neural Eng. 2009;6(3):035008.
22. Perez Fornos A, Sommerhalder J, Chanderli K, Pittard A, Baumberger B, Fluckiger M, Safran AB, Pelizzone M. Minimum requirements for mobility in known environments and perceptual learning of this task in eccentric vision. ARVO Meeting Abstracts. 2004;45(5):5445.
23. Sommerhalder J, Perez-Fornos A, Chanderli K, Colin L, Schaer X, Mauler F, Safran AB, Pelizzone M. Minimum requirements for mobility in unpredictible environments. Invest Ophthalmol Vis Sci. 2006;(47):ARVO E-Abstract 3204.
24. Cha K, Horch KW, Normann RA. Mobility performance with a pixelized vision system. Vision Res. 1992;32(7):1367–72.
25. Dagnelie G, Keane P, Narla V, Yang L, Weiland J, Humayun M. Real and virtual mobility performance in simulated prosthetic vision. J Neural Eng. 2007;4(1):S92–101.

26. Wang L, Yang L, Dagnelie G. Virtual way finding using simulated prosthetic vision in gaze-locked viewing. Optom Vis Sci. 2008;85(11):E1057–63.
27. Perez Fornos A, Sommerhalder J, Pelizzone M. Reading with a simulated 60-channel implant. Front Neurosci. 2011;5:57.
28. da Cruz L, Coley BF, Dorn J, Merlini F, Filley E, Christopher P, Chen FK, Wuyyuru V, Sahel J, Stanga P, Humayun M, Greenberg RJ, Dagnelie G. The Argus II epiretinal prosthesis system allows letter and word reading and long-term function in patients with profound vision loss. Br J Ophthalmol. 2013;97(5):632–6.
29. Sahel JA, da Cruz L, Hafezi F, Stanga PE, Merlini F, Coley B, Greenberg RG, Argus II™ Study Group. Subjects blind from outer retinal dystrophies are able to consistently read short sentences using the Argus™ II retinal prosthesis system. Invest Ophthalmol Vis Sci. 2011;(52):E-Abstract 3420.
30. Zrenner E, Bartz-Schmidt KU, Benav H, Besch D, Bruckmann A, Gabel VP, Gekeler F, Greppmaier U, Harscher A, Kibbel S, Koch J, Kusnyerik A, Peters T, Stingl K, Sachs H, Stett A, Szurman P, Wilhelm B, Wilke R. Subretinal electronic chips allow blind patients to read letters and combine them to words. Proc Biol Sci. 2011;278(1711):1489–97.
31. Stingl K, Bartz-Schmidt KU, Besch D, Braun A, Bruckmann A, Gekeler F, Greppmaier U, Hipp S, Hortdorfer G, Kernstock C, Koitschev A, Kusnyerik A, Sachs H, Schatz A, Stingl KT, Peters T, Wilhelm B, Zrenner E. Artificial vision with wirelessly powered subretinal electronic implant alpha-IMS. Proc Biol Sci. 2013;280(1757):20130077.
32. Stingl K, Bartz-Schmidt KU, Besch D, Chee CK, Cottriall CL, Gekeler F, Groppe M, Jackson TL, MacLaren RE, Koitschev A, Kusnyerik A, Neffendorf J, Nemeth J, Naeem MA, Peters T, Ramsden JD, Sachs H, Simpson A, Singh MS, Wilhelm B, Wong D, Zrenner E. Subretinal visual implant alpha IMS – clinical trial interim report. Vis Res. 2015;111(Pt B):149–60.
33. Humayun MS, Dorn JD, da Cruz L, Dagnelie G, Sahel JA, Stanga PE, Cideciyan AV, Duncan JL, Eliott D, Filley E, Ho AC, Santos A, Safran AB, Arditi A, Del Priore LV, Greenberg RJ. Interim results from the international trial of second sight's visual prosthesis. Ophthalmology. 2012;119(4):779–88.
34. Ho AC, Humayun MS, Dorn JD, da Cruz L, Dagnelie G, Handa J, Barale PO, Sahel JA, Stanga PE, Hafezi F, Safran AB, Salzmann J, Santos A, Birch D, Spencer R, Cideciyan AV, de Juan E, Duncan JL, Eliott D, Fawzi A, Olmos de Koo LC, Brown GC, Haller JA, Regillo CD, Del Priore LV, Arditi A, Geruschat DR, Greenberg R. Long-term results from an epiretinal prosthesis to restore sight to the blind. Ophthalmology. 2015;122(8):1547–54.
35. Stronks HC, Dagnelie G. The functional performance of the Argus II retinal prosthesis. Expert Rev Med Devices. 2014;11(1):23–30.
36. Jepson LH, Hottowy P, Mathieson K, Gunning DE, Dabrowski W, Litke AM, Chichilnisky EJ. Focal electrical stimulation of major ganglion cell types in the primate retina for the design of visual prostheses. J Neurosci. 2013;33(17):7194–205.
37. Jepson LH, Hottowy P, Mathieson K, Gunning DE, Dabrowski W, Litke AM, Chichilnisky EJ. Spatially patterned electrical stimulation to enhance resolution of retinal prostheses. J Neurosci. 2014;34(14):4871–81.
38. Schmid EW, Fink W, Wilke R. Operational challenges of retinal prostheses. Med Eng Phys. 2014;36(12):1644–55.
39. Habib AG, Cameron MA, Suaning GJ, Lovell NH, Morley JW. Spatially restricted electrical activation of retinal ganglion cells in the rabbit retina by hexapolar electrode return configuration. J Neural Eng. 2013;10(3):036013.
40. Abramian M, Lovell NH, Habib A, Morley JW, Suaning GJ, Dokos S. Quasi-monopolar electrical stimulation of the retina: a computational modelling study. J Neural Eng. 2014;11(2):025002.
41. Jones BW, Marc RE. Retinal remodeling during retinal degeneration. Exp Eye Res. 2005;81(2):123–37.
42. Chang MH, Kim HS, Shin JH, Park KS. Facial identification in very low-resolution images simulating prosthetic vision. J Neural Eng. 2012;9(4):046012.

43. Al-Atabany W, McGovern B, Mehran K, Berlinguer-Palmini R, Degenaar P. A processing platform for optoelectronic/optogenetic retinal prosthesis. IEEE Trans Biomed Eng. 2013;60(3):781–91.
44. Parikh N, Itti L, Humayun M, Weiland J. Performance of visually guided tasks using simulated prosthetic vision and saliency-based cues. J Neural Eng. 2013;10(2):026017.
45. Parikh NJ, McIntosh BP, Tanguay AR, Humayun MS, Weiland JD. Biomimetic image processing for retinal prostheses: peripheral saliency cues. Conf Proc IEEE Eng Med Biol Soc. 2009;2009:4569–72.
46. Fink W, Tarbell MA. Artificial vision support system (AVS(2)) for improved prosthetic vision. J Med Eng Technol. 2014;38(8):385–95.
47. Perez Fornos A, Sommerhalder J, da Cruz L, Sahel JA, Mohand-Said S, Hafezi F, Pelizzone M. Temporal properties of visual perception on electrical stimulation of the retina. Invest Ophthalmol Vis Sci. 2012;53(6):2720–31.
48. Troxler D. Ueber das Verschwinden gegebener Gegenstände innerhalb unseres Gesichtskreises. In: Himly K, Schmidt JA, editors. Ophthalmologische Bibliothek II, vol. 2. Jena: Fromann; 1804. p. 1–119.
49. De Weerd P. Perceptual filling-in: more than the eye can see. Prog Brain Res. 2006;154(1): 227–45.

Part II
Retinal Approaches

Chapter 5
Argus® II Retinal Prosthesis System

Paulo Falabella, Hossein Nazari, Paulo Schor, James D. Weiland, and Mark S. Humayun

Abstract The Argus® II epiretinal prosthesis was the first retinal implant to receive commercial approval in Europe and in the United States. To date, it is the most widely used prosthesis worldwide with over 100 implanted patients in several countries, including the United States, United Kingdom, France, Germany, Switzerland, Mexico and Saudi Arabia. The device is used as a treatment for patients with profound vision loss due to end-stage photoreceptor degenerative diseases.

Argus II works by electrical stimulation of the inner retina, retinal ganglion cells and/or bipolar cells that remain partially functional in these patients. The system is an epiretinal prosthesis, meaning that the microelectrode array is surgically implanted on the retinal surface nearest to the nerve fiber layer. Video signals are acquired by a glasses-mounted video camera and transformed into electrical pulses that are finally transmitted via the microelectrode array to the inner retina. The device is capable of eliciting visual perception in a reliable and controllable fashion through video processing and manipulation of stimulation parameters.

Argus II and its predecessor, Argus I, were the first devices tested in humans to pass safety and efficacy assessments. This chapter will summarize the history of device development, initial preclinical studies and results from clinical trials. It will also discuss several future advances needed to improve the device in order to provide a more informative visual perception to blind patients.

Keywords Argus® II • Argus I • Second Sight • Epiretinal implant • Epiretinal prosthesis • Retinal tack

---

P. Falabella (✉) • J.D. Weiland • M.S. Humayun
Department of Ophthalmology, University of Southern California, Los Angeles, CA, USA
e-mail: paulofalabella@hotmail.com

H. Nazari
Department of Ophthalmology, University of Texas Medical Branch (UTMB), Galveston, TX, USA

P. Schor
Department of Ophthalmology and Visual Sciences, São Paulo Hospital, Federal University of São Paulo, São Paulo, SP, Brazil

V.P. Gabel (ed.), *Artificial Vision*, DOI 10.1007/978-3-319-41876-6_5

Key Points

- The Argus® II epiretinal prosthesis was the first retinal implant to receive commercial approval in Europe and in the United States, and, to date, it is the most widely used visual prosthesis worldwide
- Argus II works by electrical stimulation of the inner retina, retinal ganglion cells and/or bipolar cells that remain partially functional in patients with end-stage outer retinal degeneration. Video signals are acquired by a glasses-mounted microcamera and transformed into electrical pulses that are finally transmitted via a 60-electrode microarray to the inner retina.
- The device is capable of eliciting phosphenes in a reliable and controllable fashion through video processing and manipulation of stimulation parameters.
- Human studies conducted so far have demonstrated the long-term safety of chronic stimulation with Argus® II and the potential benefits provided by the device as a visual aid for patients blinded by outer retinal degeneration.

Principal Idea

The Argus® II epiretinal prosthesis (Second Sight Medical Products, Inc., Sylmar, CA, USA) was the first retinal implant to receive commercial approval from the *Conformité Européenne* (CE Mark) in 2011 and from the United States Food and Drug Administration (FDA) in 2013. To date, it is the most widely used visual prosthesis worldwide, with over 100 implanted patients in several countries, including the United States, United Kingdom, France, Germany, Switzerland, Mexico and Saudi Arabia [1, 2].

The device is used as a treatment for patients with profound vision loss due to end-stage photoreceptor degenerative diseases [1, 2]. Although pharmacologic agents, stem cell-based and gene therapies have been proposed for the treatment of retinal degeneration, these methods are under development and, therefore, not yet commercially available and not all patients can benefit from them [3–5]. Retinal degenerative diseases, in general, start in the outer retina leaving inner retinal layers undisturbed until very late stages. In fact, post-mortem studies have shown that nearly 80 % of inner nuclear layer cells and approximately 30 % of retinal ganglion cells (RGC) are spared in patients blinded by various forms of Retinitis Pigmentosa (RP) [6, 7]. Additionally, a similar study of patients with advanced neovascular aged-related macular degeneration (AMD) also showed that 93 % of RGCs were spared [8]. Given that the inner retinal elements are relatively spared in the majority of retinal degenerations, the stimulation of inner retinal neurons has been tested and proven to be a feasible method to bypass the loss of photoreceptors and provide the perception of light [9–13].

Argus® II works by direct electrical stimulation of the inner retina, RGCs and/or bipolar cells that remain partially functional in these patients. The system is an epireti-

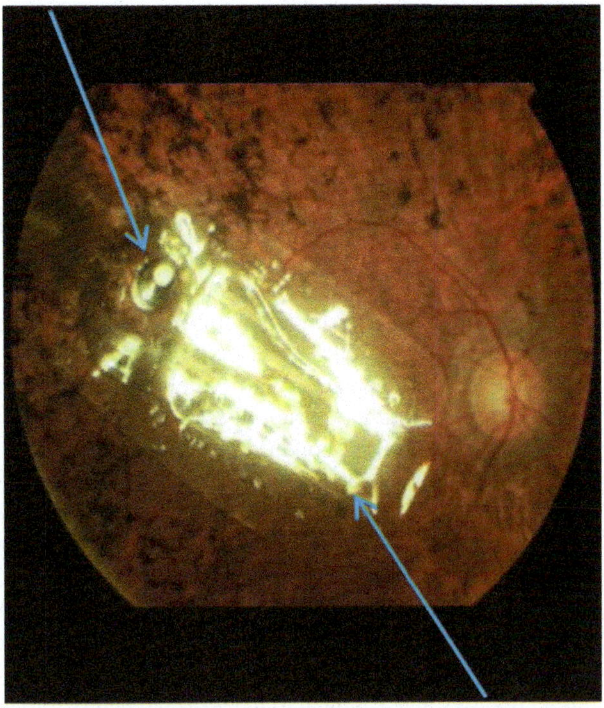

Fig. 5.1 Fundus photograph of an Argus® II retinal implant placed epiretinally over the macular region, within the retinal vessel arcades. *Arrows* indicate the microarray and the retinal tack (Reprinted with permission from Second Sight Medical Products, Inc)

nal prosthesis, meaning that the microelectrode array is surgically implanted on the retinal surface nearest to the nerve fiber layer (Fig. 5.1). Video signals are acquired by a glasses-mounted video camera and transformed into electrical pulses by a set of custom electronics that are both externally and internally implanted, linked wirelessly, and finally transmitted via the microelectrode array to the RGC and inner retina. Signals elicited from the retinal cells are sent via the optic nerve to the visual cortex, eliciting basic visual percepts called *phosphenes*. In summary, the device replaces the function (visual phototransduction) of degenerated photoreceptors in a rudimentary fashion, using the remaining natural visual pathway to induce visual responses [14].

The device is capable of eliciting phosphenes in a reliable and controllable fashion through video processing and manipulation of stimulating parameters. Patterns of stimulation in general reflect the surrounding visual scenes. Since the implanted patients have a restricted visual field of 20°, they tend to use a head scanning technique as a way of using the camera to survey an area of interest, identifying the position and the shape of an object. Studies have shown that subjects implanted with Argus® II system were able to perform practical tasks with better results than using their residual vision [1, 14].

Argus® II and its predecessor, Argus I, were the first devices tested in humans to pass safety and efficacy assessments. This chapter will summarize the history of device development and results from clinical trials. It will also discuss several future advances needed to improve the device in order to provide a more informative visual perception to blind patients.

Indication

Argus® II is designed for patients that present a combination of advanced outer retinal degeneration with relative inner retinal preservation. The device requires a significant number of viable RGCs to transmit electrical stimuli to the visual cortex in order to generate phosphene perception [1].

RP is the most common hereditary retinal dystrophy that shows the above characteristics. In fact, RP encompasses a wide range of more than 100 genetic disorders with variable molecular defects that ultimately leads to progressive visual loss due to the degeneration of rod photoreceptors. RP affects approximately 1 in 4,000 live births and more than one million patients worldwide [15]. Clinical manifestations may start at different ages, with patients presenting initial symptoms from early infancy up to adulthood. Initially, patients usually experience peripheral visual impairment in low light conditions, since rods are initially affected, and as the disease progresses the cone photoreceptor cells are also affected, and visual acuity declines. Visual loss can be profound, with 0.5 % of patients achieving no light perception while 25 % have worse than 20/200 vision in both eyes [15, 16].

In addition to RP, diseases of the retinal pigment epithelium and choroid can first affect photoreceptors and leave inner retina uncompromised. Choroideremia is an example of a choroidal vascular disease that leads to photoreceptor loss and blindness [17]. Patients with extensive geographic atrophy from dry AMD may also benefit from this technology and a clinical trial has been recently initiated to study the feasibility and potential benefits for this disease (ClinicalTrials.gov Identifier: NCT02227498).

Argus® II prosthesis is not applicable for the restoration of vision in patients who have lost their vision due to damaged RGCs and axons, which is caused by diseases such as glaucoma and optic nerve trauma. Devices that stimulate more proximal visual relay centers in thalamus (lateral geniculate body) and visual cortex may be better options for such patients.

Technical Description

The Argus® II retinal prosthesis consists of an implantable device and an external part. The latter includes a video microcamera mounted on a pair of glasses, a portable computer named the video processing unit (VPU) and a communication coil that is built into the side arm of the glasses. The coil is responsible for wireless communication through radio frequency (RF) telemetry and induction of power to the internal device. The microcamera captures video and sends it to the VPU, which digitizes the image in real time into electrical pulses, then applies image-processing filters which generate a series of commands that are transmitted via the communication coil on the glasses (Fig. 5.2) [1, 18].

The implantable part consists of a second matching coil that receives power and data from the external coil and an internal circuit that converts the commands encoded in the RF signals, sets stimulator output based on these commands, and applies stimulus output (electrical pulses) to the intraocular array. The circuit is sealed in a hermetic casing

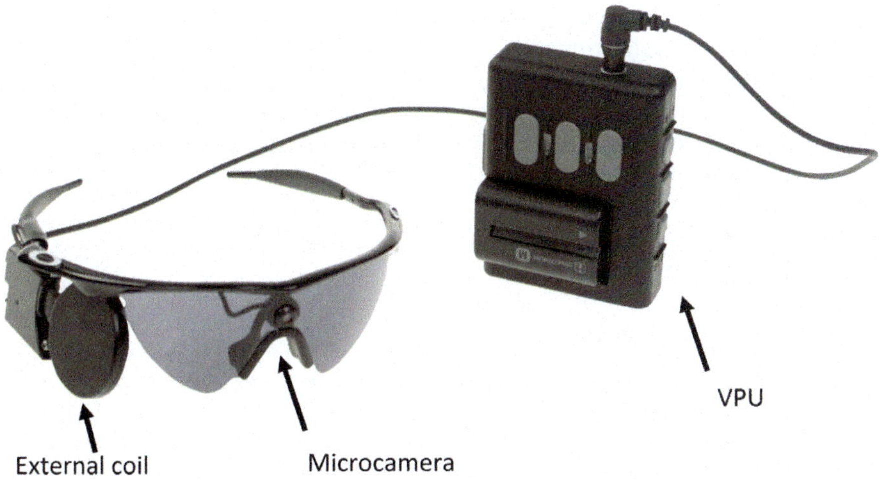

Fig. 5.2 Photograph of the Argus® II retinal prosthesis system showing the glasses-mounted microcamera, the external (inductive) coil and the video processing unit (*VPU*) (Reprinted with permission from Second Sight Medical Products, Inc.)

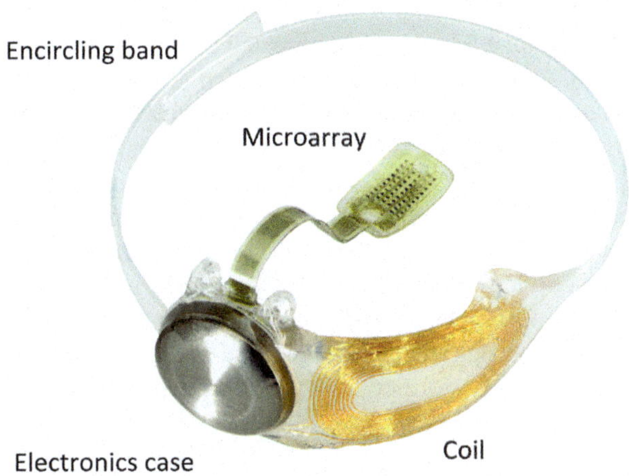

Fig. 5.3 Photograph of the implanted portion of Argus II prosthesis system showing the electrode microarray (6×10 electrodes), encircling band, electronics hermetic case and the internal (receiver) coil (Reprinted with permission from Second Sight Medical Products, Inc)

that is sutured on the scleral surface and connected to the internal microelectrode array via a cable through a 5 mm sclerotomy. All electronic components are attached to an encircling band (scleral buckle) which fits inside the orbit (Fig. 5.3). The epiretinal array includes 60 circular electrodes that are 200 μm in diameter and arranged in a 6×10 grid. The array is positioned on the macular area with one retinal tack (Fig. 5.1) [18–20]. The array measures 5.5 mm in width and 6 mm in length and spans approximately 20° in a diagonal visual angle, each microelectrode covers an area equivalent to hundreds of photoreceptors. In order to match the field of view, the image captured by the camera is cropped and down sampled to 60 pixels [1, 18, 20–22].

Argus® II is compatible with magnetic resonance imaging (MRI) up to 3-Tesla field strength, not including the external components (glasses and VPU) that must be removed during the scans. Implanted patients have been safely tested with MRI scans at 1.5 and 3-Tesla without any associated complications, change in implant position or subjective symptoms. The device, however, produces an image artifact of approximately 50 mm × 50 mm in size that obscures orbital structures. Specific instructions for MRI are provided with the Argus II patient manual and these should be followed carefully [23–25].

Surgical Methods

Argus® II can be implanted using common vitreoretinal surgical techniques in a procedure similar to a pars plana vitrectomy with an encircling buckle that takes approximately 2 to 3 h [1, 18, 19].

The procedure starts with a 360° limbal conjunctival peritomy, isolation of the rectus muscles, placement of the encircling band (containing the electronic package) under the muscles and fixed with episcleral sutures and a Watzke® sleeve (Labtician Ophthalmics, Inc., Oakville, Ontario, Canada). The episcleral inductive coil is placed under the lateral rectus muscle while the protective enclosure that contains the electronic circuit is positioned in the superotemporal quadrant [1, 18].

Vitrectomy is then conducted diligently with a posterior vitreous detachment, followed by a 5 mm incision created at 3.5 mm posterior to the limbus for the insertion of the microelectrode array and the cable. The scleral incision is sutured watertight and the array is placed and fixed on the macular region using a single custom retinal tack (Fig. 5.1) (Second Sight Medical Products, Inc., Sylmar, CA, USA). The extraocular portion of the cable is fixed with a scleral suture and the sclerotomies are closed at the end of the procedure. An allograft scleral patch (Tutoplast; IOP, Inc., Costa Mesa, CA, USA) or an alternative material (polytetrafluoroethylene patch or autologous aponeurosis graft) is sutured over the electronic package to reduce the risk of conjunctival irritation and erosion. Finally, tenon's capsule and conjunctiva are sutured [18]. A prophylactic intravitreal injection of antibiotics is performed at the end of the procedure [1, 18].

Full Clinical Study

Device Development History

It was known for almost a century that electrical stimulation of the visual cortex could elicit the perception of light spots known as phosphenes. In 1956, Australian inventor and radio engineer Graham Tassicker patented a method of implanting a light-sensitive selenium photodiode under the retina to restore light sensation; but this was never translated to a viable device that could provide visual perception to blind patients [14]. Potts and Inoue showed that stimulation of the globe with a corneal electrode could elicit visual signals in patients with RP [26]. Thus, the principle of functional electrical stimulation of the visual pathways was well established by the early 1970s. Since then, different approaches for retinal stimulation have been proposed and initially tested in animal models with the objective of ultimately restoring visual function in blind patients [14, 27].

Animal studies related to the development of Argus I and Argus® II were conducted by Humayun et al. in the early 1990s. The authors first performed electrical stimulation experiments on dissected bullfrogs' retinas, followed by rabbits with normal retinas and those with outer retinal function abolished by intravenous injection of sodium iodate [28]. These studies demonstrated that platinum electrodes were able to induce electrical evoked potentials through focal retinal electrical stimulation, which elicited phosphenes that were confined to the area of stimulation [28].

A few years later, initial experiments were conducted in humans to study the feasibility of epiretinal stimulation. A group of 5 blind volunteers with bare or no light perception were acutely implanted and tested under local anesthesia. A handheld probe with 2 or more electrodes of different sizes and shapes, was introduced via pars plana to the vitreous cavity and electrical pulses were applied to the macular region. All 5 blind volunteers perceived phosphenes consistent with the application of electrical pulses. They described visual responses of different characteristics, such as shape, size and brightness. One subject was able to distinguish phosphenes with 1.75° center-to-center distance, achieving a theoretical visual acuity of 4/200. They also showed a probable retinotopic localization of retinal responses, an important concept that would then lead to simultaneous stimulation of multiple retinal points to form geometric patterns and pixelated vision [9, 10, 29].

A study with multi-electrode arrays was then conducted with 2 blind patients possessing advanced RP, using electrodes in a 3×3 and a 5×5 spatial arrangement. Different patterns of stimulation were tested and the subjects were able to perceive corresponding shapes, such as a "box with an empty center", letter shapes ("H" and "U"), and vertical and horizontal lines when a column or a row of electrodes were activated. These findings corroborated the concept that a multi-electrode array and simultaneous stimulation could be used to elicit forms and visual function in blind patients [10].

Argus I

Argus I epiretinal prosthesis – developed by Second Sight Medical Products, Inc. – was the first epiretinal device to be chronically tested in a clinical trial between 2002 and 2006 (ClinicalTrials.gov Identifier NCT00279500). Safety and efficacy were studied in six blind patients with end-stage RP. The device consisted of 16 electrodes arranged in a 4×4 square array with alternating diameters of either 250 or 500 μm, used to evaluate how electrode size affected visual percepts [12, 30].

The Argus I electronics were based on cochlear implant technology, as such the protective enclosure for the device was placed subcutaneously in the temporal bone recess. A cable from the enclosure was tunneled along the temporal bone to reach the periorbital space via a lateral canthotomy. The retinal stimulating array was at the end of the cable. Because of this design, the surgical procedure was similar to the approach used with the cochlear implant and required the assistance of an otolaryngology/maxillofacial expert to dissect the temporal region, which resulted in a longer surgical time. The external coil would be held magnetically over the temporal bone, connecting to the internal coil. Argus® II's design, however, was modified so that the hermetic casing was implanted inside the orbit, simplifying the procedure and reducing surgical time [12].

At the end of the initial 33-month follow-up, no major adverse event was reported, thus supporting the long-term safety of the device. Additionally, electrode thresholds were evaluated within and across patients, showing that many electrodes were able to elicit phosphenes using charge densities within the safety limit [31]. Although there was variability across patients when performing visually-guided tasks (e.g. target localization, object recognition and direction of movement), the majority of tests presented better performance with the device turned ON than OFF, showing encouraging results. Subjects were able to locate and count high contrast objects, distinguish the orientation of the letter "L" on a computer screen, and identify objects such as a plate, a cup and a knife with results better than chance. One patient even managed to indicate the orientation of a high contrast square wave gratings, distinguishing directions (horizontal, vertical, diagonals right and left) better with the device enabled than disabled [12].

The study demonstrated the safety of long-term stimulation and supported the crucial concept that blind subjects were able to use an epiretinal prosthesis combined with patterned electrical stimulation to perform better in visually-guided tasks. Recently, an Argus I subject was evaluated 10 years after implantation and still had measurable perceptual thresholds. These encouraging results motivated the development of the more advanced Argus® II retinal implant [30].

Argus® II

A phase II clinical trial began in 2006 to study the safety and utility of the Argus® II System in providing visual function to blind subjects with severe to profound outer retinal degeneration. Thirty subjects were enrolled in a multicenter, single-arm, prospective and unmasked study (Clinicaltrials.gov, Identifier number NCT00407602) that was sponsored by Second Sight Medical Products, Inc., and conducted at 5 centers in the United States as well as in Mexico, France, United Kingdom, Switzerland and France. Inclusion and exclusion criteria for this study are listed in Table 5.1. Argus® II was implanted monocularly, typically in the eye with the worst vision [1].

Table 5.1 Inclusion and exclusion criteria for Argus® II System clinical trial

Inclusion criteria	Exclusion criteria
Confirmed diagnosis of retinitis pigmentosa (all centers) or outer retinal degeneration (France, U.K., Switzerland and Mexico)	Diseases or conditions that affect retinal function (CRVO, diabetic retinopathy, history of retinal detachment, trauma, infectious or inflammatory retinal diseases)
Remaining visual acuity of bare light perception (all centers) or 2.3 log MAR (France, U.K., Switzerland and Mexico) or worse in both eyes	Condition that prevents understanding or communication (e.g. cognitive decline, psychiatric disease, deafness or selective hearing loss)
History of useful vision in the worst-seeing eye	Keratitis sicca and/or ocular conditions that predisposes eye rubbing
Functional ganglion cells and optic nerve determined by a measurable electrically evoked response or documented light perception	Intolerance to implant surgery or follow-up visits
Age: 25 (USA, Switzerland) or 18 (France, U.K. and Mexico) years old	Optic nerve diseases, including history of glaucoma, or confirmed damage to visual cortex

A complete list can be found at www.clinicaltrials.gov under trial registration number NCT00407602

Patients

Surgeries were performed from 2007 to 2009 in 30 patients, of which 29 were diagnosed with RP, including one with Leber Congenital Amaurosis, and one with Choroideremia. Vision acuity was bare light perception in both eyes in 29 subjects, while one had no light perception in both eyes. At the time of surgery, patient's age ranged from 28 to 77 years (mean 57.5 ± 9.9 years); 21 being males and nine being females. All patients completed a follow-up of 3 years and each visit included complete eye examination, intraocular pressure measurement, fundus photography, fluorescein angiography and optical coherence tomography. Safety and visual function were the primary endpoints of this study, while the secondary endpoints included stability, functionality and reliability of the device, orientation and mobility tests, activities of daily living and quality of life [1].

Adverse Events

Device- or surgery-related adverse events were classified, whether or not they required medical/surgical intervention or hospitalization to prevent permanent injury, which was defined as a serious adverse event (SAE). After 3 years of implantation, the device showed an acceptable safety profile, with 11 patients (37 %) experiencing a total of 23 SAEs. Most of the SAEs (61 %) occurred within the first 6 months after surgery and only 5 SAEs (22 %) after month 12. Events were clustered within patients, with three patients (10 %) accounted for over 55 % of SAEs after 3 years of implantation. Two patients underwent an acute revision surgery (within 1 week after implantation) to re-tack the microarray to the retinal surface, and one patient's device was removed at 1.2 years due to recurrent conjunctival erosions, choroidal efusions associated with hypotony and retinal detachment that demanded multiple repairs. The most common SAEs were hypotony, conjunctival dehiscence or erosion and presumed endophthalmitis (culture negative) and apart from the explanted patient, all cases were treatable with standard ophthalmic approaches without loss of eyes (enucleation). There were three cases of sterile endophthalmitis reported in the first group of 15 surgeries that were treated and resolved with intravitreous injections of antibiotics combined with topical and systemic antibiotics [1].

A protocol adjustment was made halfway through the trial to add a prophylactic injection of intravitreal antibiotics after the surgery. After this change, no other case of endophthalmitis was reported. Modifications on the surgical technique and on the design of the device were also implemented, leading to a significant reduction of SAEs [1]. A few years later, another study by Rizzo et al. evaluated the safety outcome of six patients implanted by the same surgeon and reported no case of SAE, corroborating the importance of the refinement of surgical technique and the influence of learning curve [2]. In this study, although one patient presented high intraocular pressure postoperatively and another patient suffered from choroidal detachment, both cases were successfully managed with topical medication [2].

Functional Ouctomes

Visual Function

Considering that standard visual acuity tests, such as Snellen acuity/logMAR or contrast sensitivity could not be assessed, in general, due to the insufficient visual level provided by the prosthesis, visual function was measured by computer-based tests especially developed for low vision. Patients were objectively evaluated for basic visual skills, including target localization, motion detection, navigation, form discrimination and recognition. Since it was a single group study of a rare condition, each patient served as his/her own control, and status and performance of the implanted eye prior to surgery (residual vision) was used as a comparator [1].

In the target localization test called "square localization", patients were asked to locate and touch a white square that appeared randomly on a black touchscreen monitor. The distance between the center of the square and the patient's response was measured in centimeters, recorded and averaged after 40 trials. Another test called "direction of motion" assessed the patient's ability to draw the path of a white line that moved across a black touchscreen monitor. The difference between the patient's response and the angle of the white line was measured in degrees and averaged over 80 trials [1].

Visual acuity was evaluated using black and white gratings of various widths that were displayed randomly for 5 s on a computer screen in four orientations: horizontal, vertical, diagonal right and diagonal left. Each width corresponded to a visual acuity, on a scale that ranged from 2.9 to 1.6 logMAR (20/15887–20/756 Snellen notation, respectively). This was a 4-alternative forced-choice test, meaning that patients had to provide one of the four above alternatives, even if they could not determine the orientation of the gratings. In general, performance of these tasks increased when the device was turned ON. The results (in percent correct) for specific tasks were as follows: Square Localization (89.3 %, n=28), Direction of Motion (55.6 %, n=27) and Grating Visual Acuity (33.3 %, n=27), with mean visual acuity of 2.5 logMAR [1].

Orientation and Mobilitity Tests

The orientation and mobility tests were aimed to evaluate patients' performance in more real-world conditions, which included two indoor experiments. First, a simulated door (2.1 high × 1 m wide) made of a black cloth on a white wall was placed across a room and the patient was asked to locate and walk toward it. The "Door Task" was repeated 12 times (six times with the system ON and OFF) and the black cloth was either positioned 3 m to the right or to the left from the center of the wall. At year 3, the overall success of 28 patients in this test using the device was 54.2 ± 6.2 % versus 19.0 ± 4.3 % when the system was turned OFF. In the second test called "Line Task", a white line (15 cm wide × 6 m long) configured three different paths on a black floor made of rubber interlocking tiles. Patients were asked to walk over the path that could be a straight line or have a 90° turn to the right or to the left. The mean percentage of success of 28 patients was 67.9 ± 6.5 % with the system ON versus 14.3 ± 3.8 % with the system OFF [1].

Activities of Daily Living

Patients were also evaluated using the system in their daily lives after they had been trained to operate the device, approximately 1 month after implantation. A visual rehabilitation expert conducted interviews with patients and assessed their ability to carry out tasks of daily living such as orientation and mobility around their homes and social interactions. The impact of the system on the patients' quality of life was rated positive, mild positive, prior positive (positive effects in the past that were not present at the time of evaluation), neutral and negative. The overall effect of the device was rated positive or mild positive in 12 out of 15 subjects at year 1 (80 %) and prior positive or neutral in three subjects. At year 3, 65.2 % rated as positive and mild positive and 34.8 % as prior positive and neutral, from a total of 23 subjects [1].

In addition to the clinical trial, an increasing number of investigator sponsored studies are being reported, which provide further information on the capabilities and limitations of the Argus II. A group of 11 European subjects participated in an experiment of shapes recognition. They were asked to identify eight high contrast shapes (square, circle, triangle, rectangle, pentagon, hexagon, cross of half circle) presented in white or gray against a black background on a monitor. Each shape was shown in five different sizes (XL=22.6, L=14.3, M=9, S=5.6, XS=3.6 cm) and was either outlined or solid. The mean percentage of success using the device ON was 32.8±15.7 % versus 12.5±6.7 % with the system OFF ($p=0.02$) and chance rate of 12.5 %. When outlined shapes were presented, the percentage of success recognition was higher: 41.4±17.7 % (system ON) versus 9.4±7.5 % (system OFF). The study indicated better results when outlined shapes were used, suggesting a possible influence of total illumination on the subjetcs' performance [32].

Another study with 21 Argus® II patients investigated their ability to read high contrast letters (41.27° in height) presented on a flat LCD screen. Three groups of letters with increasing level of typographical complexity were tested: group A with the simplest form of vertical and horizontal lines (E, F, H, I, J, L T, U); group B with oblique components at the full height of the letter and minor variation on the circle (A, C, D, M, N, O, Q, V, W, Z); and group C, with oblique or curved components at half of the height of the letter (B, G, K, P, R, S, X, Y). Patients were able to correctly identify each letter group with the following mean percentage of success using the system ON versus OFF: group A, 72.3±24.6 % versus 17.7±12.9 %; group B, 55.0±27.4 % versus 11.8±10.7 %; and group C, 51.7±28.9 % versus 15.3±7.4 % ($p<0.001$ for all groups). A subgroup of 6 patients who performed well in this first experiment, identifying at least 50 % of the letters of group A under 60 s, also participated in the identification of 2-, 3- and 4-letter words with the device ON and OFF. Four of these patients were able to recognize 7 out of 10 words (mean=6.8 words) with the device ON and 0 out of 10 (mean=0.3 words) when the device was turned OFF [33].

Additionally, Luo et al. conducted an experiment with a subset of seven patients in the United Kingdom to investigate recognition of 8 daily life objects that were presented in high contrast, i.e., white or metallic objects against a black background in ambient room light. Patients were allowed 30 s per trial to give a forced-choice answer, and each object was presented twice in random order. Results once again showed a higher percentage of success when patients were using the device, with a mean correct percentage of recognition of 35.7±14.6 % (system enabled) versus 12.5±7.2 % (system disabled), and chance rate of 12.5 % [34, 35].

Human studies conducted so far have demonstrated the long-term safety of chronic stimulation with Argus® II and the potential benefits provided by the device as a visual aid for patients blinded by outer retina degeneration [1, 2, 32–35]. However, further studies are still required to better understand the underlying factors related to pattern electrical stimulation and neural interpretation at the cortical level, which may lead to device enhancements and better visual outcomes.

Future Directions

Software development and image/signal processing represent one of the most promising paths for improvement of Argus® II's performance. The use of different algorithms to interpret video signals and modulate patterned stimulation has proven to enhance visual perception without making any changes to the existing hardware.

One example of this concept is the use of maximized contrast on the edges of images to enhance object recognition and improve orientation and mobility. This adjustment was shown to be beneficial in initial patient tests and later was incorporated as an optional feature in the device [36].

Another image processing software, proposed by Sahel et al. uses magnification and minimization of the acquired image to enable a visual acuity beyond the limit set by theoretical resolution of the implanted array. Although the field of view covered by the array is about 20° diagonally, in this experiment the image was reduced or magnified in a range from 0.4× to 16× using a remote hand-held controller. One Argus® II patient was able to achieve an equivalent visual acuity of 20/200 when using 16× magnification on the gratings visual acuity test, exceeding by far the best nominal acuity achieved with the device, i.e. 20/1260. The same patient managed to read letters of 2.3 cm in height from a notebook at 30 cm, using a magnification of 4× [37].

In another experiment, Stanga et al. applied a facial recognition algorithm that resulted in a visual percept only when a human face was detected by the processor. The facial region would be extracted from the rest of the visual scene and presented by itself in a zoomed-out view. This feature enabled 5 Argus® II patients to locate faces 100 % of the time at 2–3 m distance in a significantly shorter time when using the wider field of view [38].

Apart from software development, hardware improvements have also been proposed for the next generation of epiretinal prosthesis in order to provide a more genuine visual perception. To date, the number of electrodes and the reduced visual field impose limitations to visual acuity and image resolution. An increase in the area of stimulated retina with a larger number of electrodes could potentially enhance visual function. Other approaches involve adding peripheral electrodes to the main array and adjusting the prosthesis curvature to the patient's retina, considering that electrode-retina distance has been demonstrated to be a critical factor related to perceptual threshold [21].

References

1. Ho AC, Humayun MS, Dorn JD, da Cruz L, Dagnelie G, Handa J, et al. Long-term results from an epiretinal prosthesis to restore sight to the blind. Ophthalmology. 2015;122(8):1547–54.
2. Rizzo S, Belting C, Cinelli L, Allegrini L, Genovesi-Ebert F, Barca F, et al. The Argus II Retinal Prosthesis: 12-month outcomes from a single-study center. Am J Ophthalmol. 2014;157(6):1282–90.
3. Nazari H, Zhang L, Zhu D, Chader GJ, Falabella P, Stefanini F, et al. Stem cell based therapies for age-related macular degeneration: the promises and the challenges. Prog Retin Eye Res. 2015;48:1–39.
4. Bainbridge JW, Mehat MS, Sundaram V, Robbie SJ, Barker SE, Ripamonti C, et al. Long-term effect of gene therapy on Leber's congenital amaurosis. N Engl J Med. 2015;372(20): 1887–97.
5. Sahni JN, Angi M, Irigoyen C, Semeraro F, Romano MR, Parmeggiani F. Therapeutic challenges to retinitis pigmentosa: from neuroprotection to gene therapy. Curr Genomics. 2011;12(4):276–84.

6. Santos A, Humayun MS, de Juan E, Jr Greenburg RJ, Marsh MJ, Klock IB. Preservation of the inner retina in retinitis pigmentosa. A morphometric analysis. Arch Ophthalmol. 1997;115(4): 511–5.
7. Stone JL, Barlow WE, Humayun MS, de Juan E, Jr Milam AH. Morphometric analysis of macular photoreceptors and ganglion cells in retinas with retinitis pigmentosa. Arch Ophthalmol. 1992;110(11):1634–9.
8. Kim SY, Sadda S, Pearlman J, Humayun MS, de Juan E, Jr Melia BM, et al. Morphometric analysis of the macula in eyes with disciform age-related macular degeneration. Retina. 2002;22(4):471–7.
9. Humayun MS, de Juan E, Jr Dagnelie G, Greenberg RJ, Propst RH, Phillips DH. Visual perception elicited by electrical stimulation of retina in blind humans. Arch Ophthalmol. 1996;114(1):40–6.
10. Humayun MS, de Juan E, Jr Weiland JD, Dagnelie G, Katona S, Greenberg R, et al. Pattern electrical stimulation of the human retina. Vision Res. 1999;39(15):2569–76.
11. Rizzo 3rd JF, Wyatt J, Loewenstein J, Kelly S, Shire D. Methods and perceptual thresholds for short-term electrical stimulation of human retina with microelectrode arrays. Invest Ophthalmol Vis Sci. 2003;44(12):5355–61.
12. Humayun MS, Weiland JD, Fujii GY, Greenberg R, Williamson R, Little J, et al. Visual perception in a blind subject with a chronic microelectronic retinal prosthesis. Vision Res. 2003;43(24):2573–81.
13. Yanai D, Weiland JD, Mahadevappa M, Greenberg RJ, Fine I, Humayun MS. Visual performance using a retinal prosthesis in three subjects with retinitis pigmentosa. Am J Ophthalmol. 2007;143(5):820–7.
14. Luo YH, da Cruz L. The Argus II retinal prosthesis system. Prog Retin Eye Res. 2016;50: 89–107.
15. Hartong DT, Berson EL, Dryja TP. Retinitis pigmentosa. Lancet. 2006;368(9549):1795–809.
16. Grover S, Fishman GA, Anderson RJ, Tozatti MS, Heckenlively JR, Weleber RG, et al. Visual acuity impairment in patients with retinitis pigmentosa at age 45 years or older. Ophthalmology. 1999;106(9):1780–5.
17. Coussa RG, Traboulsi EI. Choroideremia: a review of general findings and pathogenesis. Ophthalmic Genet. 2012;33(2):57–65.
18. Humayun MS, Dorn JD, da Cruz L, Dagnelie G, Sahel JA, Stanga PE, et al. Interim results from the international trial of Second Sight's visual prosthesis. Ophthalmology. 2012;119(4): 779–88.
19. Luo YH, da Cruz L. A review and update on the current status of retinal prostheses (bionic eye). Br Med Bull. 2014;109:31–44.
20. Dorn JD, Ahuja AK, Caspi A, da Cruz L, Dagnelie G, Sahel JA, et al. The detection of motion by blind subjects with the epiretinal 60-electrode (Argus II) retinal prosthesis. JAMA Ophthalmol. 2013;131(2):183–9.
21. Ahuja AK, Yeoh J, Dorn JD, Caspi A, Wuyyuru V, McMahon MJ, et al. Factors affecting perceptual threshold in Argus II retinal prosthesis subjects. Transl Vis Sci Technol. 2013; 2(4):1.
22. Roessler G, Laube T, Brockmann C, Kirschkamp T, Mazinani B, Goertz M, et al. Implantation and explantation of a wireless epiretinal retina implant device: observations during the EPIRET3 prospective clinical trial. Invest Ophthalmol Vis Sci. 2009;50(6):3003–8.
23. Cunningham S, Tjan B, Bao P, Falabella P, Weiland J. Tactile-evoked V1 responses in Argus II retinal prosthesis patients assessed with fMRI: a case study. J Vis. 2015;15(12):359.
24. Luo YH, Davagnanam I, dacCuz L. MRI brain scans in two patients with the argus II retinal prosthesis. Ophthalmology. 2013;120(8):1711. e8
25. Cunningham SI, Shi Y, Weiland JD, Falabella P, Olmos de Koo LC, Zacks DN, et al. Feasibility of structural and functional MRI acquisition with unpowered implants in Argus II retinal prosthesis patients: a case study. Transl Vis Sci Technol. 2015;4(6):6.

26. Potts AM, Inoue J. The electrically evoked response (EER) of the visual system. II. Effect of adaptation and retinitis pigmentosa. Invest Ophthalmol. 1969;8(6):605–12.
27. Brindley GS, Lewin WS. The sensations produced by electrical stimulation of the visual cortex. J Physiol. 1968;196(2):479–93.
28. Humayun M, Propst R, de Juan E, Jr McCormick K, Hickingbotham D. Bipolar surface electrical stimulation of the vertebrate retina. Arch Ophthalmol. 1994;112(1):110–6.
29. Greenberg RJ, Velte TJ, Humayun MS, Scarlatis GN, Jr de Juan E. A computational model of electrical stimulation of the retinal ganglion cell. IEEE Trans Biomed Eng. 1999;46(5): 505–14.
30. Yue L, Falabella P, Christopher P, Wuyyuru V, Dorn J, Schor P, et al. Ten-Year follow-up of a blind patient chronically implanted with epiretinal prosthesis argus I. Ophthalmology. 2015;122(12):2545–52. e1.
31. Brummer SB, Turner MJ. Electrochemical considerations for safe electrical stimulation of the nervous system with platinum electrodes. IEEE Trans Biomed Eng. 1977;24(1):59–63.
32. Arsiero M, Cruz LD, Merlini F, Sahel JA, Stanga PE, Hafezi F, et al. Subjects blinded by outer retinal dystrophies are able to recognize shapes using the Argus II retinal prosthesis system. Invest Ophthalmol Vis Sci. 2011;52(14):4951.
33. da Cruz L, Coley BF, Dorn J, Merlini F, Filley E, Christopher P, et al. The Argus II epiretinal prosthesis system allows letter and word reading and long-term function in patients with profound vision loss. Br J Ophthalmol. 2013;97(5):632–6.
34. Luo YH, Zhong JJ, da Cruz L. The use of Argus(R) II retinal prosthesis by blind subjects to achieve localisation and prehension of objects in 3-dimensional space. Graefes Arch Clin Exp Ophthalmol. 2015;253(11):1907–14.
35. Luo YHL, Zhong J, Merlini F, Anaflous F, Arsiero M, Stanga PE, et al. The use of Argus® II retinal prosthesis to identify common objects in blind subjects with outer retinal dystrophies. Invest Ophthalmol Vis Sci. 2014;55(13):1834.
36. Humayun MS, Dorn JD, Ahuja AK, Caspi A, Filley E, Dagnelie G, et al. Preliminary 6 month results from the Argus II epiretinal prosthesis feasibility study. Conf Proc: Ann Int Conf IEEE Eng Med Biol Soc IEEE Eng Med Biol Soc Ann Conf. 2009;2009:4566–8.
37. Sahel J, Mohand-Said S, Stanga P, Caspi A, Greenberg R. Acuboost™: enhancing the maximum acuity of the Argus II Retinal Prosthesis System. Invest Ophthalmol Vis Sci. 2013;54(15):1389.
38. Stanga P, Sahel J, Mohand-Said S, da Cruz L, Caspi A, Merlini F, et al. Face detection using the Argus® II retinal prosthesis system. Invest Ophthalmol Vis Sci. 2013;54(15):1766.

Chapter 6
The Subretinal Implant ALPHA: Implantation and Functional Results

Eberhart Zrenner, Karl Ulrich Bartz-Schmidt, Dorothea Besch, Florian Gekeler, Assen Koitschev, Helmut G. Sachs, and Katarina Stingl

Abstract So far there are no possibilities for restitution of vision abilities in people blind from hereditary retinal degeneration except electronic visual implants. Epiretinal and subretinal implants are already commercially available. Here the subretinal implant Alpha IMS (Retina Implant AG, Reutlingen, Germany) is presented, its technical construction, area of application, possible benefit for blind patients as well as surgical procedures including replacement, results from a clinical study in 29 patients, and safety issues. Subretinal implants are considered to have a number of advantages: the subretinal space is immunoprivileged, therefore less prone to proliferative vitreoretinal reactions; the fixation of the implant in between retina and choroid does not require scleral tacks; a retinotopically correct relation between perceived spot and retinal electrode is maintained in the visual field, thus shortening training times; natural eye movement and gaze help to localize objects; microsaccades are beneficial to avoid image fading; there are no devices attached to the face as all stimulation electronics are within the body; and resolution with 1500 pixels is the highest so far achieved.

The Alpha-IMS implant has received a CE mark for commercial use in Europe in 2013. Psychophysical testing and self-reported outcomes show restoration of useful vision in approximately half of the patients. Subretinal implantation surgery is safe. A new version (RETINA IMPLANT ALPHA AMS) with 1600 pixel and considerably improved longevity has received CE mark in March 2016 and providing centers have been recruited in several European countries.

E. Zrenner (✉)
Institute for Ophthalmic Research and Werner Reichardt Center for Integrative Neuroscience (CIN, Eberhard Karls Universität Tübingen, Tuebingen, Germany
e-mail: ez@uni-tuebingen.de

K.U. Bartz-Schmidt • D. Besch • K. Stingl
Center for Ophthalmology, University of Tübingen Medical Centre, Tuebingen, Germany

F. Gekeler
Center for Ophthalmology, University of Tübingen and Klinikum Stuttgart, Stuttgart, Germany

A. Koitschev
Department of Otorhinolaryngology, Klinikum Stuttgart, Stuttgart, Germany

H.G. Sachs
Eye Clinic, Klinikum Dresden Friedrichstadt, Dresden, Germany

V.P. Gabel (ed.), *Artificial Vision*, DOI 10.1007/978-3-319-41876-6_6

Keywords Artificial Vision • Retinal prosthesis • Subretinal implant • Retina Implant Alpha IMS • Retinitis pigmentosa • Restoration of vision

Key Points

- The Retina Implant Alpha is the only light sensitive subretinal retinal implant that has received commercial approval (presently limited to Europe). It is suited for patients blind from retinitis pigmentosa and allied diseases.
- The new version of the implant pixels with light amplifying capabilities, positioned in the immuno-privileged space between retina and choroid; thereby a stable contact is achieved between electrodes and bipolar cells without additional mechanical measures.
- The position away from the epiretinal fibres allows to use the natural image processing capabilities of the inner retina for retinotopically correct perception in the visual field which results in a short training period of only few weeks.
- As the image receiving chip moves with eye, gaze helps to localize objects and maintain a steady image; patients can adjust brightness and contrast of the perceived image.
- After implantation there are no additional technical items positioned in the facial area (except regular glasses) which is cosmetically attractive.
- Human studies in more than 50 patients have shown this implant type's safety and efficacy for regaining visual capabilities useful in daily life.
- A new version (RETINA IMPLANT ALPHA AMS) of the device with 1600 pixel and considerably improved longevity has received CE mark in March 2016 and providing centers have been recruited in several European countries.

Introduction: Principal Concept and Steps of Development

In hereditary retinal diseases such as retinitis pigmentosa the loss of photoreceptors leads progressively to blindness in the vast majority of the cases. Still, despite some reorganization of retinal circuitry, inner retina function is maintained for decades [1]. The principal idea of subretinal approaches [2–4] therefore is, to replace the photoreceptor function by technical light sensitive devices and to connect them to the inner retina to stimulate bipolar cells with local electrical currents (Fig. 6.1). This allows to utilize the inner retina's enormous power of signal processing in order to provide the brain with "natural signals" from the retina through ganglion cells and their axons (Fig. 6.1c). Moreover, as the light sensitive "camera chip" i.e. the subretinal array is implanted in the eye (Fig. 6.1b) and moves with the eye so that microsaccades and gaze information can be used for image refreshing and

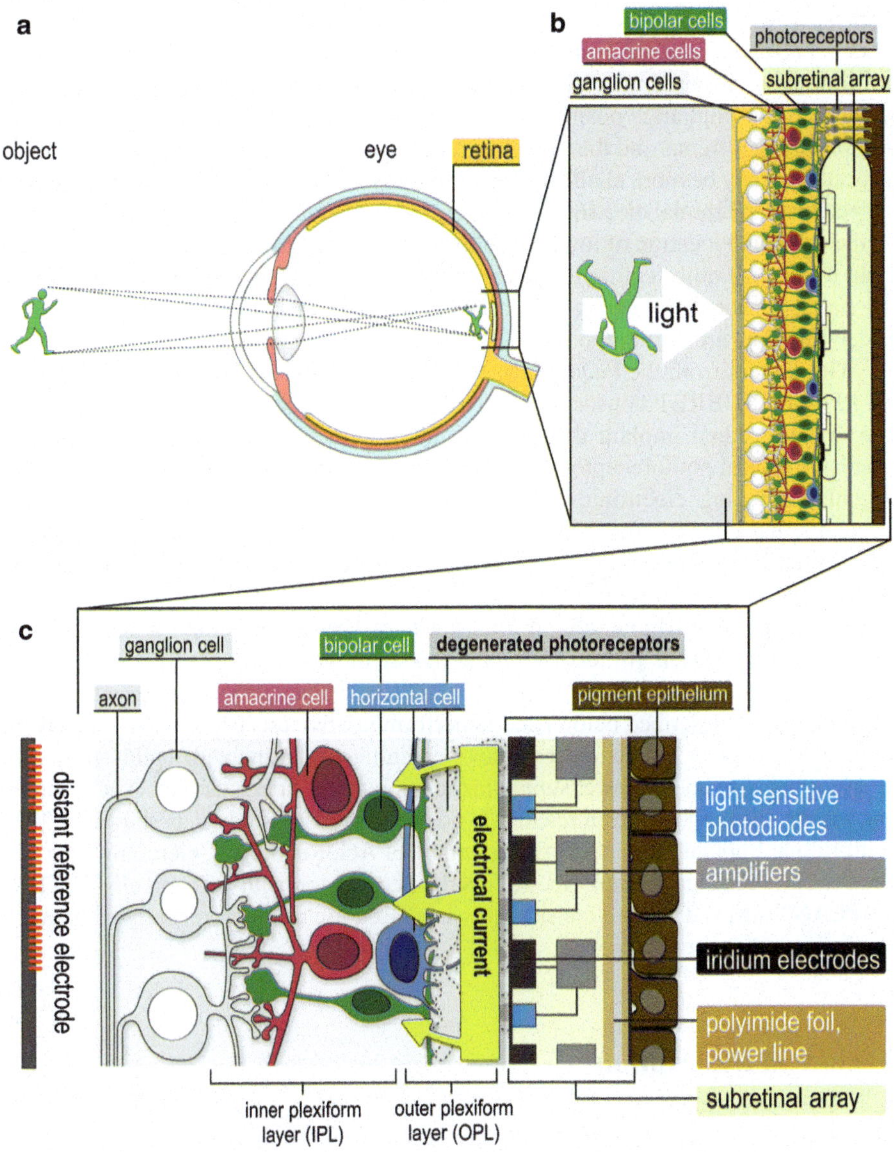

Fig. 6.1 (**a**) Sketch illustrating the principle of the subretinal approach. *Left*: the image is projected through the lens of the eye onto the subretinal implant. (**b**) The subretinal implant with its light sensitive micro-photodiode array (*bright yellow*) is positioned in the retinal layer where photoreceptor cells have been lost. (**c**) The light-induced signals from the photodiodes (*blue*) are amplified point by point by amplifiers (*grey*) and sent to the electrodes (*black*), which stimulate the bipolar cells of the inner retina directly (*green*), resulting in neuronal processing of the signals by the retinal bipolar cells, amacrine cells (*red*), and ganglion cells (*white*). Ganglion cells send the processed information via their axons to the brain. In contrast, epiretinal stimulation does not use the inner retina processing by means of the various synaptic connections but preprocesses the image in an external computer

analysis [5]. Therefore there are several good reasons to put the technical photosensors subretinally: the subretinal space is immunoprivileged, thereby less prone to proliferative vitreoretinal reactions; a stable contact to the neurons is easier to achieve if the implant is positioned in between retina and choroid than in between the wobbling vitreous and the inner limiting membrane, although subretinal surgical procedures may be more challenging; a retinotopically correct relation between perceived spot and retinal electrode is maintained in the visual field, difficult to achieve at the epiretinal location of implants, close to fibres; natural eye movement and gaze help to localize objects; microsaccades help to avoid image fading and the fact that all parts, sensors, processing electronics, electrode arrays and power and signal receiving units are within the body are cosmetically attractive.

With a grant from the Federal Ministry for Education and Research in Germany in 1995 the SUBRET consortium started a 10 year preclinical project to develop the first subretinal implant that mimics the amplification and adaptation mechanisms of natural photoreceptors in a so called multiphotodiode array (MPDA) with signal processing electronics; this is an active implant, in contrast to passive implants that just take the solar energy to stimulate retinal neurons, which turned out to provide to little energy per pixel as to excite neurons under typical lightening conditions.

This grant allowed to study all the aspects of spatial and temporal resolution in various animal models [6], do determine threshold and safety of effective electrical stimulation [7], to test materal biostability and biocompatibility [8], to develop surgical procedures (described below) and to perform in vivo tests [9]. Finally – as will be lined out below – in 2005 clinical studies were initiated starting with a pilot study with transdermal wire bound power supply to the implant in 11 patients [10]. After promising results showing that even reading is possible a pivotal study was started in 2010 with Retina Implant Alpha IMS (Retina Implant AG, Reutlingen, Germany) that had received CE certification in 2013. An overhauled version with 1600 pixels (RETINA IMPLANT AMS) that has a considerably increased life time was recently certified by the authority for use in Europe.

Technical Description

The Retina Implant Alpha IMS consists of a subretinal microchip on a polyimide foil (Fig. 6.2a) and a cable for power supply and signal control, ending in a receiver coil, housed together with electronic circuits in a small subdermal box behind the ear, similar to technology used in cochlear implants (Fig. 6.2b, c). A separate short cable connects the reference electrode to the subdermal box (Fig. 6.2a). The microchip ($3 \times 3 \times 0.1$ mm^3) consists of 1500 independent photodiode-amplifier-electrode units, each of which transforms the luminance information falling onto the particular photodiode into an electrical current that is amplified for the stimulation of the adjacent bipolar cells via a 50×50 μmm^2 iridium electrode (see Fig. 6.1c). Thus, a

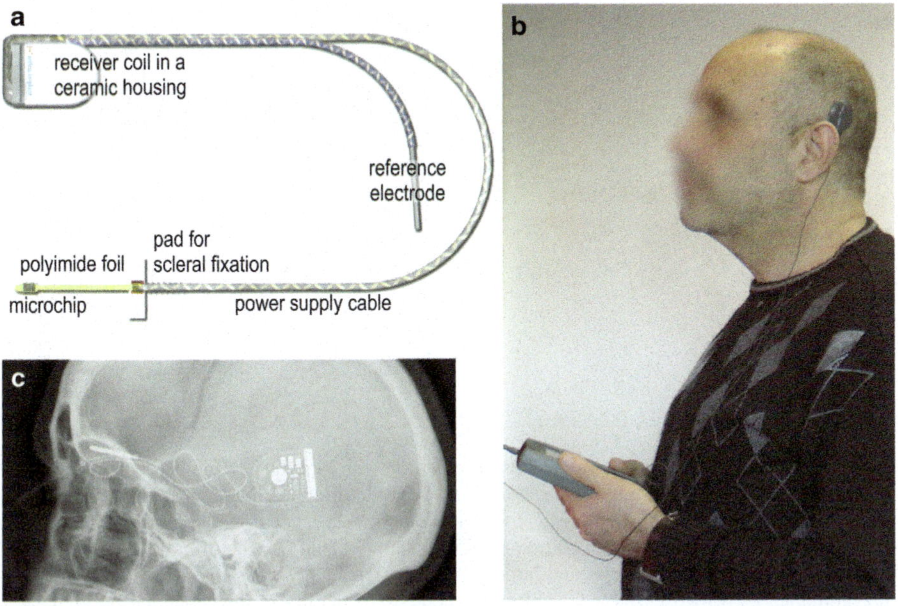

Fig. 6.2 (**a**) The Retina Implant Alpha IMS consists of the microchip (micro-photodiode array) on the tip of a polyimide foil (both placed subretinally), a power supply cable connecting the microchip with the receiver coil in a ceramic housing in the retroauricular region and the reference electrode placed subdermally near the temporal muscle. (**b**) Power and signals are sent wirelessly through the skin via a transmitter antenna coil (black) which is kept in place behind the ear with a subdermal magnet. The patient can switch on or off the device on the hand held unit, as well as adjust contrast sensitivity and brightness manually via two knobs. (**c**) As seen in the X-ray image, an implanted cable leads from the subdermal receiver coil behind the ear to the intraorbital space, where it connects to a subretinal foil. The electronic circuits in the chip are powered and controlled by electronics in the subdermal receiver coil behind the ear

point-by-point electrical image of the luminance information is forwarded to bipolar cells and processed in the inner retina and the afferent visual pathway [7]. As this process happens independently in each of the 1500 pixels and at each point exactly where the light is absorbed, the remaining visual pathway receives a retinotopical correct electrical image. Each electrode of the chip typically releases 1 ms pulses in a working frequency of the implant, usually 5 Hz, adjustable from 1 to 20 Hz. Each photodiode-electrode unit works independently from the neighbouring ones.

The polyimide foil for power and signal supply (Fig. 6.2a) lies subretinally as well and leaves the eye through the choroid and the sclera at its equator (see also Fig. 6.3c). The power supply cable runs then in a loop through the orbit and leaves it under the skin at the orbital rim, leading under the temporal muscle to the back of the ear (Fig. 6.2c), where the subdermal coil is fixed onto the skull bone. Therefore the whole implant is within the body and nothing can be seen in the facial area from the outside.

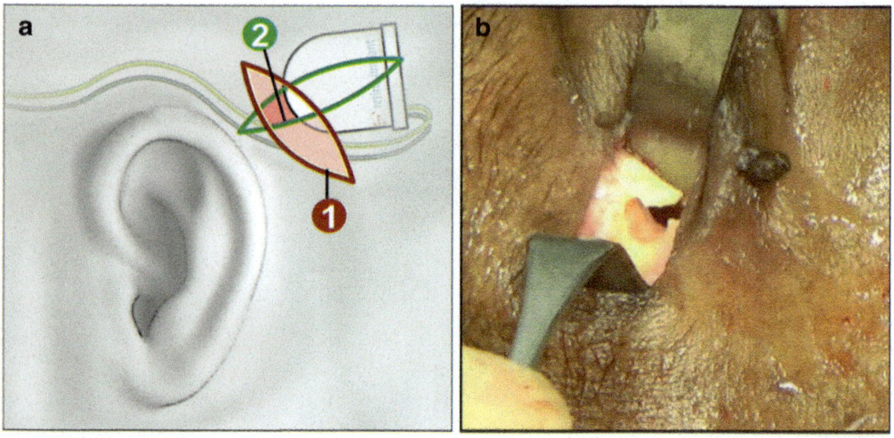

Fig. 6.3 (**a**) Illustration of the curved retroauricular incision 1 cm behind the helix of the pinna (*1*) leaving the fascia of the temporal muscle intact. A second horizontal incision nearly perpendicular to the skin incision down to the bone (*2*) provides a stabile two-layer wound closure and undermining of the periost. (**b**) In order to position the power supply cable into the orbital space, the periost is elevated around the orbital rim and into fossa temporalis, exposing the bone of the sutura frontozygomatica. A drilled L-shaped canal provides flexible stability of the cable and optimal cable angulation at the orbital rim (Modified from Koitschev et al. [15]. With permission from © 2015 to the Authors under the terms of the Creative Commons Attribution License: http://creativecommons.org/licenses/by/4.0/)

Power transmission is provided by electromagnetic induction, every time when the external primary coil is placed against the subdermal coil (Fig. 6.2b) that has a simple magnet in its center to keep the external coil in place behind the ear. A thin cable leads from the external primary coil behind the ear to a handheld box. This box serves as external battery-driven power supply equipped with electronics that are connected to the implant in the retroauricular region via a magnetic coil system. This permits an inductive transfer of energy and control signals (Fig. 6.2b, c). On the external handheld device Retina Implant Alpha IMS has two knobs for manual adjustment of contrast and brightness allowing optimal contrast vision in different luminance conditions.

The patient must switch on the external power supply box (currently approx. 12 $\times$ 5 $\times$ 2 cm^3, Fig. 6.2c) always when vision is desired; he has just to put the primary transmitter coil (seen as black in Fig 6.2b) on top of the secondary subdermal receiver coil behind the ear (Fig 6.2a). For carrying the power supply the patients use a small ba, e.g. at thr belt. During the first weeks of using the implant outdoors and beyond the clinic walls such as in the hotel, restaurant, etc. the patients are accompanied by a professional mobility trainer after having been instructed and trained in several sessions by a clinical engineer.

In the pilot study carried out in the years 2005–2009 at the University Medical Center of Tübingen (Germany), a transdermal cable with a plug was initially used experimentally for the external power supply (pilot study implant not shown here). These implants were then surgically removed again after 4 months at the latest. This study provided proof of concept that subretinal implants can restore useful visual perception up to reading capability, are well tolerated and help to master activities of daily living [10].

In the subsequent clinical study (2010–2015), the wireless, coil-based power supply described above has been used [11]. Meanwhile more than 50 patients have received such subretinal implants in clinical multicenter studies in Tuebingen, Oxford, London, Dresden, Budapest, Singapore, Hong Kong, Kiel and Hannover. The wireless system Alpha IMS has received the CE mark for commercial use in Europe in 2013, an improved version Alpha AMS with 1600 pixel and considerably improved life time was certified by the authority in 2016.

Indication for Certain Forms of Blindness

As the subretinal chip replaces principally the function of the photoreceptors this approach requires that the remaining neurons of the visual pathway function sufficiently, because the information about the image needs to be passed from the bipolar cells via ganglion cells to the brain. Not only must the remaining visual pathway function reliably, the optic media also must be clear, so that the visual information is not distorted before falling onto the chip. For this reason, cataract surgery is regularly performed at some point in time before the subretinal chip implantation. Therefore an eye with a substantial corneal opacity does not qualify for a subretinal implant.

Primarily patients with degenerations of photoreceptors, especially patients with hereditary retinal diseases such as for example retinitis pigmentosa and several related diseases (Choroideremia, Usher syndrome etc.) can benefit from subretinal chip implantation; they should not have additional eye problems, especially glaucoma, retinal detachment, uveitis, corneal opacities or diseases of the optic nerve which all are contraindications for this therapeutic approach. Also patients after a stroke with involvement of the visual brain area cannot be considered.

Another important point is that the brain has to "have learned seeing" earlier in life. Without this ability visual information cannot be processed by the brain, even if the technology and the remaining retina work optimally. That is why congenital blindness and severe amblyopia are contraindications for any electronic retinal implant.

Last but not least one must be aware of the fact that the implantation surgery can take several hours and represents one of the longest ophthalmological surgeries. If such a surgery is planned, no severe general health problems may be present, which would increase the risk of such a long anesthesia.

The patient group for whom these implants mainly have been developed for are retinitis pigmentosa patients, as well as patients with other primary rod-cone or cone-rod dystrophies in their end stage disease. These patients are born mostly with good visual functions and develop in their middle age the end stage of the disease that often leads to blindness, currently without a therapy available. Especially in the first years of the blindness the bipolar cells and the ganglion cells are functioning properly for a relatively long period, sometimes decades, as can be seen in Optical Coherence Tomography (OCT). Moreover, these patients are usually in their middle age being otherwise healthy fulfilling thus the most important condition for such an implant.

Who Can Benefit from the Subretinal Implant to What Extent?

When answering this we must realize what possibilities such a technology can provide. There are three main differences of the artificial vision by a subretinal implant to the natural vision. First, a chip area of appr. 9 mm^2 on the posterior eye pole can mediate a square-shaped visual field of approximately only 15° (across corners). Secondly, if we calculate the resolution of 1500 pixels in this area, we gain a minimal angle of resolution of 0.25° which corresponds to a maximal visual acuity of approximately 20/333–20/250. The best results for visual acuity so far reached are 20/546 for Landolt rings and 20/200 for grating acuity [11, 12]. Third, as the spectrally different photoreceptors are lost, no color discrimination is possible. All pixels of the implant have the same spectral sensitivity. The only factor distinguishable besides form is brightness, i.e. contrast, so that the perceived image is an image of areas of different levels of grey, such as in older black and white television, where the observer can adjust brightness and contrast. Indeed, the examinations could show that our patients are able to distinguish up to six and maximally nine levels of grey [10, 12].

A further difference from natural vision is the lack of spontaneous adaptation to ambient brightness such as in a healthy retina. The patient himself can adjust this manually depending on the brightness of the surroundings and the conditions of contrast. He does this with two control knobs on the power supply unit with which both contrast sensitivity and light intensity can be adjusted in order to optimize the visual image which is perceived (Fig. 6.2b). Also, based on a working frequency of the implant, usually 5 Hz (adjustable from less than 1 to 20 Hz) the image has a slightly flickering, stroboscopic character.

This technology is thus not to be understood as a complete restoration of vision, but it is to be regarded as an option for blind patients with photoreceptor degenerations to regain some useful visual information like object recognitions, localization, possibly in some cases reading of big letters or to improve their mobility or partial recognition of persons. All of these possibilities represent very important goals for severely visually impaired patients and have been achieved by many but not all patients so far (details below).

Blindness in the sense of a large central scotoma such as occurring in patients with age-related macular degeneration (AMD) could present a future condition for use of a subretinal implant in some cases; however, these patients are not completely blind in the sense as retinitis pigmentosa patients. With the central scotoma caused by dry age-related macular degeneration most patients keep almost the entire visual field in the periphery. Therefore only patients in very advanced stages of AMD may benefit. Additional problem of patients with age-related degeneration might be the state of general health which is a necessary condition for an elective surgery in long duration anesthesia.

Surgical Procedure for Subretinal Implants

The extraocular procedure [13–15] under general anesthesia a curved retroauricular incision is performed, leaving the fascia of the temporalis muscle intact; a second horizontal incision is placed along the caudal border of the temporalis muscle providing a stable two-layer wound closure (Fig. 6.3a, incision 1 and 2). A tight circumscribed subperiostal pocket and a bony well of 3–4 mm depth are created to house the implant's receiver coil capsula within the bony structures.

Subsequently an orbital rim incision is placed directly at the margo orbitalis reaching down to the bone (Fig. 6.3b). The periost is elevated around the orbital rim and shifted into the fossa temporalis exposing the bone of the sutura frontozygomatica. A drilled L-shaped canal provides flexible stability of the cable and optimal cable bending with a relatively large radius at the orbital rim. Additionally a tunnel is created to the subconjunctival space in the upper temporal quadrant.

Thereafter the retroauricular subperiostal pocket is connected to the orbital rim incision by undermining the periost under the temporalis muscle using a long, slightly curved, sharp raspatory. A custom made hollow trocar is introduced subperiosteally from the orbital rim to the retroauricular area. The implant foil with the chip is then placed safely inside the trocar tube. Subsequently the trocar is removed leaving the implant next to the orbital rim. The reference electrode remains under the temporalis muscle. The implant chip is further pulled through the subconjunctival tunnel and placed aside securely during the following intraocular surgical procedure. The power cable is placed in the bony groove at the orbital rim and fixed by a periost suture (Fig. 6.3b). Wound closure is performed after completion of the intraocular procedure allowing final adjustment of the length of the extraocular cable (see X-ray in Fig. 6.2c).

The intraocular procedure [16, 17] the chip is placed subretinally preferably directly beneath the macular region. In some patients a foveal placement is surgically difficult due to adhesions between retina and retinal pigment epithelium (RPE) in the central retinal region, which can arise as a result of the RPE degeneration in RP-patients. In these patients, a parafoveal placement of the microchip can be attempted; however, it has been shown that a parafoveal placement of the visual microchip has rather a limited functional outcome [18].

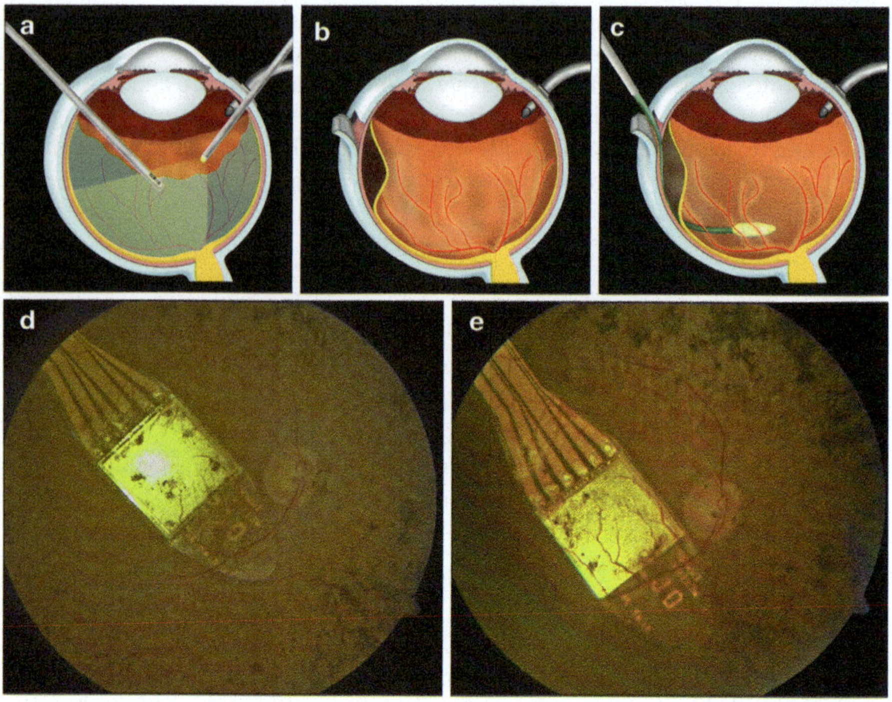

Fig. 6.4 (**a**) As a first step vitrectomy is being performed; (**b**) a subretinal bleb containing visco-elastic solution is created followed by creation of a scleral flap (4 × 5 mm^2) before choroidal penetration is performed. (**c**) The device after choroidal penetration and subretinal insertion; the guiding foil has been already removed. Implant is in subfoveal position. (**d**) Fundus photograph of subretinal Implant Alpha IMS; vessels of the transparent retina cross the 3 × 3 mm sized chip who has 1500 pixels. The six connectors provide power and control signals via a very thin foil with gold printed wires leading to a connector piece sutured to the eye ball (see also Fig. 6.2). In this patient after the first implantation procedure the device was perfectly placed directly under the fovea. Unfortunately implant suffered from malfunction several weeks after implantation. (**e**) An exchange with a second implant was performed successfully in this patient and resulted in very good visual results

The conjunctiva at that point is already open (see above) and the implant is still covered by the protective sleeve leaves in the orbit in a desired individually calculated length [19]. A standard 3-port vitrectomy is carried out and vitreous is removed as far as possible (Fig. 6.4a). One critical step is the search for suitable (choroidal) penetration site which should allow the creation of a visible subretinal fluid bleb in the equatorial region [20]. Passive rotation of the eye at that point is mandatory. The bleb which is created by injection of BSS through a 41G Teflon canula and is stabilized with viscoelastic solution (Healon) injected with a subretinal injection needle (subretinal injector, 32G), as shown in (Fig. 6.4b). Subsequently a trapezoidal scleral flap (4 × 5 mm^2) with its basis corresponding to the subretinal bleb is created. The choroid is completely exposed in a window of 2 × 4 mm^2 and radiodiathermy or conventional diathermy is applied in this region in a way that no resulting choroidal bleeding appears. This maneuver is carried out in hypotony of the eye to prevent the choroid from prolapsing. The puncturing of the choroid can then be carried out with a surgical knife without any bleeding. The subretinal space is entered by gaining access to the viscoelastic bleb from outside of the globe through the choroid in the area of the window. This small choroidal opening is widened by a specially designed lancet shaped guiding foil. Its rigidity and shape allows a safe subretinal advancement of this device into the desired subretinal posterior target area. The properties and handling of the guiding foil are decisive for an atraumatic surgical implantation procedure [21]. This tool is advanced subretinally from outside the globe through the choroid until it enters the subretinal bleb and is then subretinally advanced into the foveal region. The implant with its different zones of rigidity does not allow a one-step implantation. The role of the guiding foil is to allow for a safe and precise positioning of the implant in the subretinal space without collateral damage.

When reaching a suitable position in the subfoveal area with the guiding foil, the implant is removed out of the protective cover and gently inserted behind the guide with every care taken not to touch and harm the electronic chip with surgical instruments. Thereafter the guiding foil that had protected the retina during insertion of the implant is removed.

It is not necessary to reach the exact position within the first attempt to place the implant. As long as the guiding foil is in place there is plenty room for replacing maneuvers. When problems appear the guide can be replaced again and even a work with more than one guide can be of help to clear a difficult surgical situation

Once the subfoveal position is reached (Fig. 6.4c) the implant's foil at the scleral entry point (top of the scleral flap) is folded downwards and fixed onto the sclera in the area of the cable connection piece, sutured with 6.0 or 7.0 Prolene. At that point 5000 centistoke silicone oil is installed into the eye. A 5 cm silicone cable loop is left in the orbit to guarantee eye movement, as seen in the X-ray of (Fig. 6.2c). Donor sclera is used to cover the episcleral foil-implant part and finally the conjunctiva is carefully sutured over the donor sclera.

Replacement of Implants

Ocular implants, like any technical device, can fail or –which probably happens more often– they can be outdated if an improved version becomes available. Longevity of devices that carry circuits in the milieu of the human body is a challenge in material sciences, concerning corrosion, delamination of the subretinal foils that carry the golden connections lanes to the external parts of the device, and the millions of eye movements are stress for the moving intraorbital parts of the cable. Moreover, as the retina is not perforated during surgery, the final position of the chip at the end of an approximately 3 cm long subretinal foil can only be adjusted by manipulation from outside through the choroidal opening. Reaching the optimal position can also be prevented by retinal-RPE-adhesions which sometimes cannot be optimally separated. Finally, even when the pre-operatively defined optimal position has been reached it might turn out that the morphologically optimal region is not the functionally optimal region, concerning retinal blood supply or density of remaining inner retina neurons. In short, re-positioning or complete implant exchanges will become necessary in increasing numbers as the frequency of performed procedures increases.

In a series of meanwhile 27 implantations from October 2005 to March 2016 at the University Eye Hospital in Tübingen, Germany, four implant re-positioning procedures were done. Two were performed to improve visual function by more central localization and resulted in an increase of grating acuity from 0.3 to 1 cpd (cycles per degree) and from unmeasurable to 0.3 cpd, respectively. Two other relocations were performed when the implant had moved for 2–3 mm and a damaging touch of the optic nerve had to be prevented. All procedures were technically relatively easy as the vitreous cavity and/or the subretinal space had not to be reopened because all manipulations could be performed from externally. Another implant was removed due to technical failure and was replaced by a placeholder foil. Additionally one implant (Fig. 6.4d) was replaced 5 weeks after implantation due to technical failure and a new implant was inserted in the same explantation/re-implantation procedure [22]. The new implant (see Fig. 6.4e) was again positioned under the fovea and good visual results were obtained in grating acuity (increasing from 0.33 to 1.0 cycles per degree), albeit, with reduced form vision. In summary, re-positioning and implant exchanges are surgically feasible and anatomically tolerable and can result in improved function.

Clinical Study Results

Twenty-nine participants (13 females, 16 males) with a mean age (±standard deviation) of 53.8 ± 8.2 years (range 35–71 years) were enrolled in the clinical trial of Retina Implant Alpha IMS (www.clinicaltrials.gov, NCT01024803) and received the implant in one eye [12]. The clinical trial was a multicentric trial running in the years 2010–2014, including seven sites worldwide (Tübingen/Germany, Dresden/Germany, Budapest/Hungary, Oxford/United Kingdom, London/United Kingdom, Singapore, Hong Kong). Visual function prior to implantation was light perception without projection (20 participants) or no light perception (9 participants). The loss of vision was caused by hereditary degenerations of the photoreceptors (25 participants had retinitis pigmentosa, 4 had cone-rod dystrophy).

Primary efficacy endpoints of the study protocol were a significant improvement of activities of daily living and mobility to be assessed by activities of daily living tasks, recognition tasks, mobility, or a combination thereof. Secondary efficacy endpoints were a significant improvement of visual acuity/light perception and/or object recognition (clinicaltrials.gov, NCT01024803). According to the trial protocol, clinical and functional follow-ups extended to 1 year.

Twenty-one participants (72 %) reached the primary efficacy endpoints as set in the study protocol, twenty-five participants (86 %) reached the secondary endpoints [12]. The following paragraphs give some details on the performance for the protocol-mandated tests.

Basic visual functions of 29 participants, four could not perceive any light using the subretinal implant. The most probable reasons included an intraoperative touch of the optic nerve during device insertion, retinal edema after implant repositioning, suspected retinal perfusion problems and technical failure of the implant. The remaining 25 participants (86 %) were able to perceive light via the subretinal implant.

Basic visual functions were tested as computer screen tasks (Fig. 6.5a) using the software BaLM (Basic Light and Motion) test [23] in the two or four alternative forced condition (AFC) as shown in (Fig. 6.5b). The performance across all subjects was significantly better ($p<0.05$) with implant power on vs. off for light perception in all visits. In the test of light localization with a light wedge in four different directions the performance over all subjects was significantly better ($p<0.05$) with implant on vs. off in months 1, 2, 3 and 6. Motion detection assessed with dot patterns moving in four directions was possible for six participants, the highest speed for which the direction was correctly recognized with the implant switched on ranged from 3° to 35° per second.

Spatial resolution grating acuity and visual acuity with standardized Landolt C-rings in contrast reversal (white ring on black background), the secondary endpoints of the study (Fig. 6.5b), were tested on a screen as computer tests (AFC mode). The participant was asked to tell the orientation of the grating and the direction of the C-ring gap respectively.

The grating acuity resolutions with implant power on ranged from 0.1 to 3.3 cycles per degree. Five participants passed the grating acuity task once by reaching 75 % correct responses despite chip power being switched off; four of them indicated that it was done by guessing, whereas in all five patients the grating acuity with implant power switched off was lower than with the implant power on. Four participants successfully completed standardized visual acuity testing using contrast reversal Landolt C-rings, with visual acuities of 20/2000, 20/2000, 20/606 and 20/546.

Two activities of daily living and recognition tasks (ADL) were performed on a black table using white objects (Fig. 6.5c). Geometrical objects of about 5° visual angle each were placed in front of the participant, who was asked to report how many objects were present, point to their position, and describe what they were (shape description and localization). Thereafter, dining objects (such as white cups and cutlery) were placed around a white large plate in front of the participant, who was asked to report how many objects were present around the plate, localize them, and identify them (shape description).

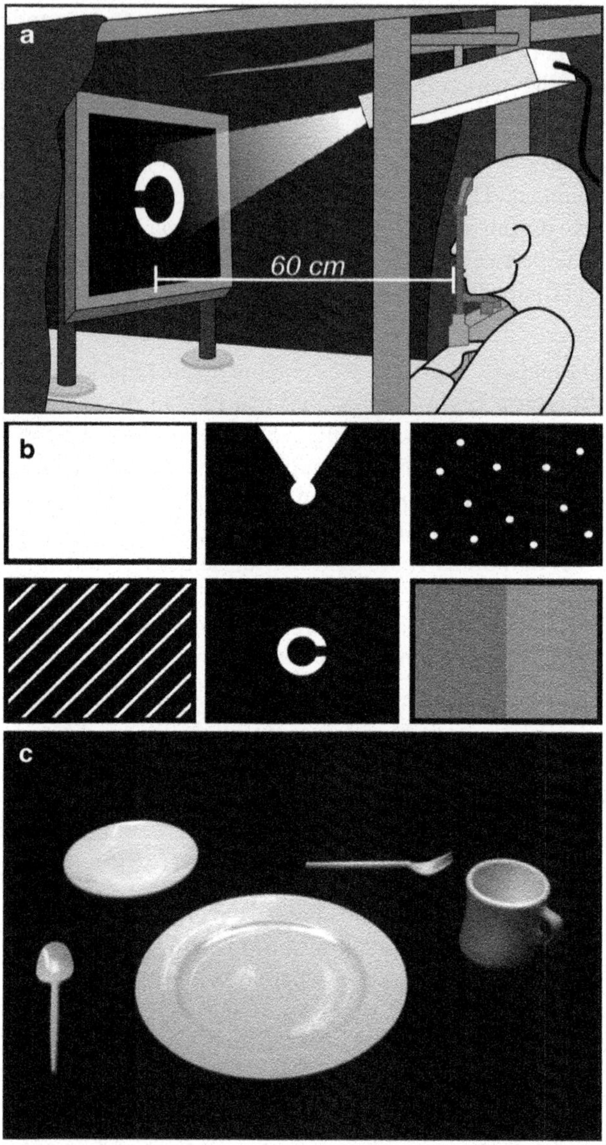

Fig. 6.5 (**a**) Set up for projecting targets on a screen. (**b**) Either areas of homogenous light, or gratings of variable width, distance and luminance, Landolt C-rings, bright wedges moving random dots or borders of various contrasts are presented individually in a 'four-alternative forced choice' mode (4AFC) to asses spatio-temporal resolution. (**c**) Activities of daily living are tested by positioning various objects around a plate in different arrangements and scaling the performance of a patient (0–4) in detecting the objects, indicating the number of objects present, and naming the objects (Modified from Stingl K, Bartz-Schmidt et al. [11]. With permission from © 2013 The Authors under the terms of the Creative Commons Attribution License: http://rspb.royalsocietypublishing.org/content/280/1757/20130077 https://creativecommons.org/licenses/by/4.0/)

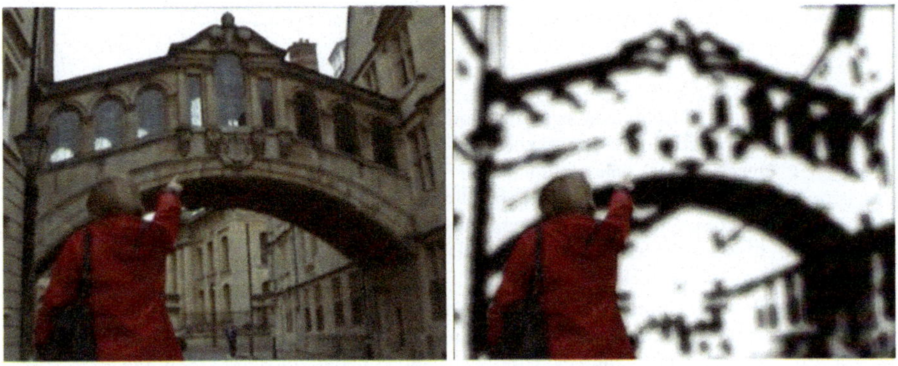

Fig. 6.6 (*Right*) sketch of the perception of a patient who described what she saw with the Retina Implant Alpha IMS when looking at the Bridge of Sighs in Oxford (*left*) i.e. reporting a blurred scene in several levels of grey consisting of an arch and neighbouring buildings (Courtesy of Prof. R. MacLaren, Oxford)

Detection, localization, and recognition of geometric shapes as well as the dining objects in a good contrast was significantly better with the implant power on compared to off during the first three months. From the month 6 visits and beyond, the statistical significance decreased ($p>0.05$) for most of the power on–off comparisons. This might be due to fewer data, as well as to a slight increase in the performance with the implant power off, as discussed below.

As recognition tasks, reading of clock hands, reading of letters and differentiation of grey tones were performed. The clock and letters tasks were performed in a good contrast, using white letters as well as white clock hands on a black background.

Five participants could read the clock hands at least once during the trial visits and tell the time. One participant passed the clock task once with the implant turned off (false positive). Four participants could read letters at least once during the trial visits. Fifteen participants (52 %) were able to recognize at least one grey level, ranging up to six (only six levels were tested in the present study), compared to an intermediate grey level. Eight participants (28 %) recognized up to three grey levels with the implant off.

Daily life experiences participants used the visual implant during their daily life, at home, outdoors, or at work, usually up to 2–3 h daily. Several participants spontaneously reported a slight improvement of the remaining light perception with the implant off during the course of the study; however, none of them could see objects without the implant power being switched on. The sketch on the right in Fig. 6.6 (from the Oxford site of the trial) illustrates the report of the patient looking at the bridge of sighs: the image is blurry, consisting of several grey levels; due to visual field size of 15 deg across corners of the chip possibly only half of the bridge's length could be perceived at a time but the patient -similar to an RP patient with such field size- could easely complete the picture by moving the eye and the head (from movie clip https://vimeo.com/93975327).

Table 6.1 Quotes from patient reports grouped for various situations

		No. of Pat.
People	Shape of head; face: eye part, mouth shape, teeth; glasses; bracelet; characteristics of dresses; heads of colleagues during work group meeting; dark hair vs. blond hair; rim of glasses; people sitting on chairs in the garden; person bending to his laptop; silhouette of a visitor on the couch; moving heads; grand daughter in white baby-dress; shoulders silhouette; face as a triangular flash; white scarf around the neck	8
Houses	Windows; house outlines; white paper sheet hanging on the door; door knob; silhouette of Tübingen town-hall; location of doors or door frames; walls; chimney margins; location of edges of steps; size of the windows; curtain stripes	10
Streets	White pile on the street; street lamps showing the direction of the street; fireworks; shop signs in darkness lit up (not reading); lines of the pavements; landmarks; arches of a viaduct	5
Cars	car reflections; car lights at night moving; bus lights; differentiating two bus companies; sitting in the car at night: car lights as "fireflies"	4
Nature	Sunflower stalk in the graden; parasol in the garden; horizon; river flowing towards the horizon (sun reflection); blooming flowers in the garden; goose swimming in the pond; outline of the dogs; dogs wagging the tail; could walk around a garden table and sit down; moon	4
Reading	Signs on the street (lighting): reading ADAC, VAPIANO	1
Own body	Own fingers in front of the TV screen; own hand; head silhouette in the mirror; own striped jacket in the mirror	3
Near/at home	Frame of a picture with texture of the image; lamp-post; fluorescent tubes; kitchen objects such as plates, etc. in good contrast; washing basin; trash can; clock on the wall (not reading hours); square-shaped carpet in the next room; frame of the TV; cup handle; small bottles; red vs. white wine; dark vs. milk chocolate; noodles vs. beef; objects on the working desk (stapler, phone, etc.); glass and cutlery on the table; picking up hot steam while cooking	9

Table 6.1 shows visual experiences that were described by patients with the implant power on (examples can be seen in video clips at https://vimeo.com/retinaimplant/videos). Patients' observations concern mainly facial and other personal features, buildings, outdoor activities, vehicles, nature, own body and indoor experiences.

Eight participants (28 %, including four who did not have any light perception via the implant) did not benefit in daily life (see Fig. 6.7). In most cases degeneration of the retina, despite layered appearance of OCT, was apparently too advanced as to allow for adequate processing of electrical signals. A further eight participants (28 %) could localize objects with a good contrast in their daily life, but could not recognize shapes or details. Seven participants (25 %) reported useful new daily life experiences with the implant, being able to see shapes and/or details of objects in grey tones; six participants (19 %) reported very good visual experiences in daily life, including recognition of letters or identified unknown shapes and objects.

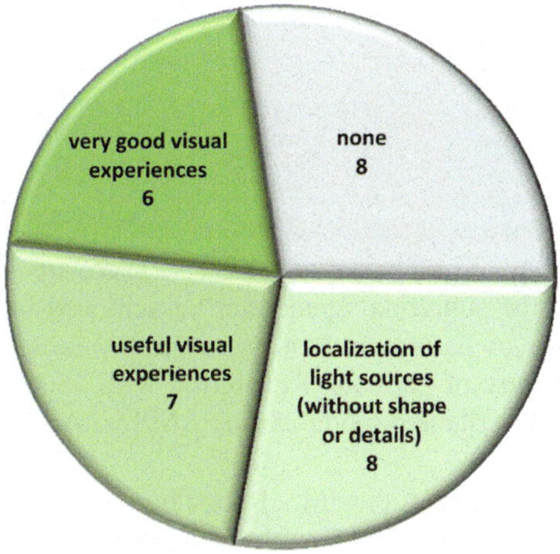

Fig. 6.7 Daily life experiences. Numbers of participants grouped according to their reports of visual experiences in daily life. Eight participants did not benefit from the visual implant in daily life. Further eight participants could only localize light sources and bright objects. Seven participants reported useful visual regained visual experiences with descriptions of shapes or details in scales of grey and six participants reported very good experiences, e.g. letters and facial expressions (Modified from Stingl et al. [12]. With permission from Elsevier under the Creative Commons Attribution License. http://www.sciencedirect.com/science/article/pii/S0042698915000784. http://creativecommons.org/licenses/by/4.0/)

Safety

Two serious adverse events (SAEs) occurred during the trial: an increase of intraocular pressure up to 46 mmHg that was successfully treated and resolved without sequelae; and a local retinal detachment near the exit point of the foil in the retinal periphery which occurred immediately after explantation of the device, was treated surgically with laser coagulation and silicone oil, and resolved with local retinal fibrotic changes. Further adverse events resolved without sequelae. Details on safety assessment of the first, monocentric part of the trial (site Tübingen/Germany in the years 2010–2012) have been published [24]; almost half of the adverse events had a relationship with the implant classified as "certain," about 80% resolved without sequelae and about the same amount were of mild intensity. However, there were some cases that needed more attention. In one subject, the implant perforated the choroid in the macular region and touched the optic nerve head during its positioning. To improve visibility of the implant and to aid in its positioning, a bluish colored guiding foil and depth marks on the implant's polyimide foil were introduced. With these developments, no further similar incidents occurred. Two subjects incurred retinal breaks during positioning of the implant: Owing to these experiences, a biometrical evaluation system was introduced that helps preventing such events [19]. Also the evaluation of subsequent study cases (publication in preparation) showed a clinically similar acceptable safety profile. In order to test the technical function of the implant in the eye of a patient, a method was developed to test the implant's response transfer characteristics via corneally recorded light responses of the implant [25].

Conclusion

Subretinal implants have a number of advantages: There are no devices attached to the face, fixation in the subretinal space can be achieved without tacks; training phases are short due to natural retinotopy, within weeks useful vision can be achieved by the majority of patients. Resolution with 1500 pixels (Model Alpha IMS) or 1600 pixels (overhauled model Alpha AMS with extended life time) is the highest so far achieved.

A subretinal visual implant (Alpha IMS, Retina Implant AG, Reutlingen, Germany) was implanted in 29 blind participants with outer retinal degeneration in an international multicenter clinical trial. During up to 12 months observation time 21 participants (72 %) reached the primary end point (improvement of activities of daily living and mobility), of which 13 participants (44 %) reported restoration of visual function which they use in daily life. Twenty-five participants (86 %) reached the secondary endpoints (significant improvement of visual acuity/light perception and/or object recognition). Measurable grating acuity was up to 3.3 cycles per degree, visual acuities using standardized Landolt C-rings were 20/546. Maximal correct motion perception ranged from 3° to 35° per second. The safety profile is good.

These results show that subretinal implants, certified as medical devices and commercially available in Europe in several centers in Germany Alpha AMS implantation is covered by the public health care insurance system can restore very-low-vision or low vision in blind (light perception or less) patients with end-stage hereditary retinal degenerations.

References

1. Santos A, et al. Preservation of the inner retina in retinitis pigmentosa. A morphometric analysis. Arch Ophthalmol. 1997;115(4):511–5.
2. Chow AY, Chow VY. Subretinal electrical stimulation of the rabbit retina. Neurosci Lett. 1997;225:13–6.
3. Zrenner E. Will retinal implants restore vision? Science. 2002;295:1022–5.
4. Zrenner E. Fighting blindness with microelectronics. Sci Transl Med. 2013;5:210 ps16.
5. Hafed ZM, Stingl K, Bartz-Schmidt KU, Gekeler F, Zrenner E. Oculomotor behavior of blind patients seeing with a subretinal visual implant. Vis Res. 2015. Online ahead of print: doi: 10.1016/j.visres.2015.04.006.
6. Zrenner E, Stett A, Weiss S, Aramant RB, Guenther E, Kohler K, Miliczek KD, Seiler MJ, Haemmerle H. Can subretinal microphotodiodes successfully replace degenerated photoreceptors? Vision Res. 1999;39:2555–67.
7. Stett A, Barth W, Weiss S, et al. Electrical multisite stimulation of the isolated chicken retina. Vision Res. 2000;40:1785–95.
8. Guenther E, Tröger B, Schlosshauer B, Zrenner E. Long-term survival of retinal cell cultures on retinal implant materials. Vision Res. 1999;39:3988–94.

9. Eckhorn R, Wilms M, Schanze T, Eger M, Hesse L, Eysel UT, Kisvárday ZF, Zrenner E, Gekeler F, Schwahn H, Shinoda K, Sachs H, Walter P. Visual resolution with retinal implants estimated from recordings in cat visual cortex. Vision Res. 2006;46:2675–90.
10. Zrenner E. Subretinal electronic chips allow blind patients to read letters and combine them to words. Proc Roy Soc B. 2011;278:1489–97.
11. Stingl K, Bartz-Schmidt KU, Besch D, Braun A, Bruckmann A, Gekeler F, Greppmaier U, Hipp S, Hörtdörfer G, Kernstock C, Koitschev A, Kusnyerik A, Sachs H, Schatz A, Stingl KT, Peters T, Wilhelm B, Zrenner E. Artificial vision with wirelessly powered subretinal electronic implant alpha-IMS. Proc Roy Soc B Biol Sci. 2013;280(1757):20130077.
12. Stingl K, Bartz-Schmidt KU, Besch D, Chee CK, Cottriall CL, Gekeler F, Groppe M, Jackson TL, MacLaren RE, Koitschev A, Kusnyerik A, Neffendorf J, Nemeth J, Naeem MA, Peters T, Ramsden JD, Sachs H, Simpson A, Singh MS, Wilhelm B, Wong D, Zrenner E. Subretinal visual implant alpha IMS – clinical trial interim report. Vision Res. 2015;111:149–60.
13. Gekeler F, Szurman P, Grisanti S, Weiler U, Claus R, Greiner TO, Völker M, Kohler K, Zrenner E, Bartz-Schmidt KU. Compound subretinal prostheses with extra-ocular parts designed for human trials: successful long-term implantation in pigs. Graefes Arch Clin Exp Ophthalmol. 2007;245:230–41.
14. Besch D, Sachs H, Szurman P, Gülicher D, Wilke R, Reinert S, Zrenner E, Bartz-Schmidt KU, Gekeler F. Extraocular surgery for implantation of an active subretinal visual prosthesis with external connections: feasibility and outcome in seven patients. Br J Ophthalmol. 2008;92: 1361–8.
15. Koitschev A, Stingl K, Bartz-Schmidt KU, Braun A, Gekeler F, Greppmaier U, Sachs H, Peters T, Wilhelm B, Zrenner E, Besch D. Extraocular surgical approach for placement of subretinal implants in blind patients: lessons from cochlear-implants. J Ophthalmol. 2015;2015:842518.
16. Sachs HG, Schanze T, Brunner U, Sailer H, Wiesenack C. Transscleral implantation and neurophysiological testing of subretinal polyimide film electrodes in the domestic pig in visual prosthesis development. J Neural Eng. 2005;2(2005):S57–64.
17. Sachs H, Bartz-Schmidt KU, Gabel VP, Zrenner E, Gekeler F. Subretinal implant: the intraocular implantation technique. Nova Acta Leopoldina NF III. 2010;379:217–23.
18. Stingl K, Bartz-Schmidt KU, Gekeler F, Kusnyerik A, Sachs H, Zrenner E. Functional outcome in subretinal electronic implants depends on foveal eccentricity. Invest Ophthalmol Vis Sci. 2013;54(12):7658–65.
19. Kusnyerik A, Greppmaier U, Wilke R, Gekeler F, Wilhelm B, Sachs HG, Bartz-Schmidt KU, Klose U, Stingl K, Resch MD, Hekmat A, Bruckmann A, Karacs K, Nemeth J, Suveges I, Zrenner E. Positioning of electronic subretinal implants in blind retinitis pigmentosa patients through multimodal assessment of retinal structures. Invest Ophthalmol Vis Sci. 2012;53: 3748–55.
20. Sachs HG, Bartz-Schmidt KU, Gekeler F, Besch D, Brunner U, Wilhelm B, Wilke R, Wrobel W, Gabel V-P, Zrenner E. Transchoroidal implantation of active subretinal implants in blind patients: experience with the new surgical implantation and explantation procedure in the first Six patients. Invest Ophthalmol Vis Sci (ARVO Abstract). 2007;48(13):4046.
21. Sachs HG, Brunner U, Gekeler F, Bartz-Schmidt KU, Wrobel W, Gabel V-P, Hekmat A, Zrenner E. The development of a guiding tool for transchoroidal chip implantation to protect the retina. Invest Ophthalmol Vis Sci (ARVO Abstract). 2008;49(13):4045.
22. Gekeler F, Sachs H, Kitiratschky V, Stingl K, Greppmaier U, Zrenner E, Bartz-Schmidt KU, Ueffing M, Dammeier S. Re-alignment and explantation of subretinal prostheses: surgical aspects and proteomic analyses. Invest Ophthalmol Vis Sci (ARVO Abstract). 2013; 54(15):1036.
23. Bach M. Basic quantitative assessment of visual performance in patients with very low vision. Invest Ophthalmol Vis Sci. 2010;51:1255–60.
24. Kitiratschky VBD, et al. Safety evaluation of 'retina implant alpha IMS' – a prospective clinical trial. Graefes Arch Clin Exp Ophthalmol Graefes Arch Clin Exp Ophthalmol. 2015; 253:381–7.
25. Stingl K, et al. Transfer characteristics of subretinal visual implants: corneally recorded implant responses. Documenta Ophthalmologica (in press). 2016. doi:10.1007/s10633-016-9557-7.

Chapter 7
The Boston Retinal Implant

Shawn K. Kelly and Joseph Rizzo

Abstract The Boston Retinal Implant Project has developed a subretinal, hermetically-enclosed, chronically-implantable vision prosthesis to restore some useful vision to people with degenerative retinal diseases, especially retinitis pigmentosa and age-related macular degeneration. Our implant attaches to the outside of the eye, with only the electrode array entering the eye, carrying over 256 independently-configurable retinal stimulation channels. Our device receives wireless power and data from an inductive link, and inbound data includes image information in the form of stimulation commands containing current amplitudes and pulse widths. Outbound data includes status information on the implant and measurements of electrode voltages. A custom-designed integrated circuit chip is packaged in an 11 mm-diameter titanium case with a ceramic feedthrough, attached to the side of the eye. The chip decodes the stimulation data, creates biphasic, charged-balanced current pulses, and monitors the resulting voltages on the stimulating electrodes. The electrode array is a thin, flexible, microfabricated film carrying hundreds of wires to exposed electrodes in the eye. The electrodes are coated with sputtered iridium oxide film to allow much greater charge transfer per unit area by means of reversible faradaic reactions. The Boston Retinal Implant is being manufactured and tested in pre-clinical trials for safety, with plans to begin clinical trials soon.

Keywords Retinal prosthesis • Retinal implant • Neural stimulation • Subretinal • Medical device • Power and data telemetry • Hermetic packaging

S.K. Kelly
Institute for Complex Engineered Systems, VA Pittsburgh Healthcare System, Carnegie Mellon University, Pittsburgh, PA, USA

J. Rizzo (✉)
Harvard Medical School and the Massachusetts Eye and Ear Infirmary, Boston, MA, USA
e-mail: Joseph_Rizzo@MEEI.Harvard.edu

V.P. Gabel (ed.), *Artificial Vision*, DOI 10.1007/978-3-319-41876-6_7

Key Points

- The Boston Retinal Implant delivers over 256 independently-configurable channels of stimulating current to create vision.
- Our device attaches to the outside of the eye, with the electrode array entering the eye, resting in the subretinal space.
- We have implemented several redundant safety features to prevent corrupted messages, overstimulation, and charge imbalance.
- Our device is being tested in preclinical studies, with plans to begin clinical trials soon.

Overview

The field of retinal prosthetics emerged in the late 1980s, and the Boston Retinal Implant Project was one of the first two research projects that were formed. The development of these implants was enabled by rapid advances in microelectronic technology [1, 2]. These devices require a large number of stimulating channels in a package small enough to conform to the eyeball. The convergence of technological improvements in integrated circuit (IC) chip fabrication, microelectromechanical systems (MEMS) fabrication, electrode materials fabrication, and hermetic packaging manufacturing has allowed implanted neural stimulators to become small enough and to have a large enough number of channels to create prostheses with a reasonable hope of restoring vision to the blind.

The overwhelming majority of patients over age 40 years in industrialized countries who are either "legally-blind" (<20/200 in their better seeing eye) or "visually-impaired" (20/40 or worse in their better seeing eye) have some form of neural blindness, usually either age-related macular degeneration (AMD), retinitis pigmentosa (RP), diabetic retinopathy, or glaucoma, and there are no satisfactory treatments to restore vision for any of these conditions. While the degenerative diseases AMD and RP cause loss of the photoreceptors in the retina, they spare the retinal ganglion cells. Electrical stimulation of these ganglion cells, or of the retinal network upstream from them, generates visual percepts that can form the basis of a visual prosthesis.

A visual prosthesis requires a number of different technological elements (Fig. 7.1). First, a method for collecting visual information is required. This is often a small electronic camera outside the body, usually mounted on a pair of glasses, but it is occasionally an implanted photodiode array. Second, the prosthesis requires a method for sending power to the implanted device, and, in the case of an external camera, for sending image data to the device. This is often accomplished with inductive coupling between wire coils, though a number of optical power transfer strategies have been explored. Circuitry is required to generate stimulating currents in a safe and controlled way, and small and charge-efficient electrodes are required that can safely deliver currents to the target tissue without creating dangerous

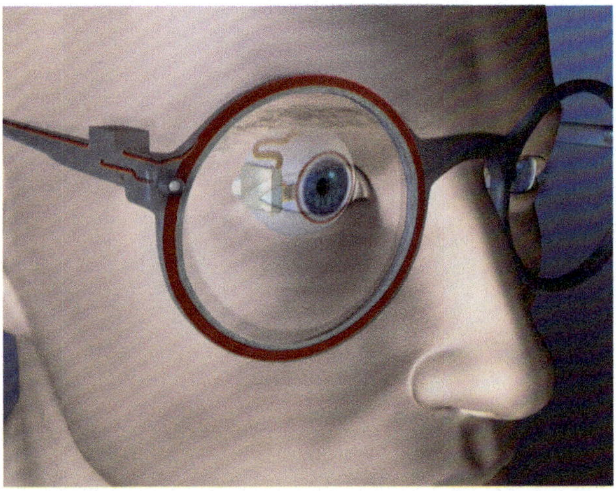

Fig. 7.1 The Boston retinal implant concept. The patient wears a camera mounted on a pair of glasses. Images are sent to a smart-phone-sized controller unit (not shown), which processes the images before sending the pertinent image data, along with power, wirelessly to the implanted device. The implant decodes the data and electrically stimulates the retinal tissue to create artificial vision

reduction and oxidation reactions. Because the implant must be quite small to attach to the eye, the circuitry is usually a custom-designed integrated circuit chip. The electrodes are often in the form of thin-film microfabricated arrays. The stimulating electrodes themselves are usually planar, but electrodes that penetrate into the retina have been explored by our group as well. Finally, a method is required for protecting the sensitive electronics from the body's saline environment. Classically, this is done using hermetic packaging, with a titanium case brazed to a ceramic block with platinum feedthroughs, but microfabricated methods are being explored.

The Boston Retinal Implant Project has chosen an approach using an external camera mounted on glasses. The image data go to a small external electronic unit that processes the image to select the most relevant few 100 pixels to send to the implant. The external unit also includes batteries and the wireless power and data transmitter. This approach provides substantial flexibility to modify image processing algorithms using external commands, or to implement multiple image processing modes, to best suit a specific patient and a specific visual situation.

The other significant design choice that we have made pertains to the specific location of the stimulating electrodes in the retina (Fig. 7.2). The electrodes may be placed on top of the inner retinal surface (epiretinal), beneath the retina (subretinal), or in a number of locations farther outward in the eye (e.g., the suprachoroidal space). We initially explored an epiretinal approach, but switched to a subretinal approach for a number of design reasons. First, the subretinal location enables an *ab externo* surgical approach, where the implant is attached to the outside of the eye, releasing its excess heat to less thermally sensitive tissues than the retina. It is possible to use an *ab externo* approach to the epiretinal surface, but it requires a relatively long electrode cable that enters the eye very near the limbus, near where the conjunctiva attaches to the eye. At this location, a device is prone to erosion through the delicate conjunctiva, and chronic hypotony of the eye has also been a complication of this approach. And, once in the eye, the electrode cable must extend to the back surface of the eye, which imposes

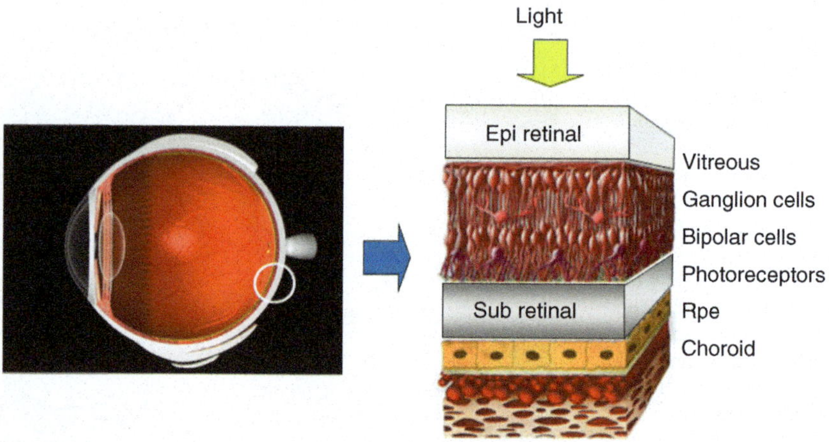

Fig. 7.2 Retinal electrode locations. Stimulating electrodes are often placed on the inner surface of the retina (epiretinal) or under the retina, between the neural cells and the retinal pigment epithelium (RPE), (subretinal). Some arrays are placed farther from the tissue, either underneath the choroid (suprachoroidal), or outside the sclera (trans-scleral)

undesirable mechanical factors that can challenge conformal alignment of the electrode array across the retina. In this regard, an epiretinal electrode requires some method of attachment to the retina, usually a tack through the retina, whereas, an array in the subretinal space is held in place without the need for external fixation. This overview of relative advantages and disadvantages of the various approaches is not intended to suggest that one approach is definitively better than the other. Ultimately, preferred methods will have to be validated with long-term human implants, and our group has yet to perform such tests.

Background

While the concept of electrically stimulating retinal ganglion cells of a patient with outer retinal degeneration seemed like a plausible therapeutic strategy, proof-of-concept experiments were a prudent step before launching into the arduous process of designing a chronic implant. In the case of BRIP, initial animal trials were performed by delivering electrical stimulation to the retina through a long connecting cable containing an electrode array, which was placed in contact with the epiretinal surface. The cable was connected to external electronics that provided stimulating current, and recording electrodes were placed into the skull over the visual cortex. This approach revealed cortical responses that were linked to photic stimuli and to electrical stimuli in separate trials, with delays consistent with synaptic transmission from the retinal ganglion cells to the visual cortex. These experiments showed that electrical stimulation of the retina can send neural signals to the cortex, but this type of experiment revealed nothing about the quality of the visual percepts.

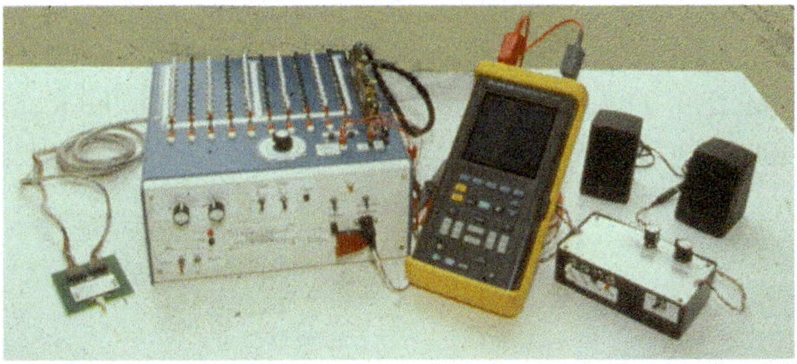

Fig. 7.3 The portable, battery powered stimulation system used in our acute human trials. The blue and white box is the 100-channel stimulator, connected via a 7-ft cable to a green circuit board containing the electrode array (at *left*). A portable battery-powered oscilloscope monitors the voltages, and a set of speakers creates a tone to alert the subjects to the timing of the stimulus

To learn something about the human perceptual response to electrical stimulation of the retina, our group performed six acute human retinal stimulation trials between 1998 and 2000 [3, 4]. In these experiments, we used the same approach developed in animal tests to deliver electrical stimulation to the retina. Subjects were chosen who had outer retinal degeneration that had progressed to a severe state, with no better than hand motion perception in the worse eye, which was always the eye studied. One subject had normal vision, but had orbital cancer, which required removal of the eye; this patient allowed us to deliver electrical stimulation to the retina just prior to enucleation. Our electrode array was a 10-μm-thick polyimide film containing between 20 and 100 planar electrodes. The use of an ultra-thin substrate like this was novel for the field of visual prosthetics. The electrodes in the first experiment were 50 μm in diameter, and in later experiments, electrodes 100 and 400 μm in diameter were added. The electrode was coated with an iridium oxide film, which is capable of safely delivering more than ten times the charge of a platinum electrode of the same size. The back end of the electrodes, outside the eye, was connected via a cable to the stimulator system (Fig. 7.3). The battery powered stimulator delivered current to up to 100 electrodes from ten current sources, allowing concurrent and/or sequential stimulation.

These human trials gave a number of important results. First, and most importantly, they showed that electrical stimulation of the retina produces distinct, perceivable visual events. These visual percepts could be combined to form recognizable lines, but more complicated structures were difficult to achieve with a severely visually impaired subject, lying on an operating room table, receiving visual percepts in their periphery for a few hours. We also learned that the thresholds for electrical stimulation of retina were reasonable, and were within the safe charge density range for iridium oxide, but that the thresholds were sensitive to the electrode position.

While the results of these human trials were encouraging, they showed the need for a chronic retinal implant, one that would allow subjects to learn to use the new visual information over time. Since then, our group has developed five generations of implantable devices, each with progressive improvements in power and data telemetry, stimulation safety, number of stimulating channels, digital controls, and hermetic packaging [5–8]. Our designs also evolved to improve surgical access for electrode array insertion and to reduce irritation of sensitive parts of the eye, especially the conjunctiva. The rest of this chapter will describe the technical details of the latest design of the Boston Retinal Implant.

Device Requirements

The Overview section above describes the technical elements of a retinal prosthesis. Here we expand upon that information to now include specific requirements for our device. The first element, the camera, is not heavily constrained in this design, except in size. With an implant driving a few hundred electrodes, the number of pixels in any camera will be too large by several orders of magnitude. However, the camera needs to be integrated into the glasses worn by the patient, so it should be small and lightweight. The wireless power and data system should be robust, first and foremost. It should be tolerant of quick movements of the eye, as well as slower shifts in the position of the glasses, and it should be able to adjust the power delivered to compensate for movements of the coil as well as changes in the power required by the chip. The telemetry system should be moderately efficient to conserve battery power, but robustness should not be sacrificed for efficiency. Finally, the telemetry system should be able to transmit at a sufficient data rate to supply stimulation information to all electrodes at the target simulation rate with appropriate systems in place to check data accuracy, and the system should be able to transmit information out from the implant, though at a slower rate.

The implanted component should include circuits with the ability to deliver precise stimulating currents, with sufficient flexibility to explore a range of stimulation parameters to create optimal visual percepts. The circuits should be small in size to fit in a package that can be attached to the eye, and should utilize low-power design to save battery life and to avoid heating the eye. In addition, the stimulating circuit should include redundant safety features to prevent dangerous electrochemical reactions and damage to the retinal tissue, and to detect and report any faults that develop over time.

The electrode array should be thin and flexible, but tough and robust enough to stand up to handling during surgery and normal movements of the eye. The stimulating electrodes should be made of a material that can convey sufficient charge to the retina to stimulate tissue with a broad dynamic range without causing irreversible reduction or oxidation reactions. The array construction should enable hundreds of connections and be small enough to pass through a relatively small incision in the eye. The materials used in the array in the electrode sites should be biocompatible, not inducing inflammation in the retinal tissue.

The implanted package should be hermetic, preventing the ingress of water over the lifetime of the device, in our case, for over a decade. This is particularly challenging due to the very small internal volume of the device. In addition, the package must be small, thinner than 2 mm in height and with a diameter on the order of 1 cm, with hundreds of feedthroughs.

The combination of these requirements is a serious engineering challenge requiring custom wireless circuit design, custom chip design, the development of new fabrication processes for electrodes, and the development of new medical device packaging technologies.

The Boston Retinal Implant

The first element in the logical stream of events, the camera and glasses, has been the last component that we have chosen to build. Small cameras are improving every year, and an off-the-shelf camera should be easily integrated into custom glasses. Therefore, our group has delayed the design and manufacturing of the camera and glasses until the more complicated implanted device is fully completed and in preclinical testing.

Wireless Power and Data

The inductive telemetry system consists of a primary coil mounted on the glasses, a secondary coil attached to the anterior surface of the eye (just posterior to the limbus and beneath the conjunctiva), and associated transceiver circuits. Approximately 30 mW is transmitted to the implant, with feedback to control the received power.

Custom Integrated Circuit Design

The retinal implant requires several unique features that demand a custom-designed integrated circuit chip. Specifically, very large numbers of current sources, as well as the associated safety features, are not available in off-the-shelf chips. Some of the digital control features could be implemented with commercially available systems, but with a cost of size that is unacceptable for an implant that needs to be small enough for this ocular application. As such, our group designed and tested a custom integrated circuit chip for our prosthesis.

The forward wireless power and FSK data link from the external controller to the implant chip that our group has built (Fig. 7.4) transmits and receives data with very high signal-to-noise ratio (SNR) and zero errors over thousands of packets to the receiver.

The more than 256 independent current sources deliver charge-balanced currents, ranging from 0 to 126 μA, in steps of 1 μA. Individual stimulation phase widths range from 17.7 to 4500 μs, in steps of 17.7 μs. Voltage supplies for the current sources can be set to ±4 V for normal operation, or up to ±8 V for higher current source compliance if needed. Stimulus commands for small numbers of

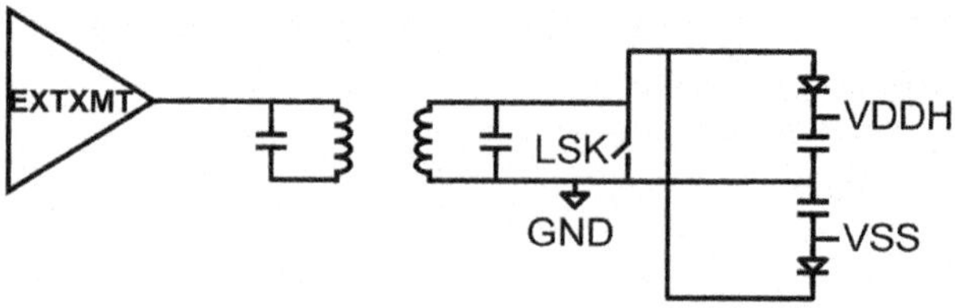

Fig. 7.4 Power and data transmission system. The transceiver block diagram shows the external transmitter and coil, secondary coil, secondary dual half-wave rectifier to establish Vddh and Vss, and LSK switch

electrodes can be sent at a stimulation refresh rate exceeding 400 Hz, or commands can cycle through groups of electrodes to drive every electrode with a refresh rate exceeding 60 Hz.

Safety features include stimulus charge limits, error checking on data transmission, comprehensive self-test and performance monitoring, and configuration pins to change operating modes or to lock out settings that might somehow cause harm. Each message from the external controller to the IC can result in a set of stimulus pulses on a subset of the electrodes, and each message generates a corresponding response from the implant IC with chip and electrode status, and any other requested data. Radio communication errors are nearly eliminated by the use of 32-bit cyclic redundancy checks (CRCs). A single data packet includes every stimulation parameter for every electrode to be stimulated in the subsequent time frame. No individual message can cause harm, and messages with a bad CRC merely result in missed stimulus pulses, drastically reducing the chances of delivering an unintended stimulation that may be dangerously imbalanced or larger than the safe limits. Several features also work to ensure operation with safe levels of electrode polarization. While allowing both high-current short-duration pulses and low-current long-duration pulses, the IC has hardware-enforced charge limits, guided by our prior electrode characterization work [5]. Configuration pins allow the limits to be changed for compatibility with a range of electrode sizes.

One particular concern is the polarization of the electrode-tissue interface. If that interface is driven outside the electrochemical water window of −0.6 to +0.8 V, charge injection occurs in the form of oxidation or reduction of water, which can be biologically damaging and mechanically damaging to the electrodes [9]. Our prosthesis uses sputtered iridium oxide film (SIROF) electrode sites, which have the benefit of allowing very high charge densities (exceeding 1 mC/cm^2) with reversible electrochemical reactions, but which have the possibility of suffering mechanical failure if the interface is repeatedly driven outside the water window. However, due to the non-linearity and distributed nature of the electrode impedance, it is very difficult to measure the electrode-tissue interface while the stimulus current is being driven [10]. Therefore, we measure the electrode polarization in the middle of the biphasic current pulse, during the interphase interval (Wip in Fig. 7.5).

During the time between biphasic pulses, each electrode is grounded (shorted to the case, which serves as a counter electrode) for at least 200 μs before any stimulus,

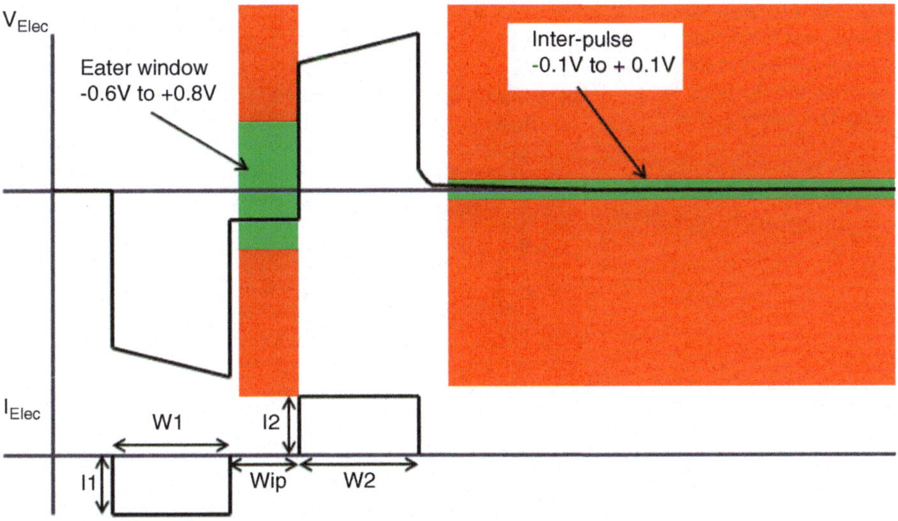

Fig. 7.5 Target ranges for safety monitoring. During the inter-phase interval, a monitor circuit ensures that the electrode-tissue interface voltage remains within the water window, the range of voltages at which water is not oxidized or reduced to release gas bubbles. During the period between biphasic pulses, a monitor circuit ensures that the electrode voltage remains very close to the counter electrode (GND) after it is shorted with a MOSFET switch

and its voltage is monitored to ensure that the electrode is fully depolarized, and monitored again between phases of the biphasic current pulse to ensure that electrode polarization is within safe limits (see Fig. 7.5) [11]. The VDDH and VSS power supplies prevent excessively large voltages from being driven on electrodes. In addition, the integrated ADCs periodically sample the voltage waveforms on each electrode, sending back detailed measurements to the external controller; this method allows open and short circuits of damaged electrodes to be detected, as well as changes in electrode-tissue impedance and responses over time.

Any subset of electrodes can be driven in a given stimulus cycle, and electrodes can be configured as sources of current or as local current sinks (returns) to provide current steering capabilities. Power consumption is minimized in a number of ways, which ultimately limits the RF energy the recipient must be exposed to while the implant is active.

Microfabricated Thin-Film Multi-electrode Array

The intimate interface between the implanted electronics and the retinal tissue is the stimulating electrode. Care must be taken in the design, material choice, and fabrication of these electrodes, to prevent mechanical damage, toxic material release, or unwanted electrochemical reactions. Our electrode arrays are microfabricated to be thin and flexible, and use biocompatible and biostable materials. The stimulation

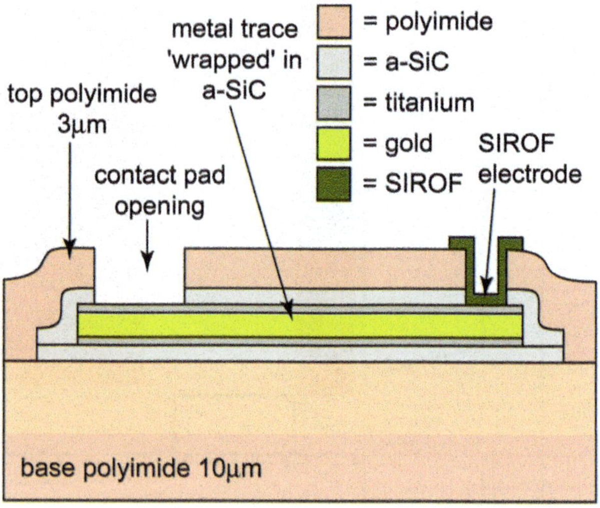

Fig. 7.6 Electrode array fabrication. Schematic cross-section diagram showing the electrode array fabrication process

sites use sputtered iridium oxide film (SIROF) to provide the capability of delivering up to 1 mC/cm^2 of stimulus charge using reversible faradaic reactions.

The electrode arrays, shown in (Fig. 7.6), were manufactured in a microfabrication facility using thin-film methods [5]. Using a silicon wafer as a foundation, layers of polyimide, titanium, and gold are created and patterned to create the wiring and openings for the electrodes. Long-term soak tests revealed that the polyimide interface can delaminate with water absorption, so layers of silicon carbide were placed above and below the metallization layers. This SiC sandwich prevented delamination during pulsing soak tests exceeding 1 year. The electrode sites were then coated with sputtered iridium oxide film (SIROF) [12–14]. The final thickness of the electrode arrays is 15 μm.

Hermetic Retinal Implant Packaging

The first retinal implant that our group implanted in an animal in 2008 was coated with poly(dimethylsiloxane) [5], allowing that device to survive up to 10 months before being explanted. However, longer-term implantation requires a barrier that is impervious to water vapor [15]. This requires the crystalline structure of a metal or ceramic. To protect the implanted circuits in the body, we have developed a small hermetic enclosure made of titanium and alumina ceramic, with more than 256 individual electrical feedthroughs [16]. The ceramic feedthrough comprises several layers of green ceramic, with punched holes filled with biocompatible conductive material. The feedthrough layers are stacked and co-fired, machined to ensure final size, and then brazed to the titanium case. The case is circular, and is roughly 11 mm in diameter, small enough to attach to the outside of the human eye in the socket.

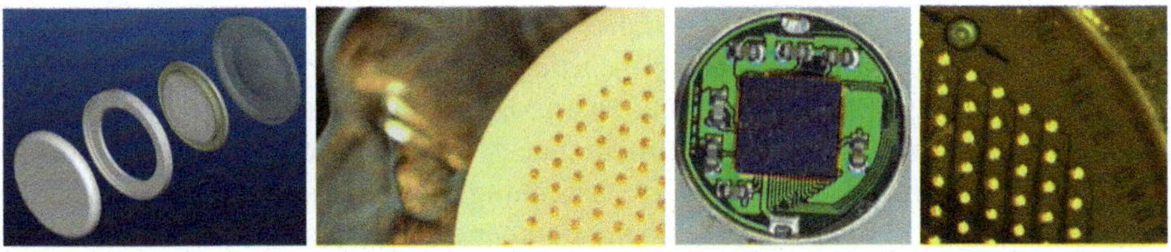

Fig. 7.7 Hermetic case assembly. From *left* to *right*: An exploded view of the case, showing titanium case pieces, feedthrough, and polyurethane header. A view of the feedthrough on a US nickel 5-cent coin. Circuit board and chip soldered into the case. Electrode array bonded to the outside of the feedthrough

A small, circular circuit board holds the chip and the small number of required resistors, capacitors, and diodes. The board is 10.6 mm in diameter and includes six metal layers with traces as small as 30 μm wide. The board contains connections between the chip and other components, as well as vias connecting the chip pads on the top layer to feedthrough pads on the bottom layer. The bare die ASIC is flip-chip assembled onto the top of the circuit board by reflowing solder bumps on the chip pads, and the off-chip components are soldered onto the board. The bottom surface of the board is attached to the inside surface of the feedthrough by reflowing solder bumps on the feedthrough pads. The titanium case is laser welded shut in a helium environment to enable hermeticity testing, and the electrode array is attached to the outside of the case by thermosonic bonding between gold surfaces electroplated onto both the array and the outside of the feedthrough. Finally, a molded polyurethane header is added over the array connections and is underfilled with epoxy. The feedthrough and hermetic package are shown in (Fig. 7.7). We expect this device to function in the body for at least the 5 years recommended by the FDA, with a target of 10 years. The device is meant to be explantable at the end of its life or in case of complications.

The co-fired ceramic feedthroughs of the package were tested for helium leakage, and measured for hermeticity. A helium leak rate of between 10^{-9} and 10^{-8} standard cc/s was measured across the devices. The moisture leak rate is typically about half that of helium, and with the internal volume of our implant, we expect a life of 5–10 years, though more careful helium leak tests need to be performed.

Current Status and Future Directions

The Boston Retinal Implant Project is currently manufacturing its chronic implant with over 256 channels. We are beginning pre-clinical animal studies required by the FDA, and we expect to enter a phase I pilot clinical trial of chronically-implanted devices in the near future.

We are also exploring a number of research directions for future implants. Our group has developed novel innovations in using varying voltages to take advantage of knowledge of the electrode impedance to reduce stimulation power [17]. We are developing circuits that can improve the safety of retinal stimulation by eliminating the residual voltage that is inherent in charge-balanced biphasic current stimulation [18]. We are exploring novel electrode shapes that may deliver stimulus current closer to the target cells, and we are beginning to examine advanced packaging techniques that will allow us to scale the number of channels up toward 1000.

References

1. Rizzo JF, Wyatt JL, Humayun M, deJuan E, Liu W, Chow A, Eckmiller R, Zrenner E, Yagi T, Abrams G. Retinal prosthesis: an encouraging first decade with major challenges ahead. Ophthalmology. 2001;108(1):13–4.
2. Humayun M, Propst R, de Juan E, McCormick K, Hickingbotham D. Bipolar surface electrical stimulation of the vertebrate retina. Arch Ophthalmol. 1994;112:110–6.
3. Rizzo JF, Wyatt JL, Loewenstein J, Kelly SK, Shire DB. Methods and perceptual thresholds for short-term electrical stimulation of human retina with microelectrode arrays. Invest Ophthalmol Vis Sci. 2003;44(12):5355–61.
4. Rizzo JF, Wyatt JL, Loewenstein J, Kelly SK, Shire DB. Perceptual efficacy of electrical stimulation of human retina with a microelectrode array during short-term surgical trials. Invest Ophthalmol Vis Sci. 2003;44(12):5362–9.
5. Shire DB, Kelly SK, Chen J, Doyle P, Gingerich MD, Cogan SF, Drohan WA, Mendoza O, Theogarajan L, Wyatt JL, Rizzo JF. Development and implantation of a minimally invasive wireless subretinal neurostimulator. IEEE Trans Biomed Eng. 2009;56(10):2502–11.
6. Kelly SK, Shire DB, Chen J, Doyle P, Gingerich MD, Cogan SF, Drohan WA, Behan S, Theogarajan L, Wyatt JL, Rizzo JF. A hermetic wireless subretinal neurostimulator for vision prostheses. IEEE Trans Biomed Eng. 2011;58(11):3197–205.
7. Shire DB, Ellersick W, Kelly SK, Doyle P, Priplata A, Drohan W, Mendoza O, Gingerich M, McKee B, Wyatt JL, Rizzo JF. ASIC design and data communications for the Boston retinal prosthesis. Transactions of the IEEE Engineering in Medicine and Biology Conference. 2012. p. 292–5.
8. Kelly SK, Shire DB, Chen J, Gingerich MD, Cogan SF, Drohan WA, Ellersick W, Krishnan A, Behan S, Wyatt JL, Rizzo JF. Developments on the Boston 256-channel retinal implant. Proceedings of the International Conference on Multimedia and Expo. 2013. p. 6.
9. Merrill DR, Bikson M, Jeffreys JG. Electrical stimulation of excitable tissue: design of efficacious and safe protocols. J Neurosci Methods. 2005;141(2):171–98.
10. Cogan SF. Neural stimulating and recording electrodes. Annu Rev Biomed Eng. 2008;10:275–309.
11. Kelly SK, Ellersick W, Krishnan A, Doyle P, Shire DB, Wyatt JL, Rizzo JF. Redundant safety features in a high-channel-count retinal neurostimulator. Transactions of IEEE Biomedical Circuits and Systems Conference. 2014. p. 216–9.
12. Klein JD, Clauson SL, Cogan SF. Reactive IrO2 sputtering in reducing/oxidizing atmospheres. J Mat Res. 1995;10:328–33.
13. Cogan SF, Ehrlich J, Plante TD, Smirnov A, Shire DB, Gingerich MD, Rizzo JF. Sputtered iridium oxide films (SIROFs) for neural stimulation electrodes. J Biomed Mat Res B Appl Biomat. 2009;89(2):353–61.
14. Mokwa W, Wessling B, Schnakenberg U. Sputtered Ir films evaluated for electrochemical perormance I. Experimental results. J Electrochem Soc. 2008;155:F61–5.
15. Jiang G, Zhou D. Technology advances and challenges in hermetic packaging for implantable medical devices. In: Implantable neural prostheses 2: techniques and engineering approaches. New York: Springer; 2010.

16. Shire DB, Salzer T, Jones W, Karbasi A, Behan S, Drohan WA, Mendoza O, Chen J, Wyatt JL, Rizzo JF. Hermetic sealing and packaging technology for the Boston retinal prosthesis. Invest Ophthalmol Vis Sci. 2012;53:5523.
17. Kelly SK, Wyatt JL. Power-efficient neural tissue stimulator with energy recovery. IEEE Trans Biomed Cir Sys. 2011;5(1):20–9.
18. Krishnan, Kelly SK. On the cause and control of residual voltage generated by electrical stimulation of neural tissue. Proceedings of the IEEE Engineering in Medicine and Biology Conference. 2012. p. 3899–902.

Chapter 8
Pixium Vision: First Clinical Results and Innovative Developments

Ralf Hornig, Marcus Dapper, Eric Le Joliff, Robert Hill, Khalid Ishaque, Christoph Posch, Ryad Benosman, Yannick LeMer, José-Alain Sahel, and Serge Picaud

Abstract Visual prostheses or Vision Restoration Systems (VRSs) aim to provide blind patients with useful visual information for face, shape, and object recognition, as well as reading and independent locomotion. VRS are specifically designed for patients having lost their photoreceptors. The loss of photoreceptors can either result from hereditary genetic retinal diseases such as retinitis pigmentosa or more complex diseases such as age-related macular degeneration. Visual restoration is achieved by electrically stimulating the residual retinal circuit. After successful clinical trials by others, Pixium Vision and its partners are developing two VRS solutions for blind patients: an epi-retinal and a sub-retinal approach. This chapter describes the specificities of the epi-retinal IRIS™ VRS that has obtained the European CE cerfication mark, and also discuss the associated innovations developed at the Vision Institute for future VRS models.

Keywords Retinal prostheses • Clinical study • Blindness • Material

R. Hornig
Pixium Vision SA, Paris, France

M. Dapper • E. Le Joliff • R. Hill • K. Ishaque
Pixium Vision, Paris, France

C. Posch • R. Benosman • S. Picaud (✉)
INSERM, Sorbonne Universités, UPMC Univ Paris 06, UMR_S968, CNRS UMR7210, Institut de la Vision, Paris, France
e-mail: serge.picaud@inserm.fr

Y. LeMer
Fondation Ophtalmologique Adolphe de Rothschild, Paris, France

J.-A. Sahel
INSERM, Sorbonne Universités, UPMC Univ Paris 06, UMR_S968, CNRS UMR7210, Institut de la Vision, Paris, France

Fondation Ophtalmologique Adolphe de Rothschild, Paris, France

CHNO des Quinze-Vingts, Paris, France

Academie des Sciences, Paris, France

V.P. Gabel (ed.), *Artificial Vision*, DOI 10.1007/978-3-319-41876-6_8

Key Points

- Epi retinal implant IRIS®II ®II with 150 electrodes.
- The IRIS®II ®II implant is designed to be explantable.
- The bioinspired, neuromorphic image sensor emulates the human retina's visual information capture process.
- A pocket processor preprocess the images and converts the image information into stimulation commands.

Introduction

Visual prostheses or Vision Restoration Systems (VRSs) aim to provide blind patients with useful visual information for face, shape, and object recognition, as well as reading and independent locomotion. VRS are specifically designed for patients having lost their photoreceptors. The loss of photoreceptors can either result from hereditary genetic retinal diseases such as retinitis pigmentosa or more complex diseases such as age-related macular degeneration. Visual restoration is achieved by electrically stimulating the residual retinal circuit. After the photoreceptor loss, the retinal circuit still contains the vertical retinal pathway from bipolar cells to retinal ganglion cells, which normally transfer visual information to the brain via the optic nerve. In fact, these retinal neurones were also shown to undergo a degenerative process following the photoreceptor loss [14]. The first acute tests had shown that electrical stimulations of the retina from blind patients can lead to the perception of phosphenes or light flashes [11]. These clinical results demonstrated that, although engaged in a degenerating process, residual retinal neurones can still convey visual information to the brain. More recently, several clinical studies have investigated different VRSs for the chronic stimulation of retinal neurones [12, 13, 23, 31]. These devices have either stimulating electrodes on the vitreous side close to the retinal ganglion cells [12, 13, 23, 31] or in the subretinal space to stimulate retinal bipolar cells [31].

Pixium Vision, together with its renowned academic and industrial partners are developing two VRS solutions for blind patients: an epi-retinal and a sub-retinal approach. We will first describe the specificities of the epi-retinal IRIS™ VRS that is in human clinical study at the time of this publication, and also discuss the associated innovations developed at the Vision Institute for future VRS models. These innovations include retinal information processing, new electrode materials and implant designs. The second VRS, a miniaturized passive sub-retinal implant, called PRIMA, that is being developed also in collaboration with Pr Palanker (Stanford University, USA), and that is in pre-clinical stage is described in a separate chapter.

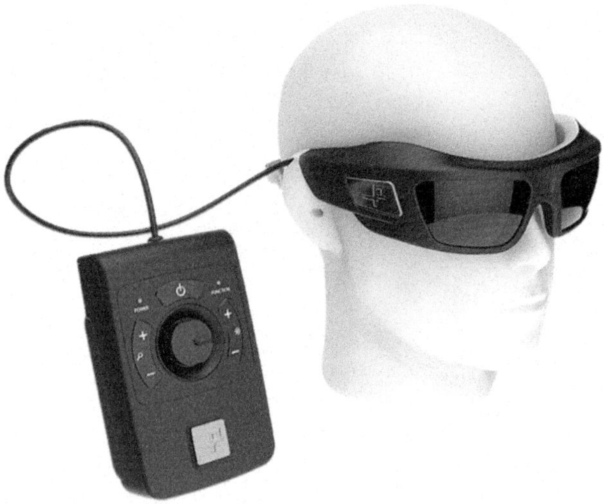

Fig. 8.1 External components of the IRIS™ VRS including the Visual Interface (goggles) and the Pocket Processor

IRIS™ System Description

Pixium Vision has developed a new VRS named the Intelligent Retinal Implant System (IRIS™) (Pixium Vision SA, Paris, France). This chapter describes its latest version that is now assessed in clinical trial (https://www.clinicaltrials.gov. Ref: NCT02670980) and has received the European CE cerfication mark. As other VRSs', our device aims at restoring a useful vision in blind patients with degenerative retinal diseases such as retinitis pigmentosa, choroideremia, cone-rod dystrophy, or Usher Syndrome.

The IRIS™ consists of three main components. These are:

- An Implant
- A Visual Interface
- A Pocket Processor

The Implant is an electronic device fixed onto the eye of a blind patient with an electrode array entering into the eye to stimulate the retinal neurons. The Visual Interface and the Pocket Processor (see Fig. 8.1) are external components designed to connect wirelessly with the implant. The Visual Interface is essentially a pair of special glasses. It incorporates a neuromorphic (ATIS) image sensor to capture visual information from the environment. This visual information is transferred via a cable to the Pocket Processor which transforms the visual data into stimulation commands. The stimulation commands are sent optically from the visual interface to the implant. The implant finally converts the stimulation commands into actual electrical stimulations to activate residual functional retinal ganglion cells. Activation of retinal ganglion cells then generates electrical signals communicated to the brain via the optic nerve, resulting in the patient's visual perception.

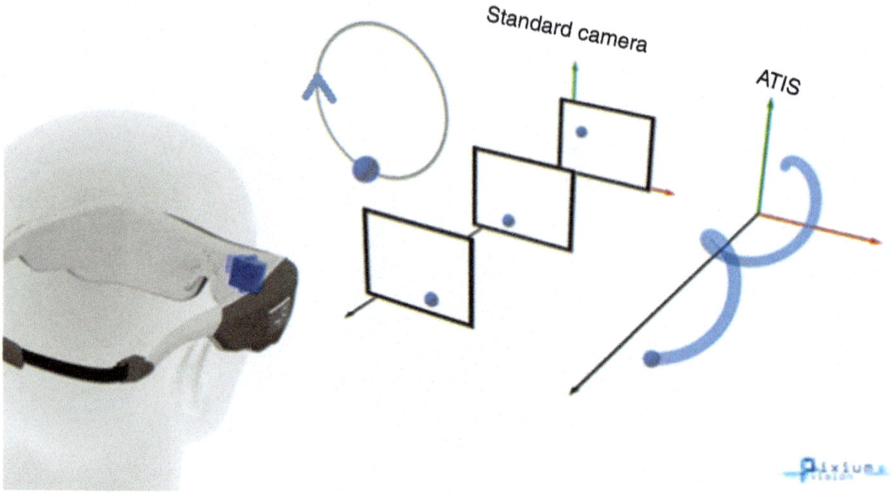

Fig. 8.2 Comparison between visual information provided by a standard camera and an ATIS image sensor. A standard camera is taking pictures at regular time intervals showing different positions of a rotating ball in front of a scene. However, the actual movement during these pictures is not known. The ATIS image sensor is measuring intensity changes in the visual scene limiting information acquisistion to the rotating ball, which is followed with a very precise timing providing thereby all its movement

External Components

The Visual Interface of the Intelligent Retinal Implant System (IRIS™) is essentially a pair of special sunglasses, with several integrated electronic elements [10]. Placed behind one of the lenses, is the proprietary neuromorphic image sensor (ATIS) that acquires the visual information. In contrast to conventional imagers classically used in the field of vision restoration, this sensor does not take series of snapshots or gray-scale image frames of the scene at arbitrary time points [26, 27]. Instead, this sensor emulates the human retina's visual information capture process. The ATIS sensor used in Pixium's VRS systems contains an array of autonomous pixels. They are autonomous because they are not driven by a shutter signal but respond in a continuous mode to the visual input they receive from the visual scene. This is the main difference with a classic camera, which takes images at regular interval with a shutter signal delimiting the acquisition period. As a consequence, a standard camera is delivering images of a complete scene as represented in Fig. 8.2 from a circling point. In the ATIS sensor, the information is not sampled on the time axis but on the intensity axis. Light intensities are divided in regular intervals, such that changes in intensity from one level to a superior or inferior threshold are encoded by a positive or negative event or spike. The information will therefore provide the coordinate of the pixel, the sign of the spike and its precise timing of occurrence. As a consequence, the ATIS sensor can provide the precise movement of the circling point (Fig. 8.2), which is the only element in the scene

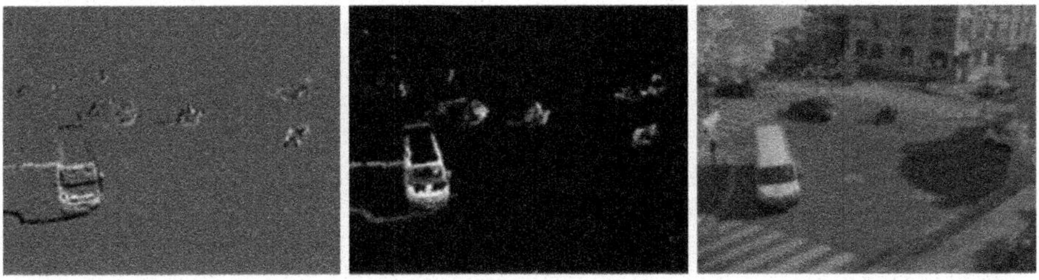

Fig. 8.3 Visual information provided by an ATIS image sensor. The ATIS image sensor provides not only the coordinates of changing pixel (*left*) but also actual light intensities at these changing pixels (*middle*). Those information enable to reconstruct the actual visual scene (*right*)

producing changes in light intensities at its borders. This precision can reach the microsecond whereas standard cameras are blind between frames (generally taken every 30 ms) and the point can move during the acquisition time resulting in a blurry picture. Pixel circuits encode transient (light change) information from the scene into the precise timing of spikes, while a second parallel mode can encode sustained (light intensity) information in a simple spike rate coding scheme. These modes provide functional models of the two major human retinal pathways, the Magno-cellular (or transient) pathway and the Parvo-cellular (or sustained) pathway. The output from the ATIS sensor was taken to advantage to model the activity of all retinal ganglion cells with their millisecond precision [18]. The output of Pixium's ATIS sensor is a continuous-time stream of spikes encoding transient and sustained visual information in a language the brain is expected to more directly interpret. As a result of this 'biologically-inspired' way of acquiring visual information, and in contrast to all conventional camera used today in other vision restoration systems, ATIS is able to provide signals at the native temporal resolution of retinal ganglion cells (~1 ms) and at a dynamic range exceeding the one of the human eye (>120 dB). Additionally, the impressive redundancy suppression performed by the human retina is reproduced by this optical sensor, ensuring that only relevant and useful signals are sent to the brain. Suppressing the redundancy in visual information is important for decreasing calculation for generating stimulations thus reducing energy consumption and increasing device autonomy.

Figure 8.2 illustrates the continuous-time acquisition of visual motion in a scene as performed by the ATIS sensor in contrast to a frame-based acquisition conducted by a conventional camera. Subsequently in Fig. 8.3, the spike-encoded output from the two pathways is shown for a natural scene. The left-most screen displays the bipolar output of changes detected in the visual scene and acquired by the transient pathway pixel circuits. The middle screen shows the sustained pathway's output encoding absolute luminance from the relevant parts of the scene in pixel-individual spike rates. The right-most screen shows the full scene content as acquired by ATIS. All visual information is encoded purely in the timing of spike pulses which constitute the basis of the stimulation signals sent to the retinal implant in Pixium's vision restoration systems.

After the visual information is transformed into digital signals, it is transferred via a cable to the pocket processor. The Pocket Processor (PP) is the brain of the IRIS™.

It can be carried on a waist belt or in a small shoulder pouch. The PP translates the image information into stimulation commands. For this processing step, in addition to the processing of the ATIS image sensor, advanced image processing algorithms are possible to use if necessary. These algorithms are designed to improve the image quality and to emphasize important elements in the images (e.g. by contrast enhancement or edge detection). Furthermore, the information from the original image is reduced to the most important elements. This is considered to be a critical processing step (and argued to be closer to more biological mode of action), given that too much or redundant information included in the stimulation signal may simply hinder the patient's ability to interpret usefully (and to mimic mode of action closer to the biological process by the receiving part of the brain). In addition to visual information processing algorithms, the visual information must be transformed into actual stimulation commands. For this step, the physiological needs of the retina and constraints of the stimulating hardware (the Implant) need to also be taken into account.

The stimulation commands – generated in the Pocket Processor – are then sent via the cable to the Visual Interface where they are transferred optically to the implant. An infrared (IR) array integrated in the Visual Interface, located directly in front of the implanted eye transmits an optical data stream through the pupil of the patient to the implant, where it is received by an optical sensor. The optical link provides the advantage of high data rates which are essential in transmitting visual information. Additionally, the optical data transmission also allows the implant to be miniaturized, since no demodulation circuit is needed to receive the data. Closing of the eye lid, similar to a normal sighted individual, would interrupt the data transmission and lead to interruption of visual perception.

In addition to visual information processing, the Pocket Processor also provides the whole system with power via a rechargeable battery. The implant is powered via high frequency electromagnetic fields (wireless RF) transmitted from the Visual Interface. This is enabled from the transmitter coil system integrated into the Visual Interface which generates an alternating magnetic field. The implant itself contains a receiver coil which is placed and secured to be within the magnetic field generated by the external Visual Interface coil. As a consequence, the implant can receive sufficient energy to transform the stimulation commands into actual currents to stimulate the retinal cells. Both this energy and the data transmission allow a certain degree of eye movement. This point becomes important for those patients who suffer also form uncontrolled eye motion (nystagmus).

The Pocket Processor comprises several control keys to:

1. switch the device on/off,
2. zoom in or out, and
3. change the brightness.

The patient also has the option to switch between different preprogrammed modes. These modes can be selected for different environmental conditions, e.g. indoor, outdoor or situation with high or low contrast. During the tuning sessions in the reeducation phase, the Pocket Processor can be connected to a laptop PC including the custom Fitting Software. With this Fitting Software, all parameters of the IRIS can be tuned and customized to the individual patient needs and preferences.

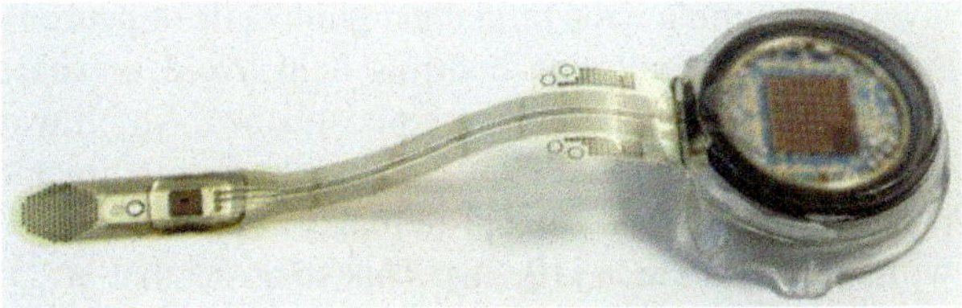

Fig. 8.4 IRIS™ Implant showing the Application Specific Integrated Circuit (ASIC) part in its circular case and the polymer foil with the electrode array at its extremity

Implant

The implant part of the IRIS™ Vision Restoration System is shown in Fig. 8.4. It is implanted into one eye of a blind patient to stimulate the remaining neurons of the retina from the epi-retinal side. It consists of an extra- and an intra-ocular part, and has no wired connection to the external components (Visual Interface and Pocket Processor). The extra ocular part is sutured onto the sclera between the musculus rectus lateralis and the musculus rectus superior. The extra ocular part is rigid and its shape is anatomically designed to adapt to the curvature of the eye. Four suture taps are used to fixate the rigid extra ocular part onto the sclera. The intra ocular part consists of a highly flexible polymer film which is introduced into the eye globe. This film passes through the sclera in the area of the pars plana into the vitreous body. The end of the polymer film is attached on the retina with a retinal tack. The tack is placed first during the intervention and the polymer film is subsequently secured on it in a way to also allow it to be removed if needed (see below). The retinal tack is placed at a position that allows the stimulating electrode array, at the extremity of the polymer foil, to cover the macula.

A tiny micro-photodiode mounted on the film of the intraocular part receives data from the external components via the optical link permitting high data transmission rates. These data contain the stimulation commands for the implant. The data stream is forwarded to the extra ocular part of the Implant, which contains the electronics to generate the stimulation currents. RF Energy is received via a coil system using an electromagnetic link to the external components. Unlike classical neurostimulation systems with configurations of implanted electrodes connected to Implanted Pulse Generators (IPG's), the IRIS™ implant itself does not contain any battery. As soon as the external components are switched off, or the Visual Interface is out of the minimum operating range of the implant, the implant is deactivated. The heart of the extra ocular part is an Application Specific Integrated Circuit (ASIC). This ASIC decodes the signals received via the optical link, process this data and generate appropriate stimulation currents. The electronics of the extra ocular part are protected from liquid ingress by a hermetic housing. The current is conducted to the electrodes via hermetic feedthroughs in the housing and tracks within the flexible polymer film. The stimulating electrodes are arranged in an array located at the distal end of the intra ocular part.

The stimulating electrodes of this epiretinal device are placed and secured close to the retinal surface in order to activate the remaining retinal neurons locally by applying electrical currents. In epi-retinal devices, the current must pass the axon layer and stimulate the retinal ganglion cells or neurons in the inner plexiform layer. Appropriate stimulation controls help avoid unwanted stimulations of the axon layer that could generate large phosphenes, which would deform the retinotopy of the visual information. However, results from clinical trials indicate that the phosphenes evoked by these epi-retinal stimulations appear to be small and localized within a certain area [10, 28]. This suggests that no axons, or only axons with cell bodies close to an electrode, are stimulated. A return electrode, distant from the stimulating electrode array, is used to lead the current applied via stimulation electrode back to the current source in the ASIC.

The intraocular part of the implant is secured on the retina using a retinal tack and a retainer ring. Retinal tacks have been proven to be efficient to fixate retinal implants [20, 30]. For fixation of the IRIS™ implant, the tack is anchored first in the sclera, the intraocular part of the implant i.e. the flexible film is positioned onto the tack and then secured and held on the tack by the retainer ring [15]. This proprietary technique carries the advantage that, in case needed, removal of the implant does not require removal of the tack. Removal of the retinal tack can lead to risk of retinal detachment and neovascularization. In case of need to explant/remove the IRIS™ implant, first the retainer ring is simply lifted off from the retinal tack, followed by the IRIS implant, and leaving the retinal tack in place, thus avoiding the risk of retinal detachment and neovascularization. Removal of an implant could become necessary if, for example, the implanted device would be defective, or would malfunction, or more importantly, if better devices would be available with potential to upgrade. The proprietary IRIS™ is designed in a such a way that, it can be removed from the retinal tack, and then if needed, a new implant can be fixed on to the same retinal tack, thus avoiding risks of retinal detachment and neovascularization associated with removal of retinal tacks.

The IRIS™ implant that has been tested in a multi-centric European clinical trial [www.clinicaltrials.gov NCT01864486] contained 49 electrodes. However the current generation of IRIS™, which in clinical trial (Ref: NCT02670980), consists of 150 electrode array.

Surgical Method

The IRIS device is implanted into one eye of a patient. Usually the eye with the worse visual function is prioritised for the implantation. However, in case the eye with the worse visual function is not considered suitable for the implant because e.g. the ganglion cell layer is damaged, the other eye would be used.

At least 3 weeks prior to implantation of the device, the patients receive a laser treatment targeting the projected tack position and planned sclerotomies. In case that cataract is present, and since it could influence the visual function, it is recommended to treat the cataract before the implantation, in order to ensure the patient fulfils the visual acuity criteria (per clinical protocol described later) without cataract.

The surgical procedure for the implantation of IRIS™ combines standard ophthalmic surgical methods along with methods specifically developed for the proprietary IRIS™ implant [29]. The implantation is carried out under general anesthesia.

The procedure starts with a 360° conjunctival peritomy. The four rectus eye muscles are fixed with sutures to easily align the eye into different position and stabilize it if necessary. Next, a scleral pocket is prepared, that is superior temporal in the area of the projected implant position, by preparing a rectangular lamella with the base on the limbus side. Thereafter the implant is placed in the orbita between the musculus rectus lateralis and musculus rectus superior, and sutured to the sclera.

A 3-port vitrectomy is performed next, with special care to completely remove the vitreous. It is recommended to use a dye to make sure all the vitreous is removed. After the vitrectomy, the retinal tack is implanted at a predefined position. Fundus photographs are used to precisely determine the tack positioning and to further ensure that the stimulating electrode array of the implant will be located in the area of the macula. For the retinal tack setting, special tack forceps are used. It is important to note that the tack is set through the port opposite to where the tack is to be positioned. This ensures that the distal electrode array will not be tilted when it is set onto the tack. During the tack setting the infusion pressure is increased to stabilize the eye. Following completion of the tack setting the infusion pressure is reduced back to the normal level.

After the tack is set accurately, the flexible film part of the IRIS™ implant can then be introduced into the eye globe. A sclerotomy is therefore performed by cutting a slit in the inner area of the scleral pocket, at 3.5 mm from the limbus. To ensure the right positioning of the electrode array the scleral incision for the implant needs to be exactly at 45° between the eye muscles *musculus rectus lateralis* and *musculus rectus superior*. The flexible intraocular part of the implant is then introduced through this slit into the eye globe, using only the silicone coated forceps to avoid damaging the flexible film. Immediately following the insertion of the wider tip of the flexible implant film, the incision is reduced by placing nylon sutures on the right and left of the film. Special care must be taken to close the incision properly and avoid leakage from the eye ball.

The next step in the procedure requires the intraocular part of the implant to be placed onto the set retinal tack. Again, to avoid damaging the flexible film and integrated wiring and electrodes, only silicone coated surgical tools should be used to handle the implant. The flexible film is grasped with the vertical vitrectomy forceps and the tack hole on the film is placed over the tack and lowering onto the tack, carefully avoiding touching the retina. The step of placing the flexible film onto the tack needs to be carried out bimanually and therefore a chandelier illumination is used. After that the film is lowered onto the tack, a silicone retainer ring is added next onto the tack using specially designed retainer fixation tool. This tool is preloaded with the silicone retainer ring and is designed to release and set the retainer ring by positioning the tool above the retinal tack. Figure 8.5 shows the extra- and intra-ocular part of the implant in implanted condition.

After the intra ocular part of the device is secured onto the tack the proximal part of the flexible film is also sutured on the sclera in the area of the scleral pocket using the four suture taps on the film. Next, the sclera flap is closed by placing at least four sutures on the edges of the flap. After suturing the sclera flap it is recommended to verify tightness. Finally all the ports are closed and the conjunctiva is sutured. Figure 8.6 shows the implanted electrode array in a human eye.

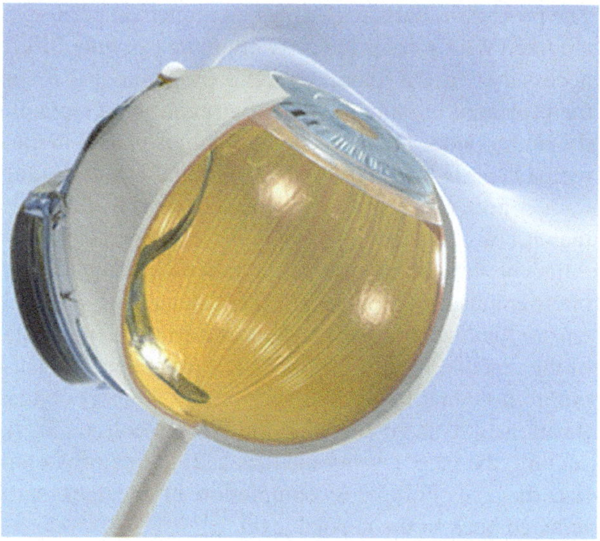

Fig. 8.5 Extra- and intraocular part of the IRIS implant

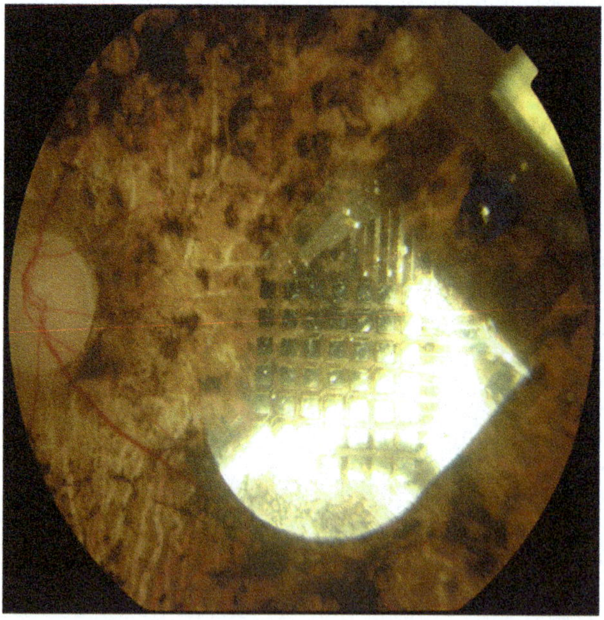

Fig. 8.6 Fundus photograph showing the electrode array of the IRIS™ implant in a human patient

The Clinical Trial

Acute Clinical Trail

To evaluate the perception patients have during stimulations, an acute trial have been performed [5, 9, 10, 17]. In this trail a handheld electrode array was place for a duration of maximum 45 min on the retina of blind patients suffering from retinal degeneration. The surgery has been performed under local anesthesia. The array was places after the vitreous of the patient was removed using vitrectomy. A special designed tool was used to place and hold the array. To reduce the risk of retinal damage, the patients were not allowed to move their head or speak. They answered to questions using push buttons in their hand. Twenty patients were enrolled in this trial.

Nineteen of the 20 patients had perception as a result of electrical stimulation. The minimum stimulation threshold to elicit visual perception was 20 nC. When activating one single electrode, the patients described the perceived objects to be similar to little stars, points, circles, triangles, rectangles, a half moon, a solar eclipse, or a hash (pound) symbol. Typically the phosphenes had sharp and clear contours. Some objects looked cloudy like a photo out of focus and only a small percentage of objects had smooth transition without edges. The typical sizes of the phosphenes were equivalent to a coin or a head of a match at one meter distance. The brightness of the perception was reported to be between a 'dark spot' and as 'bright as the sun'. Most patients described the brightness as similar to a candle or light bulb. Often the patients reported white, blue or yellow perception. Only in few cases, the color was reported to be red, green or black. In general an individual subject reported one single color. Only one patient reported perceiving a mosaic of different colors.

Chronic Clinical Trial

The IRIS™ system is currently available for the use in a multi-centric European clinical trial with sites in France, Germany and Austria (www.clinicaltrials.gov NCT01864486). Up to 20 patients are planned to be enrolled in this trial. To participate in this clinical trial and get implanted with the IRIS™ system, the patients must fulfil the following inclusion criteria.

- Is 25 years or older at the date of enrolment,
- Has a confirmed diagnosis of retinitis pigmentosa, choroideremia or cone-rod dystrophy,
- Has a visual acuity of logMAR 2.3 or worse in both the eyes as determined by a square grating scale,
- Has functional ganglion cells and optic nerve activity,
- Has a memory of former useful form vision,
- Understands and accepts the obligation to present for all scheduled follow-up visits,
- Has AP eye dimensions that are appropriate with the dimensions of the implant,
- Has head dimensions that are appropriate for the visual Interface.

The most important criteria for patient exclusion are:

- Has any eye disease that would lead to:
- Insufficient ganglion cell function,
- Adequate examination

- Has severe nystagmus
- Condition that leads to eye rubbing,
- Reduced understanding or communication,
- A history of epileptic seizure,
- General health conditions that make implantation unadvisable
- Hypotony or hypertony in the study eye,
- Has another active implanted device or any form of metallic implant in the head
- Sensitivity to the contact materials of the implant
- Is pregnant or lactating,
- Has another active implanted device or any form of metallic implant in the head that may interfere with the device function,
- Has a diagnosis requiring an active implant
- Has active cancer or a history of intraocular, optic nerve or brain cancer and metastasis,
- Is an immune-suppressed subject
- Is carrier of multi-resistant germs,
- Is participating in another investigational study

The IRIS™ clinical trial is conducted in different sites across France, Germany and Austria. In this clinical trial, the safety and performance of Pixium's IRIS™ system is being evaluated. The First patients implanted have completed their 18 months' follow-up. Study is in progress and results are not yet published. Patient reported that they are able to localize objects like a ball on a table. One patient was, for example, able to see if stairways go up or down, identify a car, a Ferris wheel, and even the Eiffel tower in Paris at night. He was also able to estimate the height of a Christmas tree. Another patient was able to localize for example, the lock on a door in a corridor. A patient reported that while the cane helps with what's on the ground, with the system she is also able to "see" obstacles (see patient testimonials: http://www.pixium-vision.com/en/clinical-trial/testimonials).

Future Technologies

Current clinical trials have demonstrated the feasibility to restore some visual perception by stimulating the residual inner retina, despite ongoing retinal degeneration. These outstanding results call for the development of new technologies to improve further the resolution of stimulating electrodes in order to increase their number and density. Indeed, psychophysical experiments have concluded for the need of at least 600 pixels to allow independent locomotion, face recognition and text reading. Different electrode distributions were shown to increase the current focalization. These distributions includes bipolar stimulation [24], a quasimonopolar stimulation using a distant return electrode in a plane above hexapolar return electrodes surrounding each stimulating electrode [22], and a ground grid surrounding all stimulating electrodes [16]. The latter ground grid configuration was found interesting for both planar [16] and 3D implant designs [3, 4]. In fact, as demonstrated by Dijilas et al. 3D designs could encode more gray levels than planar arrays, even with a distant ground [3].

Interestingly, the recent photovoltaic retinal prosthesis, named PRIMA and under development at Pixium Vision with Pr Palanker (Stanford University), has already introduced such a ground grid [21] resulting in a high visual acuity in blind rats [19]. However, the advantage of ground grids relies on very conductive materials [16]. Therefore, the development of new materials, more stable and very conductive, appears as a promising challenge for the production of very dense electrode arrays with a high resolution. In this line of research, researchers have investigated the advantage of carbon-based materials such as graphene and diamond because they have a wider electrochemical window than metals. Both materials were found to be highly biocompatible for retinal neurons, which could grow directly on them [1, 2]. We also demonstrated the in vivo biocompatibility of diamond after having developed a process for the fabrication of flexible implants with a diamond coating [3]. The efficacy of these materials at stimulating electrode depending highly on their developed surfaces, introducing a nanostructure in the diamond coating using carbon nanotubes has further enhanced the material performances [7, 8]. We further showed that these performances were very important for neuronal interfaces [25]. These new nanostructured diamonds should therefore enhance the efficacy of retinal neuron stimulation achieved with classic diamond electrodes, which had been reported by others [6].

Conclusions

The IRIS™ system has demonstrated its efficacy in restoring some visual performances in blind patients. Further development of this system continues with an increase in the number and density of stimulating electrodes. To further improve visual restoration in blind patients, other innovative technologies are being evaluated together with the Vision Institute and the Stanford University. These innovations should enable continued progress toward the goal of restoring a useful vision in blind patients for autonomous locomotion, face recognition, and text reading.

Acknowledgements The Vision Institute was supported by INSERM, UPMC (Paris VI), Foundation Fighting Blindness, the *Fédération des Aveugles de France*, *Fondation de la Recherche Médicale* (grant number DBC20101021013), the European Community's Seventh Framework Programme (FP7/2007–2013) under grant agreement no. 280433 (Neurocare project) and under the Graphene Flagship (Contract N° 604391), the LabEx LIFESENSES (ANR-10-LABX-65), which was supported by French state funds managed by the ANR within the *Investissements d'Avenir* programme (ANR-11-IDEX-0004-02).

References

1. Bendali A, Agnes C, Meffert S, Forster V, Bongrain A, Arnault JC, Sahel JA, Offenhausser A, Bergonzo P, Picaud S. Distinctive glial and neuronal interfacing on nanocrystalline diamond. PLoS One. 2014;9:e92562.
2. Bendali A, Hess LH, Seifert M, Forster V, Stephan AF, Garrido JA, Picaud S. Purified neurons can survive on peptide-free graphene layers. Adv Healthc Mater. 2013;2:929–33.

3. Bendali A, Rousseau L, Lissorgues G, Scorsone E, Djilas M, Degardin J, Dubus E, Fouquet S, Benosman R, Bergonzo P, Sahel JA, Picaud S. Synthetic 3D diamond-based electrodes for flexible retinal neuroprostheses: model, production and in vivo biocompatibility. Biomaterials. 2015;67:73–83.
4. Djilas M, Oles C, Lorach H, Bendali A, Degardin J, Dubus E, Lissorgues-Bazin G, Rousseau L, Benosman R, Ieng SH, Joucla S, Yvert B, Bergonzo P, Sahel J, Picaud S. Three-dimensional electrode arrays for retinal prostheses: modeling, geometry optimization and experimental validation. J Neural Eng. 2011;8:046020.
5. Feucht M, Laube T, Bornfeld N, Walter P, Velikay-Parel M, Hornig R, Richard G. Development of an epiretinal prosthesis for stimulation of the human retina. Der Ophthalmologe Zeitschrift der Deutschen Ophthalmologischen Gesellschaft. 2005;102:688–91.
6. Hadjinicolaou AE, Leung RT, Garrett DJ, Ganesan K, Fox K, Nayagam DA, Shivdasani MN, Meffin H, Ibbotson MR, Prawer S, O'Brien BJ. Electrical stimulation of retinal ganglion cells with diamond and the development of an all diamond retinal prosthesis. Biomaterials. 2012;33:5812–20.
7. Hébert C, Mazellier JP, Scorsone E, Mermoux M, Bergonzo P. Boosting the electrochemical properties of diamond electrodes using carbon nanotube scaffolds. Carbon. 2014;71:27–33.
8. Hébert C, Scorsone E, Mermoux M, Bergonzo P. Porous diamond with high electrochemical performance. Carbon. 2015;90:102–9.
9. Hornig R, Laube T, Walter P, Velikay-Parel M, Bornfeld N, Feucht M, Akguel H, Rossler G, Alteheld N, Lutke Notarp D, Wyatt J, Richard G. A method and technical equipment for an acute human trial to evaluate retinal implant technology. J Neural Eng. 2005;2:S129–34.
10. Hornig R, Zehnder T, Velikay-Parel M, Feucht M, Richard G. The IMI retina implant system. In: Humayun M, Weiland JD, Chader G, Greenbaum E, editors. Artifical sight: basic research, biomedical engineering, and clinical advances. New York: Springer; 2007.
11. Humayun MS, De Juan Jr E, Weiland JD, Dagnelie G, Katona S, Greenberg R, Suzuki S. Pattern electrical stimulation of the human retina. Vision Res. 1999;39:2569–76.
12. Humayun MS, Dorn JD, Ahuja AK, Caspi A, Filley E, Dagnelie G, Salzmann J, Santos A, Duncan J, Dacruz L, Mohand-Said S, Eliott D, McMahon MJ, Greenberg RJ. Preliminary 6 month results from the argus II epiretinal prosthesis feasibility study. Conf Proc IEEE Eng Med Biol Soc. 2009;1:4566–8.
13. Humayun MS, Dorn JD, da Cruz L, Dagnelie G, Sahel JA, Stanga PE, Cideciyan AV, Duncan JL, Eliott D, Filley E, Ho AC, Santos A, Safran AB, Arditi A, Del Priore LV, Greenberg RJ. Interim results from the international trial of second sight's visual prosthesis. Ophthalmology. 2012;119:779–88.
14. Humayun MS, Prince M, De Juan Jr E, Barron Y, Moskowitz M, Klock IB, Milam AH. Morphometric analysis of the extramacular retina from postmortem eyes with retinitis pigmentosa. Invest Ophthalmol Vis Sci. 1999;40:143–8.
15. Ivastinovic D, Langmann G, Nemetz W, Hornig R, Richard G, Velikay-Parel M. Clinical stability of a new method for fixation and explanation of epiretinal implants. Acta Ophthalmol. 2010;88:e285–6.
16. Joucla S, Yvert B. Improved focalization of electrical microstimulation using microelectrode arrays: a modeling study. PLoS One. 2009;4:e4828.
17. Keseru M, Feucht M, Bornfeld N, Laube T, Walter P, Rossler G, Velikay-Parel M, Hornig R, Richard G. Acute electrical stimulation of the human retina with an epiretinal electrode array. Acta Ophthalmol. 2012;90:e1–8.
18. Lorach H, Benosman R, Marre O, Ieng SH, Sahel JA, Picaud S. Artificial retina: the multichannel processing of the mammalian retina achieved with a neuromorphic asynchronous light acquisition device. J Neural Eng. 2012;9:066004.
19. Lorach H, Goetz G, Smith R, Lei X, Mandel Y, Kamins T, Mathieson K, Huie P, Harris J, Sher A, Palanker D. Photovoltaic restoration of sight with high visual acuity. Nat Med. 2015;21:476–82.
20. Majji AB, Humayun MS, Weiland JD, Suzuki S, D'Anna SA, De Juan Jr E. Long-term histological and electrophysiological results of an inactive epiretinal electrode array implantation in dogs. Invest Ophthalmol Vis Sci. 1999;40:2073–81.

21. Mathieson K, Loudin J, Goetz G, Huie P, Wang L, Kamins T, Galambos L, Smith R, Harris JS, Sher A, Palanker D. Photovoltaic retinal prosthesis with high pixel density. Nat Photonics. 2012;6:391–7.
22. Matteucci PB, Chen SC, Tsai D, Dodds CW, Dokos S, Morley JW, Lovell NH, Suaning GJ. Current steering in retinal stimulation via a quasimonopolar stimulation paradigm. Invest Ophthalmol Vis Sci. 2013;54:4307–20.
23. Menzel-Severing J, Laube T, Brockmann C, Bornfeld N, Mokwa W, Mazinani B, Walter P, Roessler G. Implantation and explantation of an active epiretinal visual prosthesis: 2-year follow-up data from the EPIRET3 prospective clinical trial. Eye (Lond). 2012;26:501–9.
24. Palanker D, Huie P, Vankov A, Aramant R, Seiler M, Fishman H, Marmor M, Blumenkranz M. Migration of retinal cells through a perforated membrane: implications for a high-resolution prosthesis. Invest Ophthalmol Vis Sci. 2004;45:3266–70.
25. Piret G, Hebert C, Mazellier JP, Rousseau L, Scorsone E, Cottance M, Lissorgues G, Heuschkel MO, Picaud S, Bergonzo P, Yvert B. 3D-nanostructured boron-doped diamond for microelectrode array neural interfacing. Biomaterials. 2015;53:173–83.
26. Posch C, Matolin D, Wohlgenannt R. A QVGA 143 dB dynamic range frame-free PWM image sensor with lossless pixel-level video compression and time-domain CDS. Solid-State Circuits IEEE J. 2011;46:259–75.
27. Posch C, Serrano-Gotarredona T, Linares-Barranco B, Delbruck T. Retinomorphic event-based vision sensors: bioinspired cameras with spiking output. Proc IEEE. 2014;102: 1470–84.
28. Richard G, Feucht M, Bornfeld N, Laube T, Rössler G, Velikay-Parel M, Hornig R. Multicenter study on acute electrical stimulation of the human retina with an epiretinal implant: clinical results in 20 patients. Invest Ophthalmol Vis Sci. 2005;46:1143.
29. Richard G, Keserue M, Zeitz O, Hornig R. Surgical aspects of a long-term implantation of a wireless chip in blind patients. I. In: Proceedings 9th EURETINA Congress Nice from 14 to 17 May 2009. p. 6:8–6:10.
30. Walter P, Szurman P, Vobig M, Berk H, Ludtke-Handjery HC, Richter H, Mittermayer C, Heimann K, Sellhaus B. Successful long-term implantation of electrically inactive epiretinal microelectrode arrays in rabbits. Retina (Philadelphia Pa). 1999;19:546–52.
31. Zrenner E, Bartz-Schmidt KU, Benav H, Besch D, Bruckmann A, Gabel VP, Gekeler F, Greppmaier U, Harscher A, Kibbel S, Koch J, Kusnyerik A, Peters T, Stingl K, Sachs H, Stett A, Szurman P, Wilhelm B, Wilke R. Subretinal electronic chips allow blind patients to read letters and combine them to words. Proc R Soc. 2011;B 278:1489–97.

Chapter 9
High Resolution Photovoltaic Subretinal Prosthesis for Restoration of Sight

Henri Lorach and Daniel Palanker

Abstract In photovoltaic subretinal prostheses, each pixel converts light into electric current to stimulate the nearby inner retinal neurons. Visual information is projected onto the implant by video goggles using pulsed near-infrared (~880 nm) light. This design avoids the use of bulky electronics and trans-scleral wiring, thereby greatly reducing the surgical complexity. Optical activation of the photovoltaic pixels allows scaling the implants to thousands of electrodes, and multiple modules can be tiled under the retina to expand the visual field.

Similarly to normal vision, retinal response to prosthetic stimulation exhibits flicker fusion at high frequencies (>20 Hz), adaptation to static images, and non-linear summation of subunits in the receptive fields. Photovoltaic arrays with 70 μm pixels restored visual acuity up to a pixel pitch in rats blinded by retinal degeneration, which is only twice lower than natural acuity in these animals. If these results translate to human retina, such implants could restore visual acuity up to 20/250. With eye scanning and perceptual learning, human patients might even cross the 20/200 threshold of legal blindness. Ease of implantation and tiling of these wireless modules to cover a large visual field, combined with high resolution opens the door to highly functional restoration of sight.

Keywords Photovoltaic prosthesis • Retina • Electrical stimulation • Retinal surgery • Blindness • Visual acuity • Safety • Restoration of sight

Key Points

- Prosthetic visual acuity with subretinal photovoltaic arrays matches the pixel pitch of 65 μm, suggesting that smaller pixels may further increase spatial resolution.
- Implants with 65 μm pixel pitch restore half of the normal acuity in blind rats. Such spatial resolution would correspond to 20/250 acuity in a human eye.

H. Lorach (✉)
Hansen Experimental Physics Laboratory, Stanford University, Stanford, CA, USA
e-mail: hlorach@stanford.edu

D. Palanker
Department of Ophthalmology and Hansen Experimental Physics Laboratory, Stanford University, Stanford, CA, USA

V.P. Gabel (ed.), *Artificial Vision*, DOI 10.1007/978-3-319-41876-6_9

- Wireless nature of photovoltaic implants allows implantation of multiple modules via small retinotomy to cover large visual field, and to follow the eye curvature.
- Intensity of NIR light required to activate the subretinal implants is safe.

Introduction

Retinal degenerative diseases, such as age-related macular degeneration and retinitis pigmentosa, lead to blindness due to gradual loss of photoreceptors, while the inner retinal neurons survive to a large extent [10, 26], albeit with some rewiring [12, 22]. Retinal prostheses aim at restoring sight by electrical stimulation of these surviving neurons. In the epiretinal approach, the primary target of stimulation are the retinal ganglion cells (RGCs) [1, 9], while subretinal stimulation elicits visual responses via inner retinal neurons (primarily bipolar cells) [2, 11, 30, 31]. Both approaches have been recently approved for clinical use, but the current systems involve bulky implanted electronics with trans-scleral cables, and require very complex surgeries. In addition, visual acuity with the epiretinal system (ARGUS II, Second Sight Inc., USA) is no better than 20/1260 [9], and the percepts are distorted due to axonal stimulation [24]. Subretinal prostheses (Alpha IMS, Retina Implant AG, Germany) provided similar acuity levels (20/2000–20/1000), except for one patient who demonstrated 20/550 [27, 28]. A third retinal implant (IRIS II from Pixium Vision, France) was recently approved for commercialization in Europe (Summer 2016) with no report on clinical results at the time of this publication.

We developed an alternative approach to retinal prosthetics, in which photovoltaic subretinal pixels directly convert pulsed light into electric current. Both the energy and information are delivered to the implant by projected images – in a completely wireless manner (Fig. 9.1). In this chapter, we describe the design and performance of this system, as well as its limitations.

System Design

Each pixel in the photovoltaic array is composed of a central stimulating electrode and a peripheral return electrode connected to 2 or 3 photodiodes in series (see [29] for details of the fabrication process). Photocurrent generated in the diodes flows through the tissue via electrodes coated with sputtered iridium oxide (SIROF). Resulting electric field in the retina polarizes the nearby neurons, leading to their stimulation (Fig. 9.1). High-density arrays are composed of 70 μm-wide and 30 μm-thick pixels separated by 5 μm trenches and arranged in a hexagonal pattern over a 1 mm diameter chip (142 pixels). Local return electrode in each pixel provides much better spatial confinement of the electric field compared to monopolar arrays, such as the Alpha IMS, and therefore yielding better contrast of the patterns [6, 13].

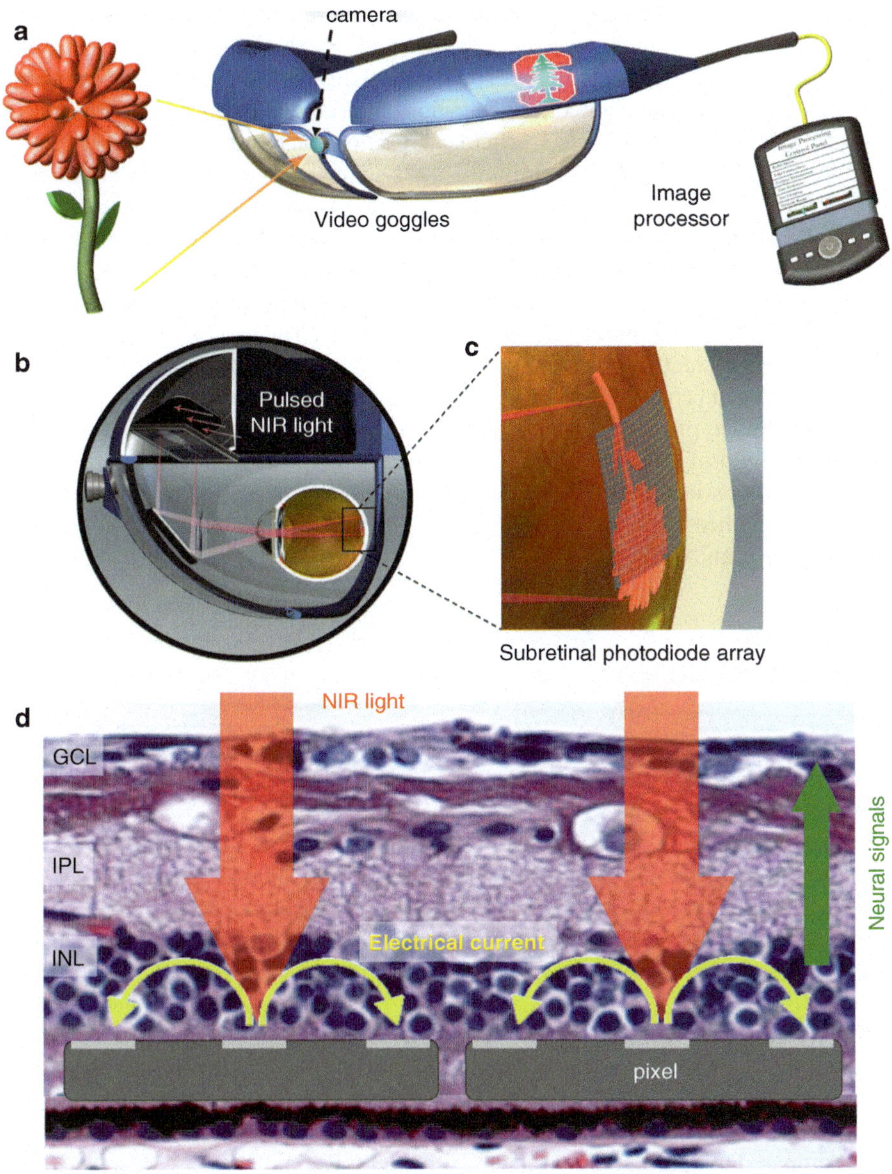

Fig. 9.1 System design. (**a**) Visual information captured by a camera is processed and displayed in the video goggles. (**b**) Images are projected via an ocular and natural eye optics onto the retina using near infrared (NIR) light (**c**) Part of the image forming over the subretinal implant is converted into stimulation pattern. (**d**) Each pixel in the implant converts the pulsed light into pulsed electric current flowing through the retina and stimulating the inner nuclear layer (INL), which then relays the response to the ganglion cells and to the brain via the optic nerve

The first attempt of using photodiodes to stimulate retinal neurons in blind patients was relying on ambient light to activate the pixels [3–5]. However, ambient light is way too dim (by at least a factor of 1000) to provide sufficient current for retinal stimulation [16], and pulsed light is required for generation of the charge-balanced electrical pulses in order to avoid irreversible electrochemical reactions on electrodes.

To provide very bright pulsed illumination, while avoiding any phototoxicity or photophobic effect due to remaining photoreceptors, we designed a goggles-based near-infrared (NIR) projection system (Fig. 9.1a). Video stream from a camera is processed in a pocket computer, and displayed in the goggles using NIR (850–915 nm) wavelengths. One design includes NIR laser source and a digital micromirror device (DMD) for image formation (Fig. 9.1b, c). The head mounted display is similar to augmented/virtual reality devices such as Google glass or night vision goggles, and can be upgraded without any modification of the subretinal implant. In particular, image-processing algorithms in the system will benefit from rapid progress in the field of computer vision and robotics. Low-level processing can allow image simplification such as edge detection, depth encoding, and object segmentation, while higher-level algorithms may include face detection, object recognition, GPS tracking, and others.

Functional Testing

To assess the stimulation capabilities and characterize the retinal response to subretinal stimulation, we performed a series of measurements ex-vivo and in-vivo in normal rats as well as in rats with retinal degeneration.

Using patch clamp recordings from individual retinal ganglion cells (RGCs), we demonstrated that anodic-first pulses with durations exceeding 1 ms selectively stimulated bipolar cells while avoiding direct activation of ganglion cells, and selectivity of such activation increased with pulse duration [2]. This approach utilizes the remaining retinal network, which results in preservation of several important features of natural vision, as will be discussed below. This observation led to design of the photovoltaic pixels with anodic wiring of the diodes to stimulating electrode [16, 17].

Retinal response to patterned stimulation was then studied ex-vivo, by placing excised rat retinas between the photovoltaic implant and a multi-electrode array recording system. Spiking of the ganglion cells in response to electrical stimulation was compared to natural responses to visible light. Retinal response decreased with increasing frequency of both, electrical and natural stimulation, diminishing to the noise level above 20 Hz. This indicates that adaptation and flicker fusion could occur with prosthetic vision, similarly to normal vision.

Mapping of electrical receptive fields of RGCs was performed by stimulating one pixel at a time in arrays with 70 μm pixels. The size of electrical receptive fields was found similar (~240 μm) to the natural visual receptive fields, which indicates that it is dominated by the signal spread in the retinal network [17]. However, measurements of the spatial resolution in the retina using alternating gratings test

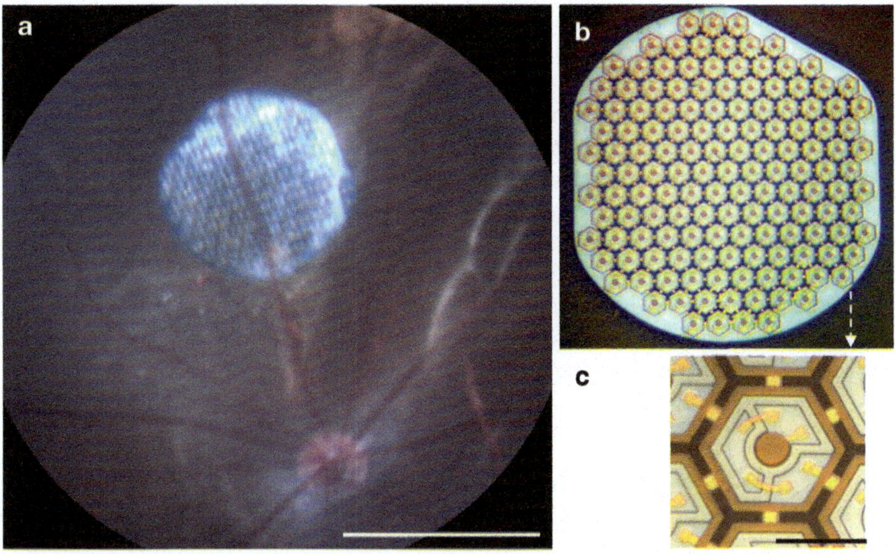

Fig. 9.2 Photovoltaic subretinal implant. (**a**) Fundus of a rat eye with subretinal implant. Scale bar is 1 mm. (**b**) Photovoltaic array is 1 mm in width and 30 μm in thickness, and is composed of a hexagonal matrix of pixels. (**c**) Each pixel is composed of 2 or 3 (shown here) diodes connected in series between the central stimulating electrode and circumferential return electrode (brown). Scale bar is 50 μm

revealed that RGCs responded to stripes of ~30 μm in width, when illuminated with visible light. With prosthetic stimulation, retinal response was limited by the pixel pitch in hexagonal array – 65 μm [17]. Both values are much smaller than the average size of the receptive field in rats. This effect can be explained by non-linear summation of sub-units in the receptive field corresponding to multiple bipolar cells connected to the same ganglion cell via non-linear synapse. Indeed, the RGCs responding at such high spatial resolution exhibited a non-linear (2nd harmonic) response to the alternating grating patterns [8, 17].

To assess visual functions in-vivo, we implanted rats blinded by retinal degeneration (Royal College Surgeon, RCS) with our photovoltaic arrays (Fig. 9.2). RCS rats undergo retinal degeneration over a few months, and their visual acuity progressively drops with the loss of photoreceptors. The implantation begins with a 2 mm sclerotomy before retinal detachment and introduction of the chip into the subretinal space. To measure cortical response to stimulation, we positioned trans-scleral electrodes over the primary visual cortex and recorded the visually and electrically evoked potentials. This signals triggered by NIR activation of the prosthesis were comparable to natural VEPs [21], but with (a) shorter latencies since prosthetic stimulation bypasses the phototransduction and (b) lower amplitude due to the limited spatial extent of the stimulus – 1 mm.

Similarly to observations ex-vivo, cortical responses decreased with increasing stimulation frequency, with a complete adaptation and flicker fusion above 40 Hz [16].

This effect allows representing a continuous percept using fast stroboscopic illumination, similarly to a conventional DLP projector or raster scanning techniques. Taking advantage of this flicker fusion, we presented alternating gratings with alternation rate of 2 Hz, illuminated by flashes at 40 Hz. At this frequency, cortical signals were correlated to the grating alternation and not to every single flash [17]. Amplitude of the response diminished with decreasing width of the grating stripes, and crossing of the noise level was defined as the acuity limit. Confirming the ex-vivo results, the acuity limit for prosthetic vision was found to be 64 μm per stripe, corresponding to the pixel pitch of the array, and twice larger than the natural acuity in rats – 27 μm per stripe. This result demonstrated that currently the acuity-limiting factor is the pixel size, and smaller pixels might improve visual acuity further. If these results were translated to the human eye, the 65 μm pixel pitch would correspond to a grating acuity of 20/250.

Surgical Technique in Human Eye

While in rodents, the implantation procedure consisted of a sclerotomy, followed by retinal detachment and subretinal insertion of the photovoltaic array, in larger eyes, the surgical procedure is very different: it begins with vitrectomy, followed by retinal detachment induced by subretinal injection of fluid. After retinal detachment, a 1–1.5 mm retinotomy is performed to provide access to subretinal space under the bleb, and the implants are placed into the retinotomy with custom forceps (Fig. 9.3). After the retinal reattachment with perfluorocarbon, retinotomy can be sealed using

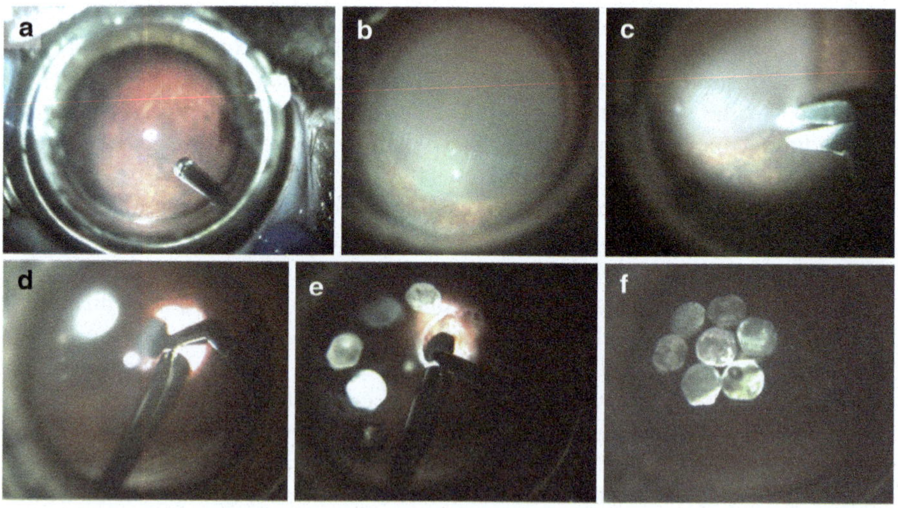

Fig. 9.3 Surgical procedure in the rabbit eye. Vitrectomy (**a**) is followed by retinal detachment with fluid injection (**b**). A small (1.5 mm) retinotomy (**c**) allows insertion of the modules into subretinal space (**d**–**e**). Retina is reattached (**f**) after injection of perfluorocarbon (Reprinted from Lee et al. [14]. With permission from SLACK Incorporated)

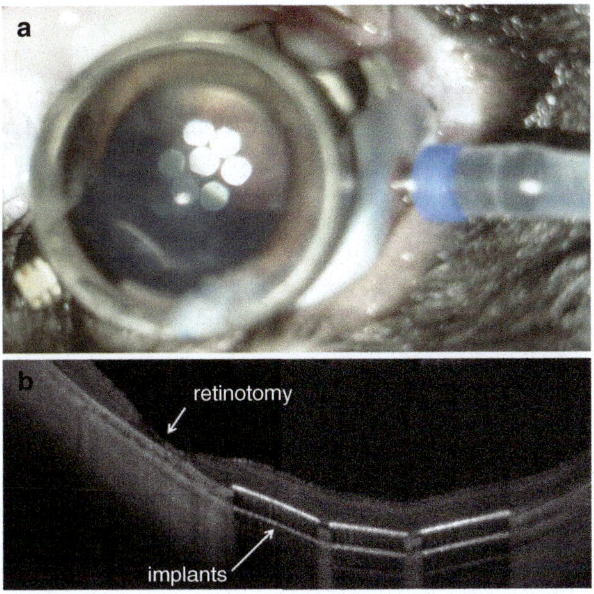

Fig. 9.4 Post-surgery imaging. (**a**) Fundus view after subretinal implantation of 7 modules of 1 mm in diameter. (**b**) OCT demonstrates complete retinal reattachment. Modules follow the curvature of the eye globe (Reprinted from Lee et al. [14]. With permission from SLACK Incorporated)

laser endo-photocoagulation. This is much simpler procedure than with any wired implants, and can be performed within 2 hours, without much custom training of the surgeon. Multiple modules placed via the same retinotomy allow expansion of the visual field, and they follow the curvature of the eye globe better than a single solid implant of the same size (Fig. 9.4).

Safety Aspects

This system is now being commercially developed in collaboration with Pixium Vision, under the product name PRIMA (Photovoltaic Retinal IMplAnt). Peak irradiance in the projection system will be limited to 5 mW/mm^2 on the retina. Operating at frequencies of 30–40 Hz to create continuous percepts with 5 ms pulses, the duty cycle will not exceed 20 %. Therefore, the average irradiance will be limited to 1 mW/mm^2 on the retina. With image sparsity not exceeding 50 % (grating pattern), the retinal temperature should not exceed 0.25 °C, which is within the noise of body temperature, and far below the thermal safety limit of 2 °C for chronic use [20].

We have demonstrated that implants were eliciting cortical responses during the 1-year follow-up – for life of the rats [16], and no damage to the inner retina has been observed within this period [19]. After explantation of the devices, however, we detected erosion of the polysilicon fillers in the device, which could cause failures in longer follow-ups. To prevent this erosion, the commercial devices are coated with silicon carbide, and demonstrated excellent biocompatibility and no erosion both, in accelerated aging tests and in-vivo [15].

Discussion

Unlike direct activation of RGCs in epiretnal approach, subretinal stimulation allows harvesting some of the natural retinal signal processing, even though degeneration often triggers some rewiring in the retinal neural network [12, 22]. Here we demonstrated that essential features of normal vision, such as flicker fusion, adaptation to static images, and non-linear summation of subunits in receptive field are preserved. However, we also demonstrated that the subretinal implantation in normal animals leads to complete loss of the photoreceptors above the implant [18], and therefore subretinal implantation should not be performed if there is still useful vision in the target area.

The wireless nature of the photovoltaic pixels enables modularity of the implant, which allows covering a large visual field via a small retinotomy by tiling. We developed the surgical technique for implantation of multiple units, as shown in Fig. 9.4. With 7 devices of 1 mm in diameter, one can cover a 10° visual field, and with 2 mm implants it could extend up to 20°. This visual field is further enhanced by eye scanning over the display. Projection of the images via the natural optics of the eye retains the natural link between eye motion and visual perception.

In prostheses where information from the camera is delivered to the retina via RF serial telemetry (EM coils), as in the Second Sight devices, the eye movements are decoupled from the image, which leads to two problems: (1) The brain expects images to shift on the retina during eye movements. In particular, stationary objects should translate with the changing direction of gaze. Since the stimulation patterns in such implants do not shift with the eye movement, the brain interprets that as motion of the object when the eye moves [25]. Similar effect has been reported with cortical visual prostheses [7]. To avoid this phenomenon, patients are asked to keep their direction of gaze steady. (2) Instead of the natural eye scanning, patients are required to scan the visual field with their heads – a very unnatural paradigm, which leads to adverse effects, such stimulus mislocalization. These limitations could be alleviated, in principle, by incorporating a fast eye-tracking mechanism in the system, which would shift the image delivered to the implant according to the direction of gaze within the physiological response time.

Additional advantages of preserving the eye scanning mechanisms include prevention of the static image fading and higher acuity due to multiple scans and averaging [23].

Conclusions and Future Directions

Commercial version of the photovoltaic retinal prosthesis (PRIMA, Pixium Vision) is being prepared for clinical trials. With 70 μm pixels, we hope to achieve visual acuity on the order of 20/250. We are also developing arrays with twice smaller pixels, which, if successful, might support twice better visual acuity – down to 20/120 level. Interactions with patients during clinical trials will help optimizing image processing and stimulation parameters (frame rate, dynamic range, etc.) for full utilization of the potential of network-mediated retinal stimulation.

References

1. Behrend MR, Ahuja AK, Humayun MS, Chow RH, Weiland JD. Resolution of the epiretinal prosthesis is not limited by electrode size. IEEE Trans Neural Syst Rehabil Eng. 2011;19(4):436–42.
2. Boinagrov D, Pangratz-Fuehrer S, Goetz G, Palanker D. Selectivity of direct and network-mediated stimulation of the retinal ganglion cells with epi-, sub- and intraretinal electrodes. J Neural Eng. 2014;11(2):026008.
3. Chow AY, Bittner AK, Pardue MT. The artificial silicon retina in retinitis pigmentosa patients (an American Ophtalmological Association thesis). Trans Am Ophthalmol Soc. 2010;108:120–54.
4. Chow AY, Chow VY, Packo KH, Pollack JS, Peyman GA, Schuchard R. The artificial silicon retina microchip for the treatment of vision loss from retinitis pigmentosa. Arch Ophthalmol. 2004;122:460–9.
5. Chow AY, Pardue MT, Chow VY, Peyman GA, Liang CLC, Perlman JI, Peachey NS. Implantation of silicon chip microphotodiode arrays into the cat subretinal space. IEEE Trans Neural Syst Rehabil Eng. 2001;9(1):86–95.
6. Djilas M, Olès C, Lorach H, Bendali A, Dégardin J, Dubus E, Lissorgues-Bazin G, Rousseau L, Benosman R, Ieng S-H, Joucla S, Yvert B, Bergonzo P, Sahel J, Picaud S. Three-dimensional electrode arrays for retinal prostheses: modeling, geometry optimization and experimental validation. J Neural Eng. 2011;8(4):046020.
7. Dobelle WH, Quest DO, Antunes JL, Roberts TS, Girvin JP. Artificial vision for the blind by electrical stimulation of the visual cortex. Neurosurgery. 1979;5(4):521–7.
8. Heine WF, Passaglia CL. Spatial receptive field properties of rat retinal ganglion cells. Vis Neurosci. 2011;28(05):403–17.
9. Humayun MS, Dorn JD, da Cruz L, Dagnelie G, Sahel JA, Stanga P, Cideciyan AV, Duncan JL, Eliott D, Filley E, Ho AC, Santos A, Safran AB, Arditi A, Del Priore LV, Greenberg RJ, A. I. S. Group. Interim results from the international trial of Second Sight's visual prosthesis. Ophthalmology. 2012;119(4):779–88.
10. Humayun MS, Prince M, de Juan E, Barron Y, Moskowitz M, Klock IB, Milam AH. Morphometric analysis of the extramacular retina from postmortem eyes with retinitis pigmentosa. Invest Ophthalmol Vis Sci. 1999;40(1):143–8.
11. Jensen RJ, Rizzo 3rd JF. Thresholds for activation of rabbit retinal ganglion cells with a subretinal electrode. Exp Eye Res. 2006;83(2):367–73.
12. Jones BW, Marc RE. Retinal remodeling during retinal degeneration. Exp Eye Res. 2005;81(2):123–37.
13. Joucla S, Yvert B. Improved focalization of electrical microstimulation using microelectrode arrays: a modeling study. PLoS One. 2009;4(3):e4828.
14. Lee DY, Lorach H, Huie P, Palanker D. Implantation of modular photovoltaic subretinal prosthesis. Ophthalmic Surg Lasers Imaging Retina. 2016;47(2):171–4.
15. Lei, X, Kane, S, Cogan, S, Lorach, H, Galambos, L, Huie, P, Mathieson, K, Kamins, T, Harris, J & Palanker, D. 'SiC protective coating for photovoltaic retinal prosthesis'. Journal of Neural Engineering. 2016;13(4) DOI 10.1088/1741-2560/13/4/046016
16. Lorach H, Goetz G, Mandel Y, Lei X, Kamins TI, Mathieson K, Huie P, Dalal R, Harris JS, Palanker D. Performance of photovoltaic arrays in-vivo and characteristics of prosthetic vision in animals with retinal degeneration. Vision Res. 2015;111(Pt B):142–8.
17. Lorach H, Goetz G, Smith R, Lei X, Mandel Y, Kamins T, Mathieson K, Huie P, Harris J, Sher A, Palanker D. Photovoltaic restoration of sight with high visual acuity. Nat Med. 2015;21:476–82.
18. Lorach H, Kung J, Beier C, Mandel Y, Dalal R, Huie P, Wang J, Lee S, Sher A, Jones BW, Palanker D. Development of animal models of local retinal degeneration. Invest Ophthalmol Vis Sci. 2015;56(8):4644–52.
19. Lorach H, Lei X, Galambos L, Kamins T, Mathieson K, Dalal R, Huie P, Harris J, Palanker D. Interactions of prosthetic and natural vision in animals with local retinal degeneration. Invest Ophthalmol Vis Sci. 2015;56(12):7444–50.

20. Lorach H, Wang J, Lee DY, Dalal R, Huie P, Palanker D. Retinal safety of near infrared radiation in photovoltaic restoration of sight. Biomed Opt Express. 2016;7(1):13–21.
21. Mandel Y, Goetz G, Lavinsky D, Huie P, Mathieson K, Wang L, Kamins T, Galambos L, Manivanh R, Harris J, Palanker D. Cortical responses elicited by photovoltaic subretinal prostheses exhibit similarities to visually evoked potentials. Nat Commun. 2013;4:1980.
22. Marc RE, Jones BW, Watt CB, Strettoi E. Neural remodeling in retinal degeneration. Prog Retin Eye Res. 2003;22(5):607–55.
23. Martinez-Conde S, Macknik SL, Hubel DH. The role of fixational eye movements in visual perception. Nat Rev Neurosci. 2004;5(3):229–40.
24. Nanduri D, Fine I, Horsager A, Boynton GM, Humayun MS, Greenberg RJ, Weiland JD. Frequency and amplitude modulation have different effects on the percepts elicited by retinal stimulation. Invest Ophthalmol Vis Sci. 2012;53(1):205–14.
25. Sabbah N, Authie CN, Sanda N, Mohand-Said S, Sahel JA, Safran AB. Importance of eye position on spatial localization in blind subjects wearing an Argus II retinal prosthesis. Invest Ophthalmol Vis Sci. 2014;55(12):8259–66.
26. Santos A, Humayun M, de Juan E, Greenberg RJ, Marsh MJ, Klock IB, Milam AH. Preservation of the inner retina in retinitis pigmentosa: a morphometric analysis. Arch Ophthalmol. 1997;115(4):511–5.
27. Stingl K, Bartz-Schmidt KU, Besch D, Chee CK, Cottrial C, Gekeler F, Groppe M, Jackson TL, MacLaren RE, Koitschev A, Kusnyerik A, Neffendorf J, Nemeth J, Naeem MA, Peters T, Sachs H, Simpson A, Singh MS, Wilhelm B, Wong D, Zrenner E. Subretinal visual Implant Alpha IMS – clinical trial interim report. Vision Res. 2015;111(Pt B):149–60.
28. Stingl K, Bartz-Schmidt K-U, Gekeler F, Kusnyerik A, Sachs H, Zrenner E. Functional outcome in subretinal electronic implants depends on foveal eccentricity. Invest Ophthalmol Vis Sci. 2013;54(12):7658–65.
29. Wang L, Mathieson K, Kamins TI, Loudin JD, Galambos L, Goetz G, Sher A, Mandel Y, Huie P, Lavinsky D, Harris JS, Palanker DV. Photovoltaic retinal prosthesis: implant fabrication and performance. J Neural Eng. 2012;9(4):046014.
30. Zrenner E. Fighting blindness with microelectronics. Sci Transl Med. 2013;5:210–6.
31. Zrenner E, Bartz-Schmidt KU, Benav H, Besch D, Bruckmann A, Gabel V-P, Gekeler F, Greppmaier U, Harscher A, Kibbel S, Koch J, Kusnyerik A, Peters T, Stingl K, Sachs H, Stett A, Szurman P, Wilhelm B, Wilke R. Subretinal electronic chips allow blind patients to read letters and combine them to words. Proc R Soc B: Biol Sci. 2011;278(1711):1489–97.

Chapter 10
Suprachoroidal Retinal Prostheses

Lauren N. Ayton, Gregg J. Suaning, Nigel H. Lovell, Matthew A. Petoe, David A.X. Nayagam, Tamara-Leigh E. Brawn, and Anthony N. Burkitt

Abstract Visual prostheses are currently being developed by a number of international teams for the restoration of basic visual function to those with profound vision impairment or blindness. In this exciting field of research and development, a number of unique device designs and surgical placements have been developed.

This chapter discusses the engineering specifications, preclinical testing and clinical trial outcomes for suprachoroidal prostheses. These implants are placed between the posterior blood supply of the eye (choroid) and the outer white layer of the eye (sclera), with this surgical location primarily being chosen for stability and safety. In the pilot study of a prototype suprachoroidal implant, which was held in Australia between 2012 and 2014, there were no unexpected intraocular serious adverse events in the three implanted participants. Future trials will examine safety and efficacy of implants with larger numbers of electrodes in larger cohorts of participants with profound vision loss from retinitis pigmentosa. It is also hoped that in the future suprachoroidal prostheses may be able to be used in people with some residual vision (such as in age-related macular degeneration).

L.N. Ayton, PhD, B.Optom, FAAO, FACO (✉)
Centre for Eye Research Australia, The University of Melbourne, Royal Victorian Eye and Ear Hospital, East Melbourne, VIC, Australia
e-mail: lnayton@unimelb.edu.au

G.J. Suaning, BSc, MSc, PhD • N.H. Lovell, BE (Hons), PhD
Graduate School of Biomedical Engineering, University of New South Wales, Sydney, NSW, Australia

M.A. Petoe, BSc, BEng (Hons), PhD • D.A.X. Nayagam, BSc, BE(ElecEng)(Hons), PhD
Bionics Institute, The University of Melbourne, Melbourne, VIC, Australia

T.-L. E. Brawn, BA, BBSc, PostGradDip Ed, MBA
Bionic Vision Australia, University of Melbourne, Parkville, VIC, Australia

A.N. Burkitt, PhD, BSc (Hon), BSc
Department of Electrical and Electronic Engineering, The University of Melbourne, Melbourne, VIC, Australia

V.P. Gabel (ed.), *Artificial Vision*, DOI 10.1007/978-3-319-41876-6_10

The work described in this chapter, conducted by the Bionic Vision Australia (BVA) consortium, deals exclusively with suprachoroidal implantation of a stimulating array. Data are presented from the surgical implantation and psychophysical responses of a 24-channel percutaneously connected prototype device implanted in three subjects. The architecture of two future-generation fully-implantable suprachoroidal prostheses, a 44-channel device and the 99-channel 'Phoenix' device are also presented.

Keywords Suprachoroidal • Retinal stimulation • Retinal prosthesis • Vision restoration • Retinitis pigmentosa • Medical bionics

Key Points

- Suprachoroidal retinal prostheses are placed in the suprachoroidal space, between the sclera and the choroid.
- A prototype suprachoroidal prosthesis was trialled in a pilot study of three patients in Melbourne, Australia between 2012 and 2014.
- This prototype study showed that the device was safe and effective, and further clinical trials are now being planned.

Principal Idea

Vision is the most feature-rich and complex of the senses and visual cues are critical for many activities of daily living. Vision impairment results in significant social and economic burdens, both to individuals and to our broader society. The increasing and aging population has led to an increase in the number of people living with vision impairment, and this number will continue to rise. For this reason, a number of vision restoration techniques are being developed, including stem cells, gene therapy, optogenetics and visual prostheses. Of the intervention options currently under development, visual prostheses or 'bionic eyes' are the most clinically advanced, which has led to the regulatory approval of two commercial retinal prosthetic devices.

The site of insult or injury to the visual pathway will dictate the range of possible target locations for a visual prosthesis. These possible implantation sites span the visual system and include the visual cortex, the lateral geniculate nucleus (LGN), the optic nerve and various locations proximal to the retina. Retinal prostheses have been implanted in patients with retinal degeneration epiretinally [1], subretinally [2, 3], suprachoroidally [4], and intra-sclerally [5].

A key advantage of the suprachoroidal location (Fig. 10.1) is that the electrodes do not contact the neural retina, and hence the device has a reduced risk of retinal damage. In addition, the surgical technique is such that the implant does not need to enter the vitreous cavity at all, negating the need for corneal incisions, intraocular lens extraction, vitrectomy and retinal surgery. The device is instead slid into the

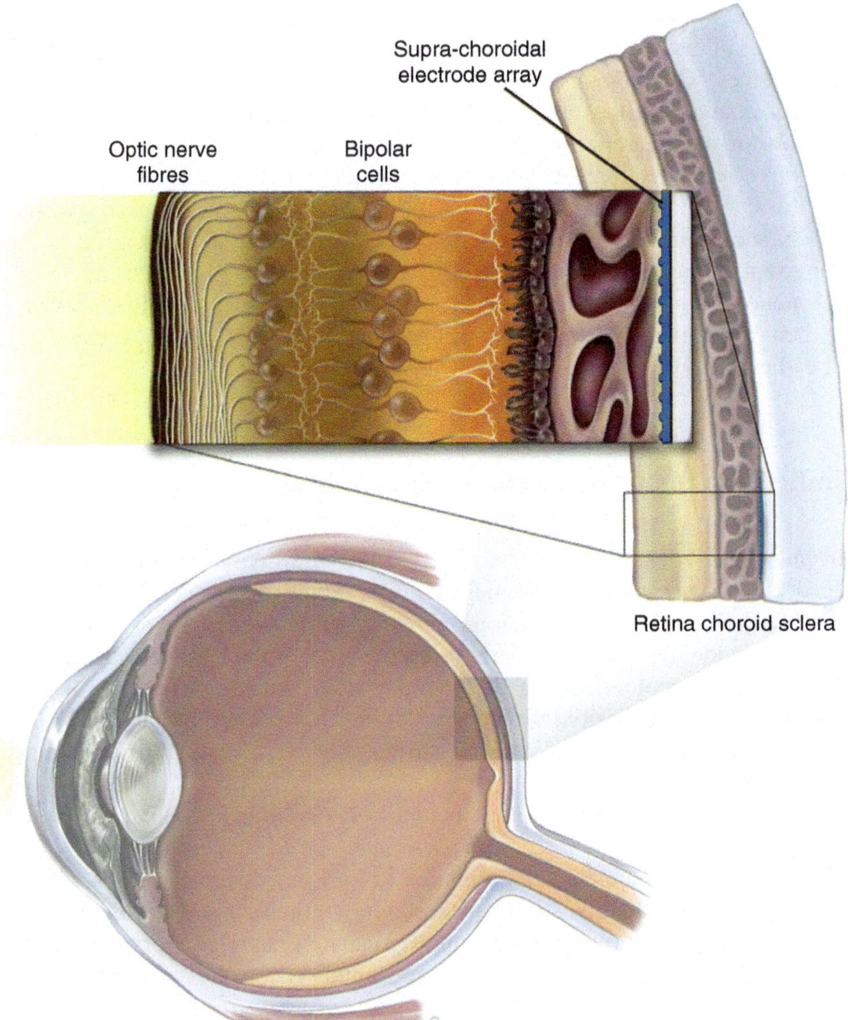

Fig. 10.1 Schematic of the human eye showing the location of the suprachoroidal implant, which is located between the choroid and the sclera (Image courtesy of Bionic Vision Australia, copyright Beth Croce)

natural cleavage plane of the suprachoroidal space via a scleral incision, and has been shown to be a relatively simple and a safe procedure [4].

The distance between electrodes placed in the suprachoroidal space and the retinal ganglion cells does come at the expense of higher stimulation thresholds, and may impact on the upper limit of the useful electrode densities that can be implemented with this approach. However, these issues are likely to be eclipsed by the overriding importance of the long-term stability and functionality of the therapy.

The suprachoroidal position also means the device does not interfere with the existing optics of the eye and therefore could co-exist with residual vision (unlike epiretinal devices, which block areas of natural vision).

This chapter outlines the work completed by Bionic Vision Australia (BVA), a consortium of research teams in Australia,[1] between 2010 and 2015. Over this time, BVA has developed three devices: a 44-channel (which was tested in participants in the form of a 24-channel prototype prosthesis in the 2012 pilot study) and a 99-channel suprachoroidal prosthesis (both to be trialled in the near future) and an epiretinal diamond electrode array. This chapter will focus on the technology, clinical outcomes and future directions for suprachoroidal devices alone;further information regarding the epiretinal technology developed by BVA can be found elsewhere [6–9].

Indication for Certain Forms of Blindness

In industrialised nations, approximately 29 % of all cases of blindness in people aged 29–40 are caused by the degenerative retinal disorder, retinitis pigmentosa (RP) [10]. This disease affects approximately 1 in 4000 people, or 1.5 million people worldwide. RP typically begins with the death of the light-sensitive cells of the retina (photoreceptors) in the peripheral vision, and progresses at varying rates towards the central vision, ultimately leading to profound blindness. There is no known effective treatment for RP. For those affected, a visual prosthesis may offer significant hope.

A retinal prosthesis (that is implanted next to or within the retinal layers) requires a viable optic nerve and, accordingly, is not suitable for all forms of blindness. Retinal prostheses substitute the function of light-sensitive nerve cells with electrical impulses to directly stimulate surviving retinal neurons from a surgically implanted electrode array. The most appropriate first candidates for retinal prostheses are those with end-stage RP, with profound vision loss (usually bare light perception).

However, the possibilities for a device that co-exists with residual vision (such as a suprachoroidal implant which does not block incident light) are exciting. A device that allows the coexistence of prosthetic vision and residual vision would have the potential to treat conditions like age-related macular degeneration (AMD). AMD is the leading cause of adult blindness in western nations and affects more than 1.75 million people in the United States of America alone, where some 200,000 new

[1] The Bionic Vision Australia consortium consists of the University of Melbourne, the University of New South Wales, The Centre for Eye Research Australia, The Bionics Institute and NICTA. Supporting participants are the Royal Victorian Eye and Ear Hospital, the National Vision Research Institute of Australia and the University of Western Sydney. The BVA consortium was funded between 2010 and 2015 by the Australian Research Council, through its Special Research Initiative in Bionic Vision Science and Technology Program.

cases are diagnosed each year [11, 12]. This number is set to grow significantly with an aging population. Recent pharmacological anti-vascular endothelial growth factor (VEGF) treatments have been shown to reduce vision loss from neovascular AMD [13]. However, up to 15 % of patients will not respond to these drugs, and will continue to lose vision despite anti-VEGF treatment [13], and many people still suffer from atrophic AMD, for which there is no effective treatment at this time.

In the vast majority of AMD cases, useful peripheral vision remains intact. Accordingly, there is much at risk in the implantation of a visual prosthesis into AMD-affected eyes until more is known of the long-term effects of the therapy – its effect on residual vision in particular. An analogous situation applied in the early stages of cochlear implants, and it took many years before surgical techniques were developed that ensured that the devices could both deliver benefit and coexist with residual hearing. When this was shown, the number of people who could gain benefit from the device multiplied several-fold. Should the same be found to be true for AMD, the potential number of indications of a visual prosthesis could increase significantly. For the time being however, the majority of visual prostheses are being developed and tested for severely visually impaired people suffering from end-stage RP.

Technical Description of the BVA 24-Channel Prototype Prosthesis

To minimise risk, the BVA suprachoroidal prostheses only use materials that have a robust historical record of prior use in regulatory approved, chronically implanted medical devices. These include: platinum, silicone rubber, titanium and a braze alloy (TiCuNi) first used in pacemaker hermetic encapsulation. While these choices do not circumvent or obviate the need for preclinical testing, their employment does mitigate a number of key risks associated with the safety of the prosthesis and have served to expedite the clinical trials.

The suprachoroidal approach was first implemented in a pilot clinical trial conducted by BVA between 2012 and 2014 (www.clinicaltrial.gov, #NCT01603576). The BVA pilot trial implanted three participants with end-stage RP and bare light perception with a 24-channel prototype prosthesis (Fig. 10.2) manufactured by the Bionics Institute. The electrode array was 19 mm long × 8 mm wide; and composed of a medical grade silicone substrate with 33 platinum electrodes (diameters: 30 × 600 μm, 3 × 400 μm) and two large return electrodes (diameter: 2 mm). A remote platinum return electrode was implanted under the skin behind the ear. The outer ring of electrodes was electrically coupled to provide a fourth alternate return configuration, meaning that there remained a total of 20 electrode channels that could be individually stimulated. In this study, a direct electrical connection with the array was made possible through the use of a percutaneous connector, which allowed flexible neurostimulation and electrode monitoring without the need for any implanted electronics.

Electrical stimulation parameters were determined for each participant in a psychophysics setting to address inter-participant differences and obtain clear and

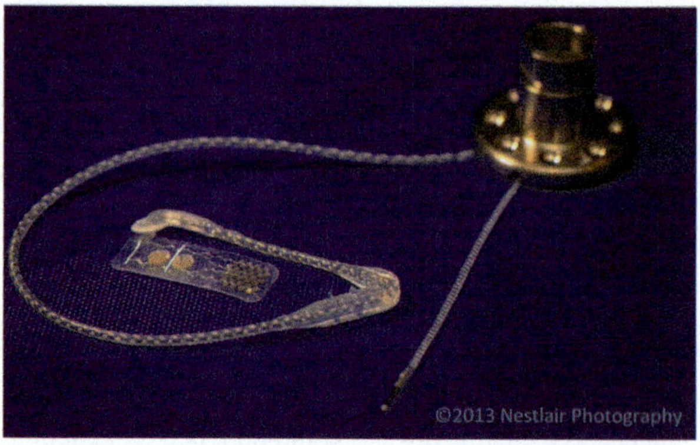

Fig. 10.2 The clinical suprachoroidal electrode array (*left*) and percutaneous lead system (*right*) used for research purposes in the initial BVA pilot study (2012–2014) (Courtesy of Dr. David Nayagam, Bionics Institute Australia)

reliable 'phosphenes' (electrically evoked visual percepts) on all electrodes in each participant. These were generated in the form of a phosphene map for each participant which specified the number of available electrodes that could be used for stimulation, the pulse width (PW), interphase gap (IGP) and stimulation rate (pulses-per-second, PPS) for each electrode, the threshold current for each electrode and the maximum current for each electrode. During camera-based tasks, stimulation was interspersed with intervals of no stimulation to alleviate brightness fading and adaptation observed in continuous stimulation [14, 15].

Testing incorporated a head-mounted video camera with a manufacturer stated field-of-view of 67° × 50.25° (Arrington Research Inc., Scottsdale AZ, USA) and a pixel dimension of 320 by 240 pixels. Within the implant, the 20 stimulating electrodes were arranged in a staggered grid measuring 3.5 mm × 3.46 mm, corresponding to a visual field projection on the retina of approximately 12.4° × 12.2° [16]. A similarly sized sub-region of the camera image was presented to the electrodes after vision processing. Participants were trained to utilize head movements to explore a wider field-of-view.

Surgical Methods

One of the main advantages with the suprachoroidal implant location is the relative simplicity of the surgical procedure. Whilst epiretinal and subretinal surgeries require multiple steps, often including a vitrectomy, intraocular lens extraction, and retinal fixation techniques, the suprachoroidal surgery is simpler and less invasive. The suprachoroidal surgical procedures were developed using cadaver studies (feline and human), and acute and chronic implantations in a feline model [17]. In addition, BVA surgeons were able to trial the surgery on a human patient who was undergoing enucleation due to an unrelated ocular condition [17].

To date, implantation of an active suprachoroidal implant has been completed in three participants in Australia (in 2012), and took 3–4 h in each case [4]. The participants were administered general anesthesia and standard surgical preparation was undertaken (Betadine wash, instrument and device sterilization etc.). A lateral canthotomy was performed and an orbitotomy was created with 1 mm burrs to allow lead stabilization. Once the wall of the eye was exposed, a temporal peritomy was performed and the lateral rectus muscle removed. The scleral incision, through which the device is implanted, was made underneath the insertion point of the lateral rectus muscle. A full thickness scleral incision was made, and the suprachoroidal space was dissected with a blade and then a lens guide. The electrode array was inserted into this space, and the wound was closed using nylon sutures and a Dacron patch. After the scleral wound was closed, the lateral rectus muscle was reattached and all skin wounds closed.

With the 24-channel prototype prosthesis, a percutaneous connector was used to allow direct stimulation of the array. For implantation of this connector, an incision was made through the posterior temporalis muscle to expose a flat section of bone, to which the connector was attached. A tunnel was created below the fascia macula to allow a lead wire to run from the percutaneous connector to the electrode array. The electrode array was then passed forward from this behind-ear incision within a custom-built trochar to protect the device during implantation, and placed into the suprachoroidal space.

In future clinical trials of the 44-channel and 99-channel prostheses, the percutaneous connector will be replaced with a fully implantable stimulator, utilising the same surgical techniques as used to implant the neurostimulator coils in cochlear implants.

Experimental Results

The suprachoroidal prostheses [18–21] were further developed by a multidisciplinary team from BVA, through a series of iterative preclinical studies (2009–2012) of safety and efficacy, surgical development and form factor optimisation [22, 23].

Acute electrophysiological studies were performed to verify the efficacy of suprachoroidal stimulation [24–26]. Passive chronic implantation, removal and replacement studies demonstrated the implant biocompatibility and stability [27, 28]. These studies culminated in an active implantation study, which showed that long-term stimulation of the retina with a suprachoroidal array was both safe and efficacious [29]. Following these studies, the clinical prototype was specified based on measurements made in cadavers, the various implant and lead components were tested in accelerated bench tests, and a custom trochar was developed for the surgical implantation [17].

Clinical Pilot Study (24-Channel Prototype Prosthesis)

The 2012 BVA pilot study was the first assessment of suprachoroidal retinal prostheses in humans. The pilot study followed three participants during weekly research visits for 2 years to assess safety and efficacy of the suprachoroidal surgery, device design and stimulation strategies.

The three participants all had baseline visual acuity of light perception only, and a documented medical history of RP. Two of the subjects had rod-cone dystrophy, and one had Bardet-Beidl syndrome. All subjects had at least 10 years of light perception vision, and all had form vision when they were younger. This is important in retinal prosthesis studies, as it is not clear whether the devices would work as effectively in people with malformed visual pathways.

The suprachoroidal device was implanted successfully in all three participants, in a surgery which took between 3 and 4 h. The intraocular array was positioned below the fovea. Due to the thinned choroid [30] and retina in the participants secondary to their RP, the array was easily imaged using fundus photography and optical coherence tomography (Fig. 10.3).

In all participants, a subretinal hemorrhage was noted 3–4 days postoperatively, which was an expected adverse event due to the proximity to the vascular choroidal layer. This resolved without intervention in all cases, although one subject did retain

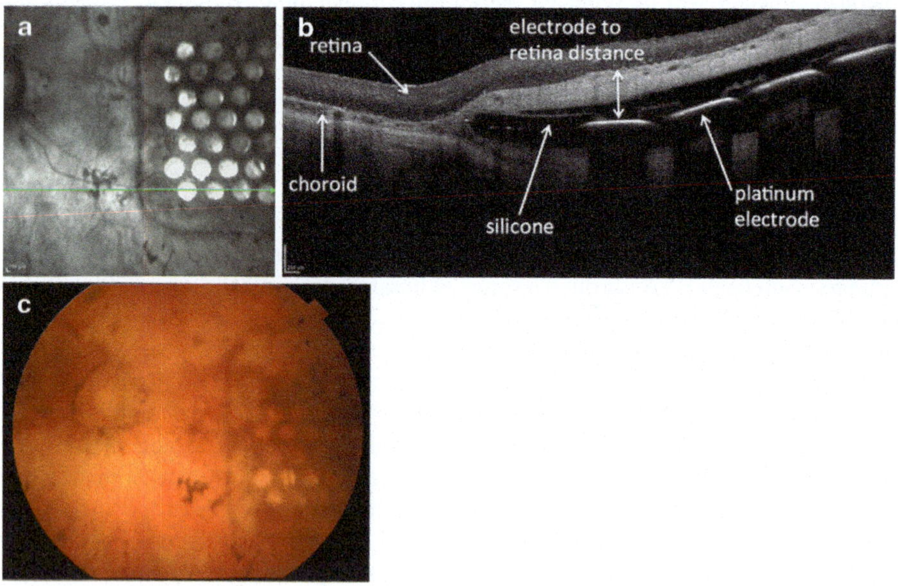

Fig. 10.3 An infrared image (**a**), optical coherence tomography scan (**b**) and fundus photograph (**c**) showing the suprachoroidal intraocular electrode array in situ in a trial participant. The horizontal *green line* in the infrared image (**a**) shows the location of the OCT scan (**b**) (**a**, **b** Reprinted from Ayton et al. [4]. With permission from PLOS ONE)

some retinal fibrosis from this event. Participants remained in hospital for up to 5 days of postoperative care before being discharged, and only required mild analgesia and routine antibiotic and steroid eye drops. The other serious device-related adverse events that occurred during the study period were related to infection of the external percutaneous connector, and were managed with antibiotics and revision surgery for correction of the placement of the connector in one case. The replacement of the percutaneous connector with an implanted stimulator in the next generation devices will eliminate the risk of these types of adverse events.

Mapping of phosphene locations, shape, and size was achievable using a motion-tracking device affixed to the participant's finger, and an eye-facing camera to track gaze position. Phosphene appearance was found to be varied depending on subject, electrode position and stimulation parameters, but were controllable (in terms of size and, brightness and complexity), retinotopically placed and locatable in the visual field by two of the subjects [31]. The third subject reported transient phosphenes that looked like short curved lines that swept quickly from right to left. Although phosphene intensity increased with stimulation level for this subject, there was no clearly discernible difference between phosphenes from different electrodes.

In the other two subjects, electrodes close to the fovea produced somewhat complex shapes, whereas electrodes at the periphery were punctate. There was overlap of phosphenes from adjacent electrodes, and marginal overlap from electrodes two electrode-spacings apart, although the participants were able to use the characteristic shapes of each phosphene to discriminate them. The reasons for these shapes and overlap are likely to be a combination of the higher charge required to stimulate from the suprachoroidal position (resulting in a spread of current) and the retinal structure at the fovea when compared to the periphery (i.e. greater retinal ganglion cell representation at the fovea). There was also a temporal element to evoked phosphenes, which has been well-described in other human studies [14]. Phosphenes appeared bright at the onset, but were described by the participants as having a 'waviness' quality to them throughout sustained stimulation. Some electrodes also produced a bright flash at stimulus offset.

The full results of the prototype study have been published previously [4], and provided promising evidence of the effectiveness of stimulation of a suprachoroidal electrode. The study was designed to be a proof-of-concept Phase 1 safety study, and hence the prototype was simple with only 20 individually stimulating electrodes. Despite this, participants were able to use the prosthesis to complete tasks such as light localisation (using the Basic Assessment of Light and Motion test, BALM), optotype recognition (Landolt C), grating acuity (using the Freiburg Visual Acuity Test, FrACT), identification of a subset of Sloan letters, and basic activities of daily living tasks, such as locating objects on a table and navigating obstacles whilst walking [32].

The best possible Landolt-C score measured using the prototype was 20/4451 (logMAR 2.35), which is similar to the best-measured grating acuity score of 20/4250 (logMAR 2.33). Both of these results approach the calculated limit of 20/4242 (logMAR 2.33) based on electrode separation and size [16]. Identification of a subset of Sloan letters was also successful in a four-alternate-forced-choice letter recognition task. With the device off, subjects were not able to perform above chance on any of the acuity tasks. This improvement in acuity is promising given the low number of stimulating electrodes in the prototype, and suggests that future suprachoroidal prostheses may be able to improve letter recognition for patients.

However, the most likely use for retinal prostheses in the immediate future is to assist patients with mobility and simple activity of daily living tasks. We have developed a series of tasks known as the Low Vision Assessment of Daily Activities (LoVADA) protocol, which have been shown to detect small changes in vision [32–34]. These tasks were used in the prototype study, and showed that the prosthesis improved the subjects' ability to localize objects on a table [32], and to navigate around obstacles whilst walking. The resolution of the prostheses is not yet sufficient to allow subjects to reliably name the objects that they see, but there is hope that future devices will allow this level of vision.

Future Directions

In addition to the success of the BVA 24-Channel prototype clinical trial, two next-generation prostheses are being developed. Both of these next-generation prostheses are implanted in the suprachoroidal space, but they differ in the number of electrodes, device design and available stimulation strategies.

The 44-Channel Fully Implantable Device

The next BVA device to be trialed in patients will include a 44-channel electrode array, with a similar footprint and array design as the 24-Channel prototype. The main differences will be an increase in the number of electrodes to increase the horizontal field of view, an increase in electrode size (to 1000 μm diameter) and the inclusion of implanted stimulating electronics. Additionally, the 44-Channel device will be capable of simultaneously activating two distinct channels of stimulation, which will allow for more controllable visual percepts and an enhanced dynamic range. Importantly, as it will be fully implantable, the participants will be able to use the device outside of the laboratory environment.

The electrode array will be connected by 46 fine platinum wires (which includes 2 wires for the large return electrodes), formed into a helical lead, to a pair of implanted stimulators. Each stimulator will control 22 individual electrodes in the array with precise control of timing and level. These stimulators will be surgically implanted under the skin behind the ear, in a similar position to that used for bionic ear patients. Standard magnetic induction coils will couple the implanted stimulators to a body worn vision processor, which in turn receives input from a small camera mounted on a pair of spectacles. The vision processor will send instructions via the inductive coils to the implanted stimulators as well as receive telemetry relating to the status of the electrode array and stimulators.

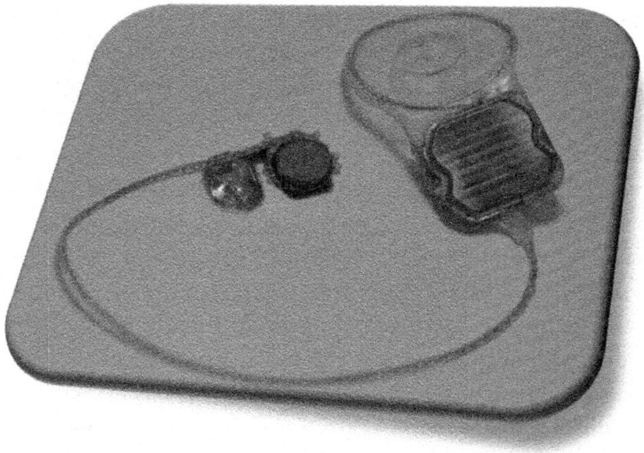

Fig. 10.4 A prototype Phoenix 99 implant system showing the intra-ocular components of electrode array and stimulating electronics (*left*) and the electronics and wireless coil (*right*) for transfer of data and power, joined by a 2-wire interface

As this device will be able to be used by participants in their normal home and work environments, we anticipate that the functional vision outcomes will be improved through neural plasticity. This next clinical trial will also allow increased vision rehabilitation and training on how to use the new prosthetic vision, which will maximize potential benefit.

The 99-Channel Fully Implantable Device ('Phoenix-99')

The third generation suprachoroidal prosthesis is a fully implantable device with 99 electrodes and embedded, hermetically encapsulated electronics. This device, known as the Phoenix-99 (Fig. 10.4), is currently undergoing pre-clinical testing at UNSW Australia as part of the BVA consortium.

In addition to the Phoenix-99 device offering more than four times the number of stimulation sites, it differs from the previously tested 24 channel prototype device in several ways. The Phoenix-99 is fully implantable – containing its own stimulation circuitry contained within a hermetically-sealed chamber that is wirelessly configured by external image processing hardware.

The Phoenix-99 device possesses a number of unique stimulation features that aim to provide focused and meaningful perceptions. Electrodes are arranged in a hexagonal mosaic – that is, electrodes arranged in clusters of seven electrodes taking the form of a hexagon with six electrodes at the corners, and one stimulating electrode at the hexagon's centre. Stimulation current is delivered to the single electrode at the centre of the hexagon and the return path for the current is directed into the six, surrounding electrodes – each of which carries approximately 1/6th of the stimulating current. This approach is very effective in limiting current spread and containing the stimulation to an area of retina near the stimulating electrode [35, 36]. As a result of the limited current spread, multiple hexagons may be stimulated simultaneously without significant ‘cross-talk’ between stimulation sites. This approach allows the visual scene to be conveyed more rapidly than with series stimulation.

With the suprachoroidal space being somewhat distant from the targeted retinal neurons, stimulation thresholds are known to be relatively high in hexapolar stimulation. The Phoenix-99 implant addresses this issue by combining the focused activation achieved by hexapolar stimulation with the threshold-reducing attributes of monopolar stimulation in a strategy we describe as ‘quasi-monopolar’ stimulation (QMP). In QMP stimulation, monopolar and hexapolar stimulation are delivered to the same stimulating electrode concurrently: one sub-threshold, monopolar stimulation to increase the propensity of the tissue to be activated by a second, hexapolar stimulation of low amplitude relative to hexapolar stimulation alone. The result is a substantial reduction in stimulation threshold with no significant reduction in focusing benefits from the hexapolar stimulation [37–39].

Conclusion

The initial proof-of-concept 24-channel prototype suprachoroidal implant clinical trial (2012–2014) has provided important information on the safety and efficacy of this approach. In particular, the work from Bionic Vision Australia has shown that it is possible to elicit useful phosphenes with a device that is further away from the retinal ganglion cells than an epiretinal array. Future work will now focus on providing a “take-home” device which will enable participants to benefit from training and rehabilitation, and devices with an increased number of electrodes and advanced stimulation capabilities.

References

1. Humayun MS, Dorn JD, da Cruz L, et al. Interim results from the international trial of Second Sight’s visual prosthesis. Ophthalmology. 2012;119(4):779–88.
2. Stingl K, Bartz-Schmidt KU, Besch D, et al. Artificial vision with wirelessly powered subretinal electronic implant alpha-IMS. Proc Biol Sci. 2013;280(1757):20130077.
3. Palanker D, Vankov A, Huie P, et al. Design of a high-resolution optoelectronic retinal prosthesis. J Neural Eng. 2005;2(1):S105–20.
4. Ayton LN, Blamey PJ, Guymer RH, et al. First-in-human trial of a novel suprachoroidal retinal prosthesis. PLoS One. 2014;9(12):e115239.
5. Fujikado T, Kamei M, Sakaguchi H, et al. Clinical trial of chronic implantation of suprachroidal-transretinal stimulation system for retinal prosthesis. Sensor Mater. 2012;24(4):181–7.
6. Hadjinicolaou AE, Leung RT, Garrett DJ, et al. Electrical stimulation of retinal ganglion cells with diamond and the development of an all diamond retinal prosthesis. Biomaterials. 2012;33(24):5812–20.
7. Garrett DJ, Saunders AL, McGowan C, et al. In vivo biocompatibility of boron doped and nitrogen included conductive-diamond for use in medical implants. J Biomed Mater Res B Appl Biomater. 2016;104(1):19–26.

8. Ganesan K, Garrett DJ, Ahnood A, et al. An all-diamond, hermetic electrical feedthrough array for a retinal prosthesis. Biomaterials. 2014;35(3):908–15.
9. Lichter SG, Escudie MC, Stacey AD, et al. Hermetic diamond capsules for biomedical implants enabled by gold active braze alloys. Biomaterials. 2015;53:464–74.
10. Buch H, Vinding T, La Cour M, et al. Prevalence and causes of visual impairment and blindness among 9980 Scandinavian adults: the Copenhagen City Eye Study. Ophthalmology. 2004;111(1):53–61.
11. Friedman DS, O'Colmain BJ, Munoz B, et al. Prevalence of age-related macular degeneration in the United States. Arch Ophthalmol. 2004;122(4):564–72.
12. Bressler NM. Age-related macular degeneration is the leading cause of blindness. JAMA. 2004;291(15):1900–1.
13. Rosenfeld PJ, Brown DM, Heier JS, et al. Ranibizumab for neovascular age-related macular degeneration. N Engl J Med. 2006;355(14):1419–31.
14. Perez Fornos A, Sommerhalder J, da Cruz L, et al. Temporal properties of visual perception on electrical stimulation of the retina. Invest Ophthalmol Vis Sci. 2012;53(6):2720–31.
15. Ray A, Lee EJ, Humayun MS, et al. Continuous electrical stimulation decreases retinal excitability but does not alter retinal morphology. J Neural Eng. 2011;8(4):045003.
16. Dacey DM, Petersen MR. Dendritic field size and morphology of midget and parasol ganglion cells of the human retina. Proc Natl Acad Sci U S A. 1992;89(20):9666–70.
17. Saunders AL, Williams CE, Heriot W, et al. Development of a surgical procedure for implantation of a prototype suprachoroidal retinal prosthesis. Clin Experiment Ophthalmol. 2014;42(7):665–74.
18. Sakaguchi H, Fujikado T, Fang X, et al. Transretinal electrical stimulation with a suprachoroidal multichannel electrode in rabbit eyes. Jpn J Ophthalmol. 2004;48(3):256–61.
19. Zhou JA, Woo SJ, Park SI, et al. A suprachoroidal electrical retinal stimulator design for long-term animal experiments and in vivo assessment of its feasibility and biocompatibility in rabbits. J Biomed Biotechnol. 2008;2008:547428.
20. Wong YT, Chen SC, Seo JM, et al. Focal activation of the feline retina via a suprachoroidal electrode array. Vision Res. 2009;49(8):825–33.
21. Fujikado T, Kamei M, Sakaguchi H, et al. Testing of semichronically implanted retinal prosthesis by suprachoroidal-transretinal stimulation in patients with retinitis pigmentosa. Invest Ophthalmol Vis Sci. 2011;52(7):4726–33.
22. Shepherd RK, Shivdasani MN, Nayagam DA, et al. Visual prostheses for the blind. Trends Biotechnol. 2013;31(10):562–71.
23. Villalobos J, Allen PJ, McCombe MF, et al. Development of a surgical approach for a wide-view suprachoroidal retinal prosthesis: evaluation of implantation trauma. Graefes Arch Clin Exp Ophthalmol. 2012;250(3):399–407.
24. Cicione R, Shivdasani MN, Fallon JB, et al. Visual cortex responses to suprachoroidal electrical stimulation of the retina: effects of electrode return configuration. J Neural Eng. 2012;9(3):036009.
25. Shivdasani MN, Fallon JB, Luu CD, et al. Visual cortex responses to single- and simultaneous multiple-electrode stimulation of the retina: implications for retinal prostheses. Invest Ophthalmol Vis Sci. 2012;53(10):6291–300.
26. Shivdasani MN, Luu CD, Cicione R, et al. Evaluation of stimulus parameters and electrode geometry for an effective suprachoroidal retinal prosthesis. J Neural Eng. 2010;7(3):036008.
27. Villalobos J, Nayagam DA, Allen PJ, et al. A wide-field suprachoroidal retinal prosthesis is stable and well tolerated following chronic implantation. Invest Ophthalmol Vis Sci. 2013;54(5):3751–62.
28. Leung RT, Nayagam DA, Williams RA, et al. Safety and efficacy of explanting or replacing suprachoroidal electrode arrays in a feline model. Clin Experiment Ophthalmol. 2015;43(3):247–58.
29. Nayagam DA, Williams RA, Allen PJ, et al. Chronic electrical stimulation with a suprachoroidal retinal prosthesis: a preclinical safety and efficacy study. PLoS One. 2014;9(5):e97182.

30. Ayton LN, Guymer RH, Luu CD. Choroidal thickness profiles in retinitis pigmentosa. Clin Experiment Ophthalmol. 2013;41(4):396–403.
31. Shivdasani MN, Sinclair NC, Dimitrov PN, et al. Factors affecting perceptual thresholds in a suprachoroidal retinal prosthesis. Invest Ophthalmol Vis Sci. 2014;55(10):6467–81.
32. Ayton LN, McSweeney SC, O'Hare F, et al. A prototype suprachoroidal retinal prosthesis enables improvement in a tabletop object detection task. Invest Ophthal Vis Sci. 2015;56(7):4782.
33. Ayton LN, Finger RP, Deverell L, et al. Developing a very low vision orientation and mobility test battery as part of the Low Vision Assessment of Daily Activities (LoVADA) protocol. Optom Vis Sci. 2016. [Epub ahead of print].
34. Finger RP, Tellis B, Crewe J, et al. Developing the impact of vision impairment-very low vision (IVI-VLV) questionnaire as part of the LoVADA protocol. Invest Ophthalmol Vis Sci. 2014;55(10):6150–8.
35. Suaning GJ, Hallum LE, Preston P, et al. An efficient multiplexing method for addressing large numbers of electrodes in a visual neuroprosthesis. Conf Proc IEEE Eng Med Biol Soc. 2004;2:4165–8.
36. Lovell NH, Dokos S, Cheng E, et al. Simulation of parallel current injection for use in a vision prosthesis. Conf Proc IEEE Eng Med Biol Soc. 2005; 458–61.
37. Matteucci PB, Chen SC, Tsai D, et al. Current steering in retinal stimulation via a quasimonopolar stimulation paradigm. Invest Ophthalmol Vis Sci. 2013;54(6):4307–20.
38. Abramian M, Lovell NH, Habib A, et al. Quasi-monopolar electrical stimulation of the retina: a computational modelling study. J Neural Eng. 2014;11(2):025002.
39. Habib AG, Cameron MA, Suaning GJ, et al. Spatially restricted electrical activation of retinal ganglion cells in the rabbit retina by hexapolar electrode return configuration. J Neural Eng. 2013;10(3):036013.

Chapter 11
Retinal Prosthesis by Suprachoroidal-Transretinal Stimulation (STS), Japanese Approach

Takashi Fujikado

Abstract The Consortium for Retinal Prosthesis in Japan has developed a new method to stimulate the retina called suprachoroidal-transretinal stimulation (STS). The original plan for the STS retinal prosthesis was to insert the stimulating electrode array in the suprachoroidal space and the return electrode in the vitreous cavity. The transretinal currents would then stimulate the functioning retinal neurons. However, experiments showed that the stability of the electrode array was better when it was fixed inside a scleral pocket so currently we implant the electrode array in a scleral pocket which is adjacent to the suprachoroidal space. The semichronic clinical trial was done using the first generation STS system by nine active electrodes on two patients with advanced RP. The results showed that grasping an object task is possible by prosthetic vision using STS ststem. At present we are doing clinical trial using second generation STS system using 49 channel electrode on three patients with advanced RP. In future, we are planning to implant multiple electrode array using STS system to expand the visual field for walking.

Keywords STS system • Retinal implant • Retinitis pigmentosa • Multiple electrode array • Walking

Key Points

- A new method of retinal prosthesis called suprachoroidal-transretinal stimulation (STS) inserts the stimulating electrode array in the scleral pocket and the return electrode in the vitreous cavity.
- The semichronic clinical trial for advanced retinitis pigmentosa by STS system using nine active electrodes showed that grasping an object task was possible.
- Clinical trial by second generation STS system using 49 channel electrodes is underway.

T. Fujikado, MD, PhD
Department of Applied Visual Science, Osaka University Graduate School of Medicine, Suita, Osaka, Japan
e-mail: fujikado@ophthal.med.osaka-u.ac.jp

V.P. Gabel (ed.), *Artificial Vision*, DOI 10.1007/978-3-319-41876-6_11

Principal Idea

The Consortium for Retinal Prosthesis in Japan has developed a new method to stimulate the retina called suprachoroidal-transretinal stimulation (STS) [1, 2]. The orignal plan for the STS retinal prosthesis was to insert the stimulating electrode array in the suprachoroidal space [3] and the return electrode in the vitreous cavity. The transretinal currents would then stimulate the functioning retinal neurons. However, experiments showed that the stability of the electrode array was better when it was fixed inside a scleral pocket so currently we implant the electrode array in a scleral pocket which is adjacent to the suprachoroidal space (Fig. 11.1a, b).

The total system is schematically shown in Fig. 11.2. In the external system, a charge-coupled device (CCD) video camera is attached to spectacles. The camera records the images of the outside world, and the signals created by the images are transmitted wirelessly to the internal system. The position of the internal system is shown in Fig. 11.3 in the X-ray image taken after implanting the internal system. The electric power is also transmitted by the same wireless system. In the internal system, the transmitted signals are decoded to analogue signals and electrical

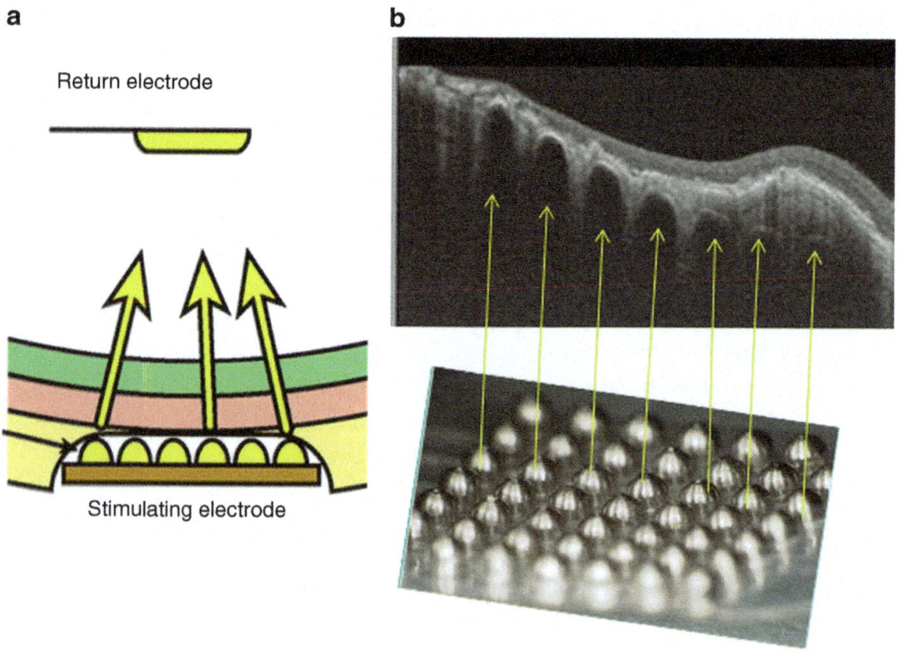

Fig. 11.1 Schema (**a**) and Optical coherence tomographic (OCT) image (**b**) of the STS retinal prosthesis. (**a**) The stimulating electrode array is inserted in a scleral pocket adjacent to the suprachoroidal space and the return electrode is inserted into the vitreous cavity. The retinal currents then pass through the retina and stimulate the functioning neurons effectively. (**b**) OCT image of an eye implanted with electrode array 6 months after surgery. Each electrode is embedded at posterior pole and held tightly in the scleral pocket with the tip adjacent to the suprachoroidal space

currents are sent to the individual electrodes using with the strength of the currents related to the signal strength.

In our STS system, the return electrode is placed in the vitreous cavity so the transretinal electrical current can be confined and stimulate the functional retinal neurons effectively. We developed an optical imaging system in the retina to identify the retinal activated area by the electrical current [4]. The results of a cat study with an implanted STS system and an optical imaging system showed that the area of retinal activation was 20–30 % smaller when the return electrode was set in the vitreous cavity than in an extraocular position (Fig. 11.4). In addition, the threshold current for eliciting a potential from the visual cortex by the STS was comparable to that by other electrode systems in animals [2].

The resolution of the images might be lower with the STS prosthesis because the electrodes were located some distance from the retina. However, the advantage of the STS prosthesis over epi- or sub-retinal prostheses is the safety of the surgical procedures because the electrodes do not touch the retina and are stably fixed in the

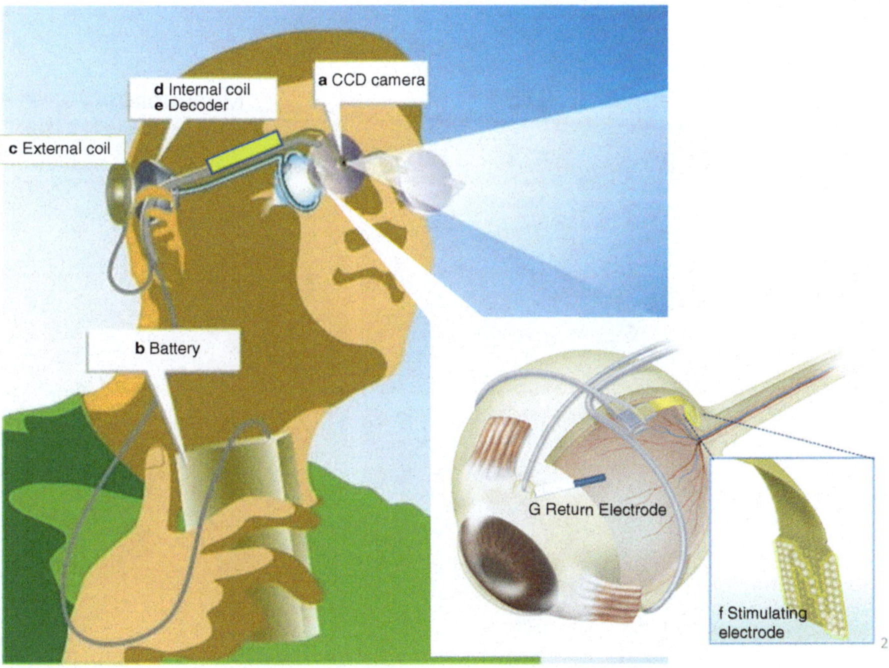

Fig. 11.2 Schema of the external and internal system of STS prosthesis. (**a**) A charge-coupled device (CCD) video camera is mounted on spectacles records the objects in the visual field, and the signals are processed by a small computer which is attached to the temple of spectacles. (**b**) The battery pack is suspended from the shoulder or neck of the patients. (**c**) The external coil is attached to an area behind one ear using a magnet. (**d, e**) Internal coil and decoder are fixed to the temporal bone. (**f**) Stimulating electrode array is implanted in the scleral pocket. (**g**) Return electrode is implanted in the vitreous cavity

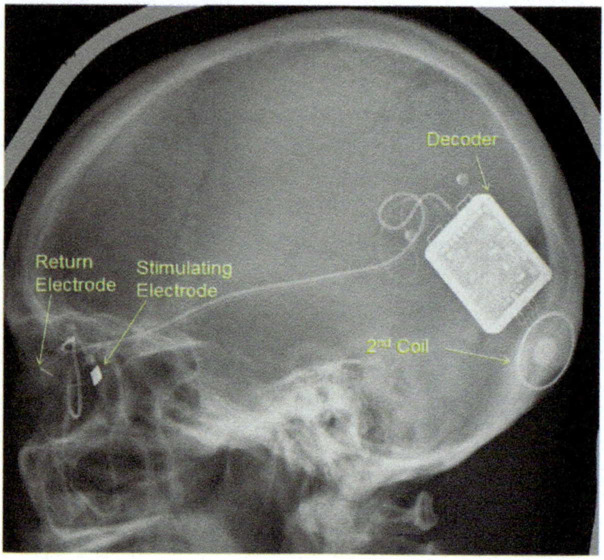

Fig. 11.3 Lateral view of the skull XP after implantation surgery. Decoder and internal coil are fixed on the temporal bone and the stimulating and return electrodes are implanted in the eye

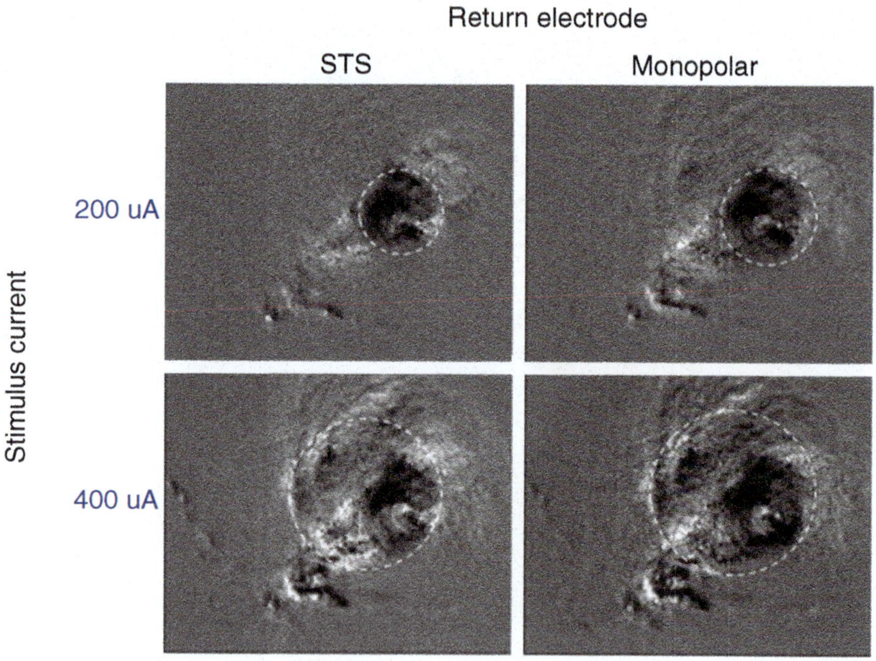

Fig. 11.4 Retinal activated area using optical imaging (STS vs Monopolar) Retinal reflectance change by near infrared light was recorded in response to the electrical stimulation using single electrode attached to the fenestrated sclera in a cat. The dark area represents the area of retinal activation. The activated area was restricted in cases with return electrode inserted in the vitreous cavity (STS) compared with it attached to the skin of the forehead (Monopolar)

scleral pocket. Based on the safety of this approach, the STS system has been adopted by several other groups [5, 6].

Indications for Certain Forms of Blindness

Because the number of electrodes is limited to 49 in the current STS model prosthesis in Japan, the spatial resolution is not high. Therefore, the implantation is limited to patients whose visual acuity is equal to or less than hand motion (HM) vision in both eyes.

A common requirement for the implantation of the STS retinal prosthesis is that the retinal neurons other than the photoreceptors should be functioning. Therefore, retinal diseases such as advanced retinitis pigmentosa (RP), advanced Stargardt disease, and advanced autoimmune retinopathy are diseases in which the STS system might be useful.

We are planning to implant multiple electrode arrays to enlarge the visual field (Fig. 11.5) [7]. For this, the indications for STS prosthesis may be expanded to those patients with advanced RP with only a small residual visual field. Patient could use the artificial vision for identifying the location of objects quickly and use the residual vision for identifying things thereafter.

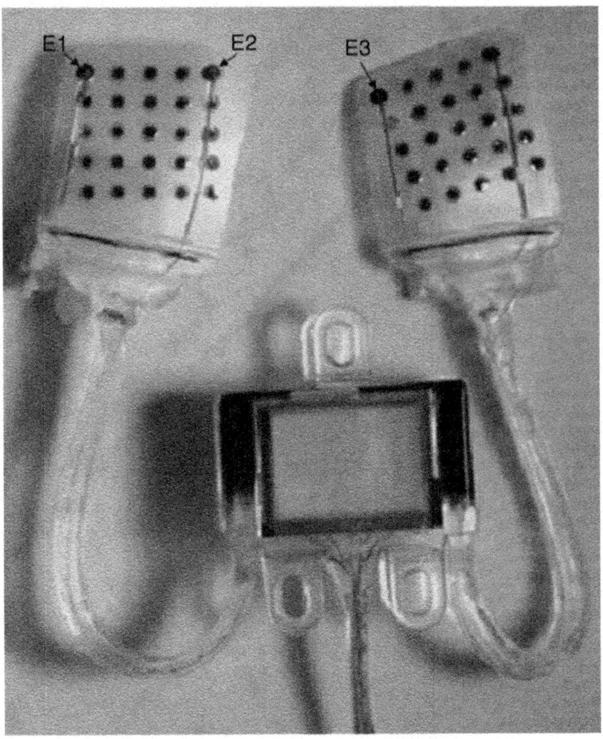

Fig. 11.5 Photographs of wide-field, dual-array STS devices (Photograph showing dual-array STS electrodes used in the animal experiments)

Technical Description

The implanted electronic devices consist of a secondary coil which receives signals from the external coil and a decoder which generates biphasic pulses to deliver to the individual electrodes sequentially (Fig. 11.6). The size of the electrode array is 5.7×4.6 mm (Nidek, Gamabori, Japan) and consisted of 49 electrodes made of 0.5 mm diameter platinum wire. The center-to-center separation of a pair of electrode was 0.7 mm. Each electrode protruded from the silicon base by 0.5 mm. The return electrode was a 0.5 mm diameter, 6 mm long platinum wire that is insulated except for 3 mm of the tip.

Surgical Procedures

To determine the optimal site to implant the internal STS array, the lateral rectus muscle is dissected at its insertion under local anesthesia. Then, transscleral monopolar stimuli were delivered to determine the scleral area that consistently evoked low threshold phosphenes [8]. After identifying and marking the low threshold area, the patient was placed under general anesthesia. The skin over the left temporal bone was incised to insert the electronic devices. A second skin incision was made

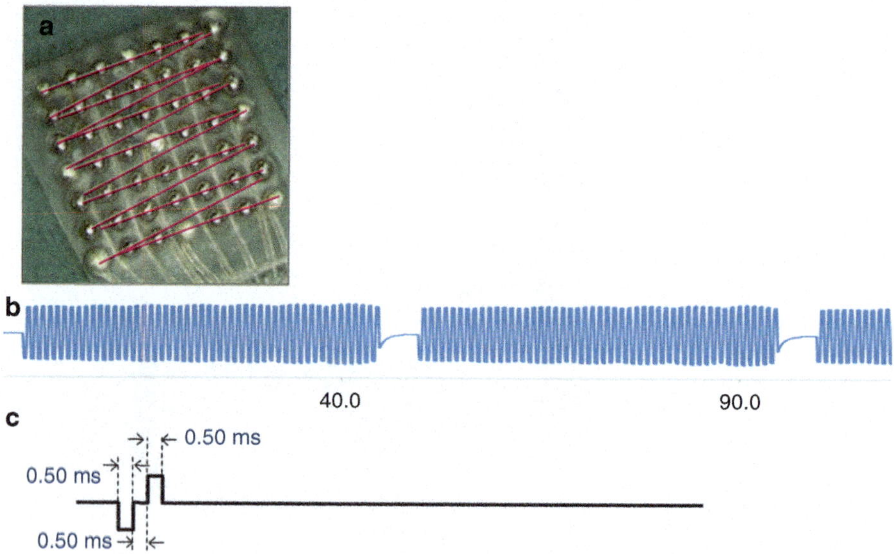

Fig. 11.6 Stimulus sequence of 49-channel electrode array. (**a**) Photograph of a 49-channel electrode array superimposed by bars representing the stimulus sequence. Stimulation starts from the upper left electrode and ends at the lower right electrode. (**b**) Representative waveforms of the stimulus artifacts derived from each of 49 electrodes sequentially at the cornea in an animal experiment. (**c**) Time scale of the biphasic pulse applied to each electrode

over the left zygomatic bone to fix the cable. The electrode array and the return electrode were passed under the fascia of the temporal muscle from the first incision to the second incision through a trocar catheter.

Before the electrode array was implanted in the scleral pocket, the bone of the lateral orbital wall was drilled, and the return electrode and cable were passed into the periocular space using a trocar catheter. The cable with its protective covering was fixed by a titanium plate below the second incision. The electrode array and cable were circled around the equator of the eye passing under the four recti muscles.

A scleral pocket of 6×5 mm was made at the temporal to lower-temporal scleral area where the phosphenes were elicited. The 49 electrode array was placed in the scleral pocket [9] (Fig. 11.7) and secured with sutures that passed through the protective silicone cover around the junction of the electrode array and the cable [9]. The return electrode was inserted into the vitreous cavity through the upper nasal pars plana area.

After suturing the conjuntival incision, the electronic device was fixed to the temporal bone and the skin was sutured.

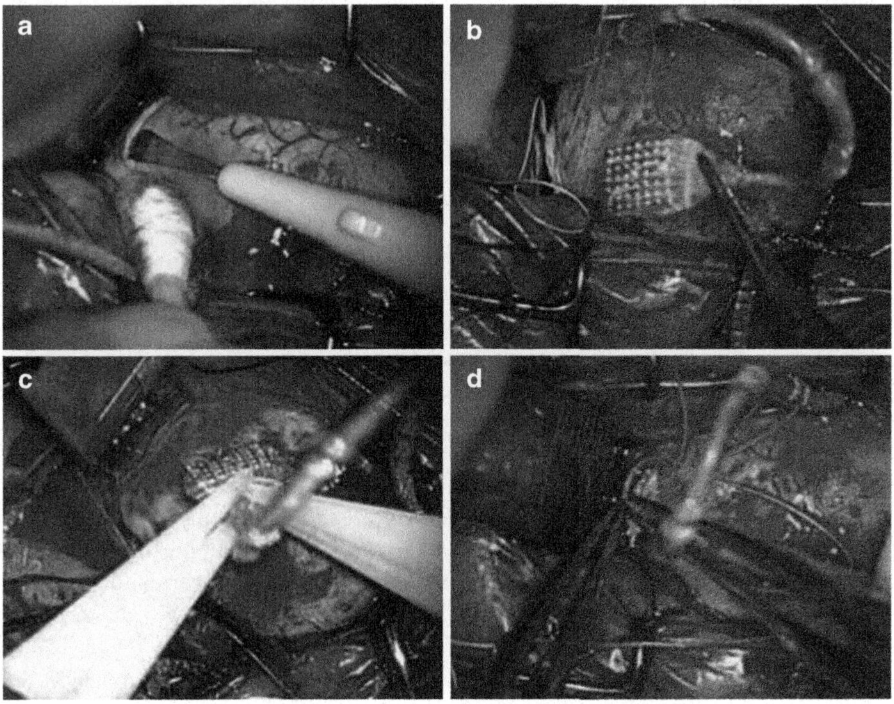

Fig. 11.7 Photographs of surgical procedures during the implantation of the electrode array. (**a**) Creating a scleral pocket. (**b**) Holding the electrode array. (**c**) Grasping the electrode array for insertion. (**d**) Inserting the electrode array into the scleral pocket (Reprinted from Fujikado et al. [9]. With permission from Association For Research In Vision And Ophthalmology)

Pilot Clinical Study

Two eyes of two patients with advanced RP have had the STS retinal prosthesis implanted for 1 month [8]. The visual acuity of both eyes before the implantation was light perception.

Functional Testing of Each Electrode

Nine of the 49 electrodes were tested to determine that they were able to stimulate retinal neurons. The distance between adjacent active electrode was 2.1 mm. To identify the position of the phosphene, a plastic board (65 × 65 cm) was set in front of a patient at a distance of 40 cm. The patient was instructed to put her right index finger on the position of the perceived phosphene while the left index finger was positioned on a pad glued to the center of the board (Fig. 11.8).

Electrical pulses from any one of the 9 electrode array elicited localized phosphenes which were reproducible for each of the 6 channels in Patient 1 and for 4 channels in Patient 2 with current ≤ 1 mA. The size of the phosphene varied from the size of pea to a quarter coin at arm's distance depending on the channel stimulated in both patients. The phosphenes were perceived mostly in the upper nasal field, which is consistent with the position of the stimulating electrodes in the inferior temporal quadrant (Fig. 11.8).

Functional Testing with Video Camera

The patients performed visual tasks using a commercial video camera as the detector of the visual objects. The camera was attached to a headband, and an eye mask was placed over the both eyes during the testing. Because the field of view of the camera was approximately 16.7° and the implant covered 14.3°, the visual angle subtended by an object on the retina was reduced by a factor 1.2.

The objects viewed by the camera were converted to a 3 × 3 squares with 40 × 40 pixels, and if the light level was above threshold, the square was expressed as white (on), and when the light level was below the threshold, the square was expressed as black (off). The information of the square was converted to an electrical signal and sent to the secondary coil through the external coil. The activated electrodes were channels (Chs) 2 to 8 (7 electrodes) in Patient 1, and Chs 1, 2, 3, 4, and 7 (5 electrodes) in Patient 2. Both patients scored better than chance in the object detection and object discrimination tasks with head scanning. Patient 2 scored (90 %) better than chance in detecting the direction of motion task but Patient 1 scored (60 %) which was not significantly better than chance. The task of grasping objects was carried out by Patient 2 because the elicited phosphene was

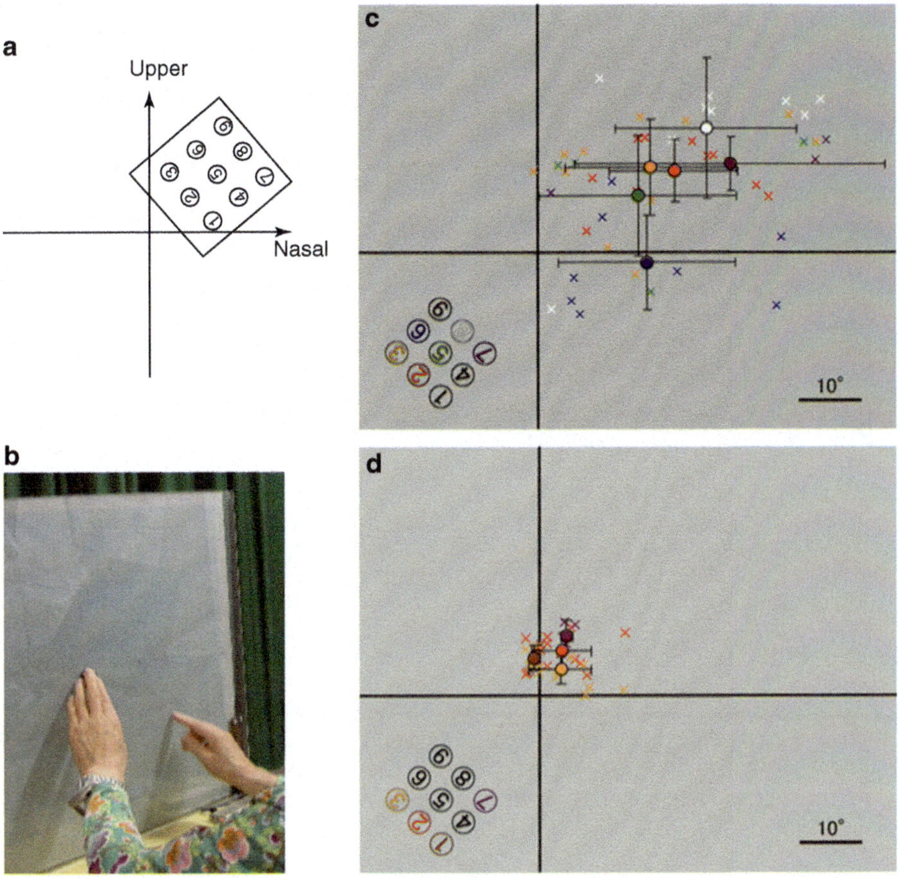

Fig. 11.8 Mapping the position of the perceived phosphenes. (**a**) Schematic map of the perceived phosphenes in response to the stimulation of individual electrodes. The estimated position of the phosphenes when each electrode is stimulated and normal topographical organization exists between the retina and visual cortex. (**b**) Method of recording the position of the phosphenes in relation to the center of the body. The left index finger is positioned at the center of the board, and the right index finger is placed at the position of the perceived phosphene. (**c**) The phosphene maps of Patient 1. The results of multiple trials are superimposed. The *colored circles* indicate the gravitational center of the responses to the stimulation of the individual channels. The *bars* indicate the standard deviations. (**d**) The phosphene map of Patient 2 (Reprinted from Fujikado et al. [9]. With permission from Association For Research In Vision And Ophthalmology)

located close to the subjective center. The score (90 %) was significantly better than chance. The success rate of behavioral tasks with the electrical stimulator off was less than the chance level for each task in both patients. The touch panel task was applied to only Patient 2. The subjective phosphene was perceived slightly to the right of the bar when presented on the right side and shifted to the left of the bar when presented on left side. The success rate increased with repeated testing (Fig. 11.9).

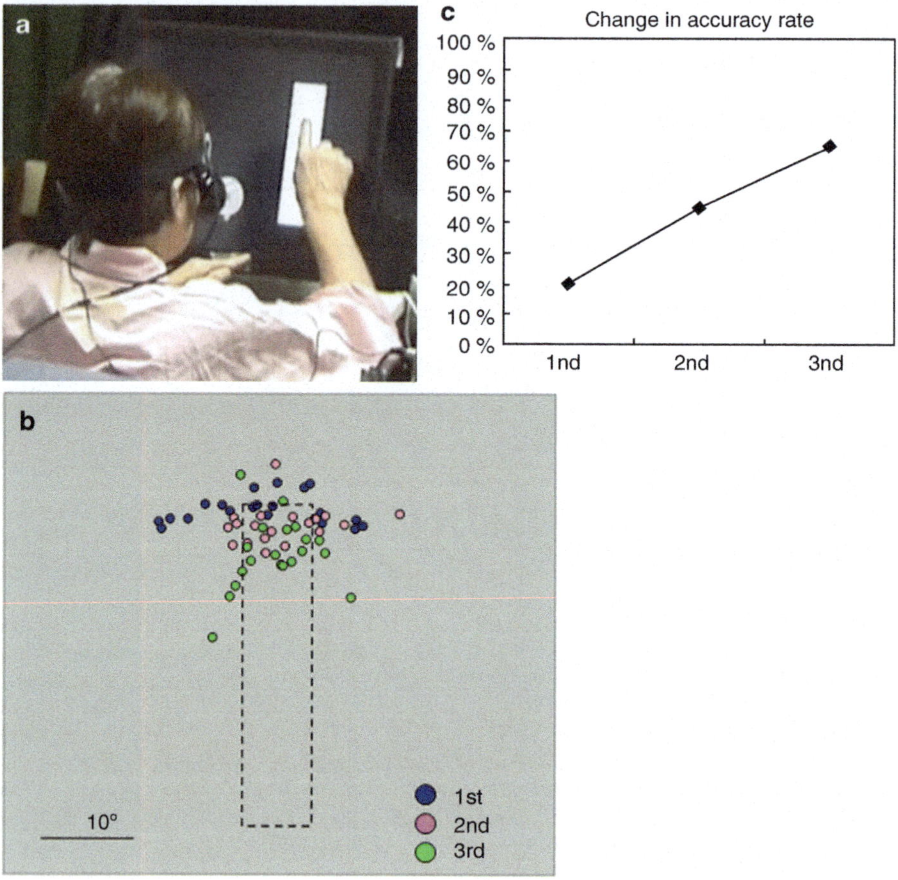

Fig. 11.9 Results of the touching the panel task in Patient 2. (**a**) Patients are instructed to touch the white bar presented on the touch panel. The panel has an auditory system and if a patient touch the bar, a sound comes from the panel. (**b**) The touched positions of patient 2. The *dashed rectangular area* represents the position of the white bar. *Blue dots* represent the touched position at first 20 trials, *pink dots* represent at the second 20 trials, and the *green dots* represent at the third 20 trials. (**c**) The success rate increased with the repetition of the trials. (**b**, **c** Reprinted from Fujikado et al. [9]. With permission from Association For Research In Vision And Ophthalmology)

Future Direction

49-Channel STS System

At present, we are performing a clinical trial using a second generation STS System in three patients with advanced RP. In this system, the number of electrode was increased from 9 (first generation) to 49 by introducing a multiplexer system [10]. The surface of the electrodes were fabricated by a femtosecond laser to enlarge the surface area, and each electrode protruded from the silicon base by 0.3 mm, which is 0.2 mm less than the first generation STS system.

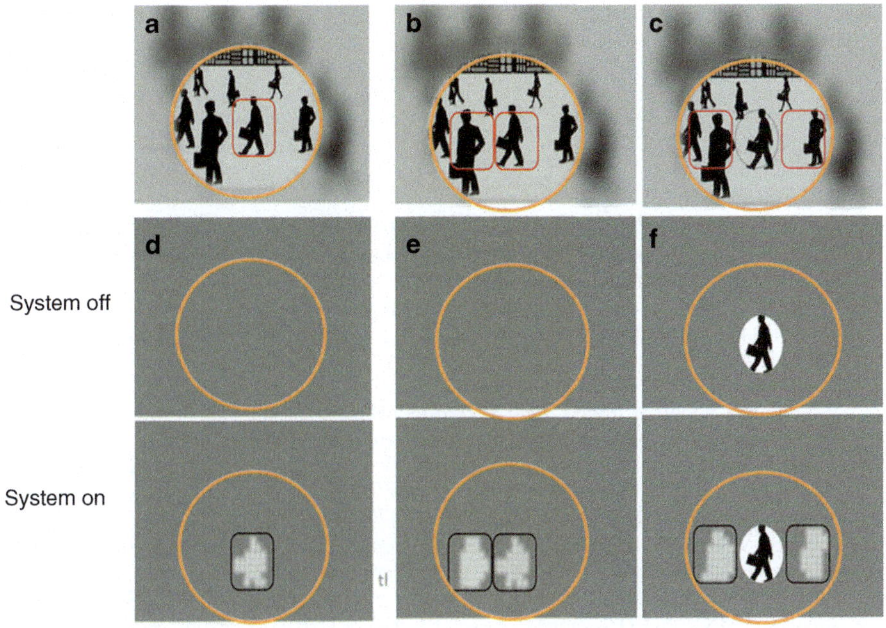

Fig. 11.10 Schematic drawing of images perceived by patients with advanced RP with implanted STS retinal prosthesis. (**a**–**c**) Images recorded by CCD camera. *Orange circle* represents the scene recorded by a CCD camera and *red square* represents the area to stimulate the electrode array using single array in a total blind patient (**a**), dual array in a total blind patient (**b**), and dual array in a patient with residual visual field (**c**). *Blue circle* in (**c**) represents the residual visual field. (**d**–**f**) Simulated images perceived by patients with system off (*upper column*) and system on (*lower column*). Visual field is enlarged in a case with dual array compared with single array. In patients with residual visual field, dual array enlarges the peripheral visual field adjacent to the residual visual field. *Black square* represents the visual field obtained by prosthetic vision

Multiple Array System

In the third generation STS system, we are planning to increase the number of electrode array from one to two (Fig. 11.5). The results of animal experiments showed that two electrode arrays can be implanted safely in the scleral pocket and the electrical current can stimulate retinal neuron using multiplexer system [7]. With this system, the visual field of patients can be expanded from about 15° (1 array) to about 30° (2 arrays), which allows patients to walk without head scanning. When implanted in patients with small residual visual filed, patients can use the residual vision for the central target and get information of the peripheral visual field using prosthetic vision (Fig. 11.10). Under these conditions, the eye tracking system is necessary to match the residual vision and the prosthetic vision.

Acknowledgements We appreciate Drs. Motohiro Kamei, Hirokazu Sakaguchi, Kentaro Nishida, Takeshi Morimoto, Haruhiko Kishima, Tomoyuki Maruo to develop the surgical method for implanting the STS prosthesis (Osaka University). We appreciate Takao Endo, Hirokazu Hirota to develop the evaluation system of phsphene. We appreciate Drs. Motoki Ozawa, Kunihiko konoma,

Koji Osawa to supply the STS devises (Nidek Company). We also appreciate Dr. Hiroyuki Kanda for the preparation of figures (Osaka University).

References

1. Kanda H, Morimoto T, Fujikado T, Tano Y, Fukuda Y, Sawai H. Electrophysiological studies on the feasibility of suprachoroidal-transretinal stimulation for artificial vision in normal and RCS rat. Invest Ophthalmol Vis Sci. 2004;45:560–6.
2. Nakauchi K, Fujikado T, Kanda H, et al. Transretinal electrical stimulation by an intrascleral multichannel electrode array in rabbit eyes. Graefes Arch Clin Exp Ophthalmol. 2005;243:169–74.
3. Sakaguchi H, Fujikado T, Fang X, Kanda H, Osanai M, Nakauchi K, Ikuno Y, Kamei M, Yagi T, Nishimura S, Ohji M, Yagi T, Tano Y. Transretinal electrical stimulation with a suprachoroidal multichannel electrode in rabbit eyes. Jpn J Ophthalmol. 2004;48:256–61.
4. Okawa Y, Fujikado T, Miyoshi T, Sawai H, Kusaka S, Mihashi T, Hirohara Y, Tano Y. Optical imaging to evaluate retinal activation by electrical currents using suprachoroidal-transretinal stimulation. Invest Ophthalmol Vis Sci. 2007;48:4777–84.
5. Zhou JA, Woo SJ, Park SI, Kim ET, Seo JM, Chung H, Kim SJ. A suprachoroidal electrical retinal stimulator design for long-term animal experiments and in vivo assessment of its feasibility and biocompatibility in rabbits. J Biomed Biotechnol. 2008;2008:547428.
6. Shivdasani MN, Luu CD, Cicione R, Fallon JB, Allen PJ, et al. Evaluation of stimulus parameters and electrode geometry for an effective suprachoroidal retinal prosthesis. J Neural Eng. 2010;7:036008.
7. Lohmann TK, Kanda H, Morimoto T, Endo T, Miyoshi T, Nishida K, Kamei M, Walter P, Fujikado T. Surgical feasibility and biocompatibility of wide-field dual-array suprachoroidal-transretinal stimulation prosthesis in middle-sized animals. Graefes Arch Clin Exp Ophthalmol. 2016;254:661–73.
8. Fujikado T, Morimoto T, Kanda H, et al. Evaluation of phosphenes elicited by extraocular stimulation in normals and by suprachoroidal-transretinal stimulation in patients with retinitis pigmentosa. Graefes Arch Clin Exp Ophthalmol. 2007;245:1411–9.
9. Fujikado T, Kamei M, Sakaguchi H, Kanda H, Morimoto T, Ikuno Y, Nishida K, Kishima H, Maruo T, Konoma K, Ozawa M, Nishida K. Testing of semi-chronically implanted retinal prosthesis by suprachoroidal-transretinal stimulation in patients with retinitis pigmentosa. Invest Ophthalmol Vis Sci. 2011;52:4726–33.
10. Fujikado T, Kamei M, Sakaguchi H, Kanda H, Morimoto T, Nishida K, Kishima H, Maruo T, Oosawa K, Ozawa M, Nishida K. Feasibility of 2nd generation STS retinal prosthesis in dogs. Conf Proc IEEE Eng Med Biol Soc. 2013;2013:3119–21.

Chapter 12
A Fully Intraocular Approach for a Bi-Directional Retinal Prosthesis

Peter Walter

Abstract Because cable connections between a retinal stimulator inside the eye and external electronic components may be hazardous we developed a fully wireless intraocular retinal prosthesis and performed a clinical trial to prove the concept. We also developed concepts and tools to improve the stimulation efficacy and specificity by simultaneous recording of neural activity in the retina with such a device. This chapter demonstrates the technical and surgical concepts of the fully intraocular prosthesis, results from the clinical trial and experimental results form the development of a bi-directional retinal stimulator.

Keywords Action potentials • Amacrine cells • Animal models • Bi-directional retinal prosthesis • Blindness • Capacity coupled electrical stimulation • Extracellular recording • Retinal ganglion cells • Retinitis pigmentosa

Abbreviations

ASIC	Application specific integrated circuit
ASK	Amplitude shift keying
BIMEA	Bi-directional multielectrode array
CMOS	Complementory metal oxide semiconductor
PDMS	Polydimethylsiloxane
RGC	Retinal ganglion cell
RIS	Retina Implant System
RP	Retinitis pigmentosa
VLARS	Very large array retina stimulator

P. Walter
Department of Ophthalmology, University Hospital RWTH Aachen, Aachen, NRW, Germany
e-mail: pwalter@ukaachen.de

V.P. Gabel (ed.), *Artificial Vision*, DOI 10.1007/978-3-319-41876-6_12

Key Points
- Retinal stimulators can be fabricated as fully intraocular devices without any cable connection between the implant and external components.
- Recording of retinal neural activity with implants used for stimulation can help to improve stimulation algorithms and to adapt the stimulation parameters to the individual situation
- Prototypes for implantable bi-directional multielectrode arrays and the corresponding complex electronics are under development

Principle Idea

Retinal prostheses are intended to electrically stimulate the retina in situations where the photoreceptors are lost due to inherited diseases such as Retinitis pigmentosa (RP) or other causes of outer retinal degeneration. The basic concepts for retinal prostheses were designed some 20 years ago and after successful preclinical tests and functional experiments the first devices were approved for clinical use and are now being implanted in a number of blind patients [1–10].

For all currently approved and for the majority of discussed retinal stimulators the electrode arrays inside the eye are physically connected with a cable to electronic components outside the eye to provide the implants with energy and/or with data. Such a cable connection may cause adverse events such as infection or conjunctival erosion and in some instances these problems may be a reason to remove such an implant. Furthermore, in case of severe infections the globe may be lost due to the consequences of endophthalmitis. Therefore we designed a retinal stimulator without any cable connection between the parts inside the eye and the parts outside the eye. In brief, the electrode array placed onto the retinal surface is connected to an artificial intraocular lens carrying some miniaturized electronic components together with a receiver coil for capturing signals sent from a transmitter coil in front of the eye. The connection between the transmitter and implant is fully wirelessly. The transmitter received its data from a video processing unit calculating stimulation pulses based on a camera picture. The system provides the technology platform for a bi-directional enhancement. In this scenario the electrodes are not only stimulating but also recording network activity of neurons within the degenerated retina. Data on the network activity is used to modify the stimulation algorithm to achieve a much better stimulation efficacy and specificity (Fig. 12.1).

Indication for Certain Forms of Blindness

As any other epiretinal or subretinal retinal implant this device is designed to treat blindness resulting from photoreceptor degeneration such as in Retinitis pigmentosa (RP) or similar diseases.

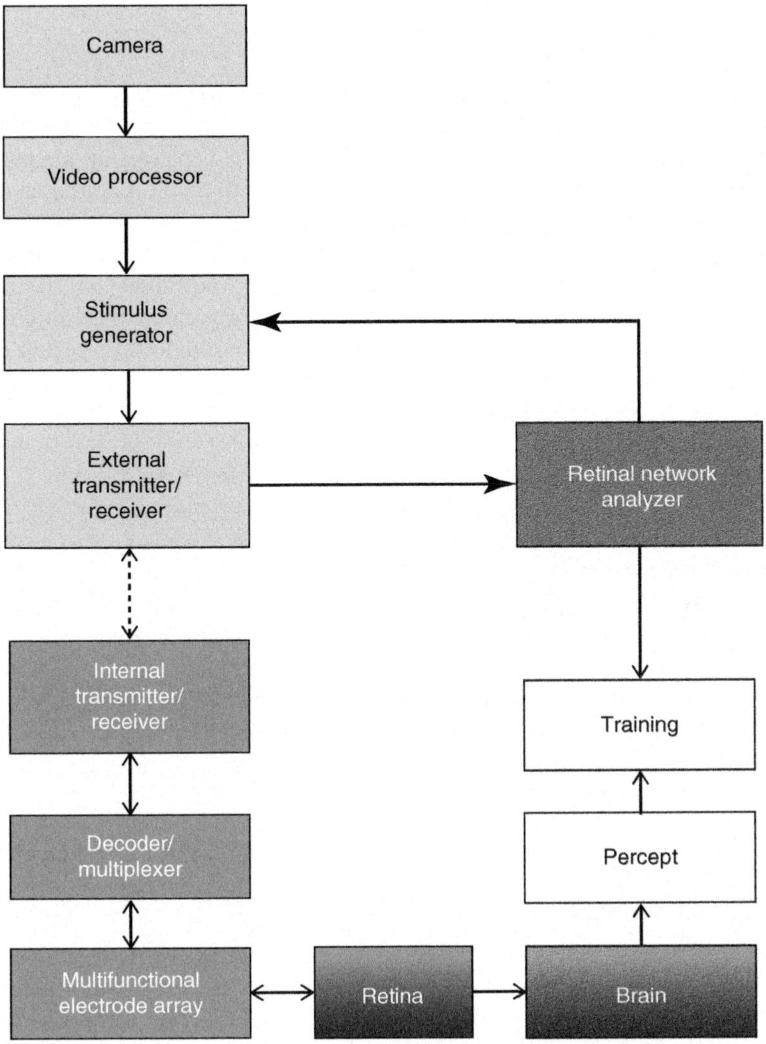

Fig. 12.1 Block diagram of the enhanced EPIRET concept for a fully intraocular retinal prosthesis. Visual data is captured by a video camera. The signal is processed by a Video Processor calculating the spatiotemporal stimulus pulse pattern for the implanted electrode array. This data package is sent wirelessly to the implant via an external transmitter/receiver. The implant itself consists of another receiver/transmitter module capturing the stimulation pattern information. It is decoded, stimulus pulses are generated within the implanted electronics and the pulses are distributed to the electrode array via a multiplexer. Thus the retina is stimulated leading to activation of the visual cortex in the brain. The percept is analyzed in a training process and matched to the visual stimulus. The implanted electrode array is also able to record action potentials and field potentials from the retina. This data is sent back from the eye to the external electronics where it is used in a Retinal Network Analyzer. The processed data is then used to modify the algorithm how the camera data is transferred to the stimulus pattern

Technical Description

The basic system is based on the EPIRET technology which is a fully intraocular epiretinal retina implant system. It consists of a CMOS camera to capture the visual information, a visual processor to extract and calculate a spatiotemporal pattern of stimulation pulses, a wireless transmission system with a coil working as a transmission antenna in front of the eye, and the intraocular implant. The implant itself consists of a receiver embedded into a semiflexible artificial intraocular lens with a diameter of 11 mm. The inductive link between the transmitter and the receiver provides enough energy to drive the implant. The information concerning the spatiotemporal stimulation pulse pattern is realized by amplitude shift keying (ASK). The receiver antenna is also integrated into the lens. The receiver is placed into the posterior chamber of the eye and is connected with a flexible cable to the stimulator. The stimulator itself is placed onto the inner surface of the retina. It is fixated here using one or more retinal tacks. The base material of the implant is polyimide, the stimulating electrodes are gold electrodes covered by plasma activated iridium oxide. For the proof of concept study in blind human volunteers the system was provided with 25 active electrodes. The housing of the receiver was PDMS (Polydimethylsiloxane) and a secure insulation was achieved with Parylene C [11].

As a new innovative method we designed and fabricated a circuit for pulsed charge controlled stimulation. The method is based on pumping very small charge quanta into the tissue with ultrahigh frequencies [12]. By this approach we prevent large stimulation artifacts when simultaneously recording retinal activity during or directly after the stimulation. These responses give insight into the type of responses obtained upon stimulation in certain retinal areas (Fig. 12.2).

Surgical Methods

The EPIRET device is a fully intraocular device. It requires removal of the natural lens or of a previously implanted artificial lens. It further requires a full vitrectomy with removal of epiretinal membranes if necessary. Triamcinolone could be helpful to identify cortical vitreous still left on the retina after a core vitrectomy. Because of possible tractional forces in the anterior vitreous during the insertion process we strongly recommend to remove the anterior vitreous s much as possible under indentation. Then a limbal corneal incision is made or enlarged to insert the 11 mm lens type receiver in the sulcus ciliaris. In certain cases it could be helpful to fixate the receiver with supporting transscleral sutures, e.g. after removal of intraocular lenses with a fibrotic capsular bag where it is not possible to keep the capsular structures. Then the cable with the stimulator head is pushed underneath the receiver into the eye's cavity. The stimulator is guided through an opening in the posterior capsula in those cases where the posterior capsula is still intact. The corneal incision is closed and the stimulator head is moved onto the retinal surface. Once the

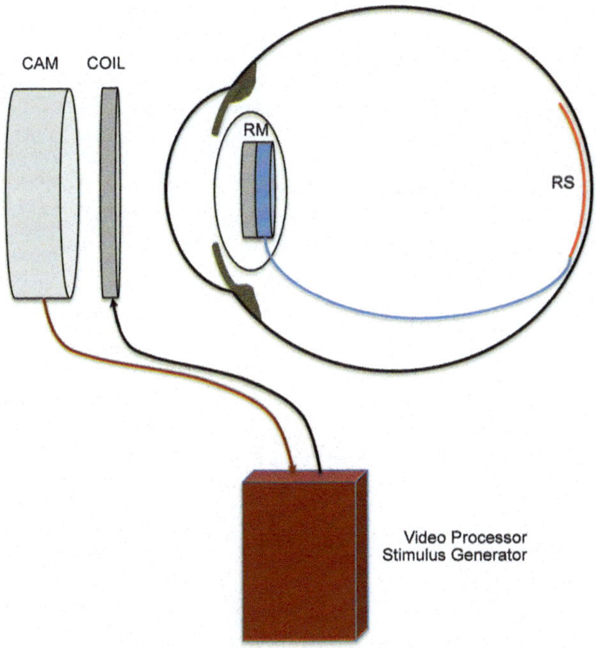

Fig. 12.2 General concept of the EPIRET technology platform. The camera is connected to the Video Processor linked to a Stimulus generator. Information on the stimulus pattern is transmitted via an external coil to the receiver module (RM) of the implant. RM consists of the receiver antenna or coil, the receiver electronics for decoding of the information and a programmable stimulus generator. The stimulus generator is connected to each of the electrodes in the Retina Stimulator RS placed onto the retinal surface

stimulator is in place it is fixated here using standard retinal tacks. The stimulator head offers several openings in its base structure to place the tacks. Surgery should be finished with a fluid air exchange. Figure 12.3 explains the major steps of the implantation procedure.

Clinical Study

The basic EPIRET system was implanted in one eye of six blind volunteers with RP. The trial was registered within the German Clinical Trial Register under DE/CA21/A/07/Dr. Schmidt IOL/EPIRET III. In all six patients the implantation was done without any intraoperative complications. In all cases the stimulator was placed on the central retina and two tacks were used to achieve a stable position onto the retina. Postoperatively in one case a culture negative hypopion was seen. It responded quickly to local and systemic steroids and antibiotics. Activation of the system was done after 1 week, after 2 weeks and after 4 weeks. The system

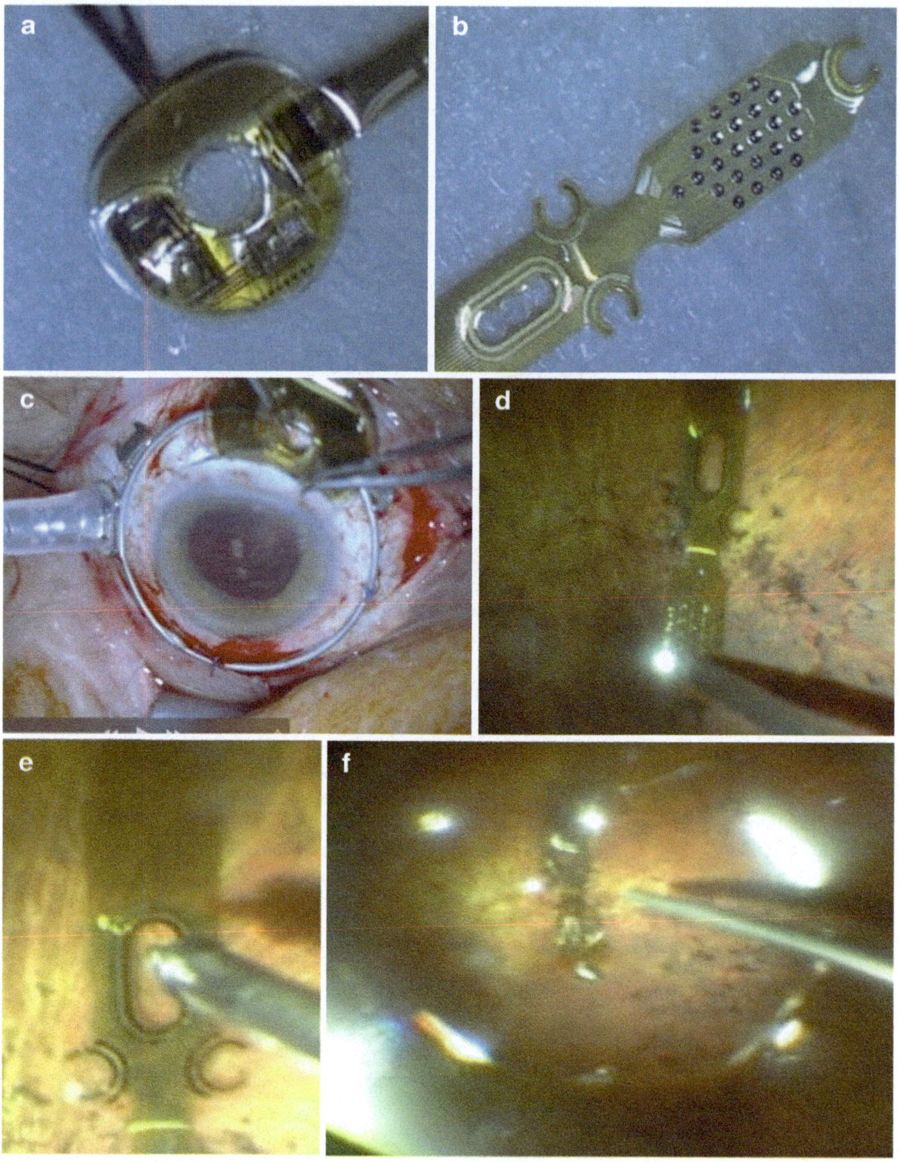

Fig. 12.3 Major steps of the EPIRET implantation. (**a**) Semiflexible receiver system with microfabricated coil and two microASICS for signal extraction and pulse generation. (**b**) Stimulator head with 25 IrOx electrodes on a polyimide base. (**c**) Insertion of the receiver lens through a 11 mm corneoscleral incision in the posterior chamber. The eye is stabilized with the pp infusion and an additional Fliringa ring. (**d**) The stimulator head is positioned onto the central retina using a soft tip fluid needle. (**e**) Fixation is done with a standard retinal tack. (**f**) The eye is closed after fluid air exchange

had received approval for a 4 week experimental phase according to the German Medical Law. It was removed after 4 weeks. The removal was done without complications except in one case where a large retinal tear developed requiring additional steps (Perfluorocarbon fluid installation, Endolaser, Silicone oil fill) to prevent subsequent retinal detachment. In all six patients patterned phosphenes could be elicited despite the fact that the patients were already blind for many years. The thresholds were surprisingly low [13–15]. Patients reported single round or oval shaped usually bright phosphenes corresponding to the site of the electrical stimulation. In some cases patients also reported colored phosphenes. Even with very similar stimulation parameters patients reported a large variation of visual sensations obviously depending on the individual status of their retinal degeneration. In a series of experiments in one of the patients the electrodes were activated in a pattern such as a circle or a line or an angle. This patient was able to identify very well the circle as an oval shape but the line pattern was identified as an arc.

Experimental Results

The EPIRET technology platform was fabricated based on several experimental findings. In the first phase of the development biocompatibility and feasibility studies were performed. It could be demonstrated in rabbits and in pigs that the materials are well tolerated within the eye and that tack fixation is a useful tool to accomplish a stable connection between the implant and the retinal surface [16, 17]. In the second phase functional tests were performed in rabbits as demonstrated by electrical evoked potentials [18]. Wireless EPIRET devices were also implanted in the cat's eye. Field potential responses were obtained from the visual tract and the visual cortex. Cortical activation was also measured by visualizing intrinsic metabolic activity by optical imaging techniques. With these techniques it was shown that local electrical stimulation of the retina with the device elicited local activity of neurons in the visual cortex of the cat corresponding to a potential visual acuity of approximately 20/400 [19, 20] (Fig. 12.4).

For the bi-directional enhancement we characterized the electrical properties of retinal ganglion cells RGCs in several animal models of retinal degeneration resembling human RP. We could demonstrate that in contrast to normal retina the susceptibility of the degenerated retina for electrical stimulation is worse. It seems that in the same retina several types of spontaneous activity exists. In recording experiments in mouse models of RP using multielectrode arrays areas of normal firing of retinal ganglion cells can be found adjacent to areas where slow oscillations or burst activity are present. The spatial distribution of these areas is unpredictable. The type of spontaneous electrical activity may be an important factor preventing successful stimulation of the retina. Slow oscillations and burst activity coupled to the negative phase of the oscillations are predictors of a less successful stimulation. We could demonstrate that electrical stimulation of the inner

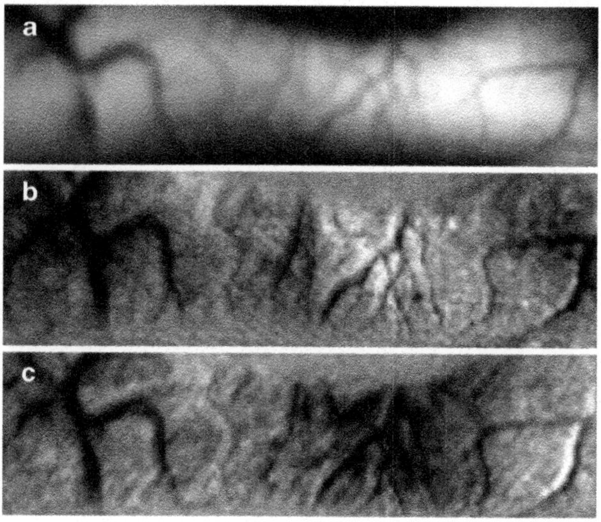

Fig. 12.4 Optical imaging in the cat's visual cortex after electrical stimulation of the retina. (**a**) Camera picture of the exposed visual cortex of the cat. (**b**) Infrared sample in control condition. (**c**) Infrared recording after electrical stimulation of a defined area of the retina. The *black area* represents that cortical area in which the oxygen consumption is significantly elevated

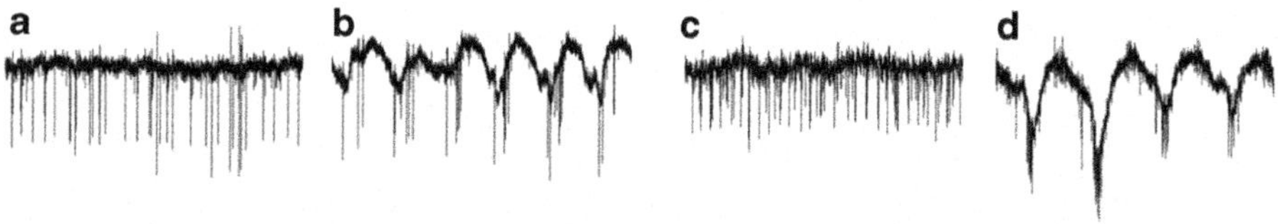

Fig. 12.5 Electrical manipulation of disease driven pathologic intrinsic activity of retinal ganglion cells. (**a**) Regular pattern of spontaneous electrical activity of RGCs in a healthy mouse. (**b**) Slow oscillations and burst activity of RGCs in a mouse model of RP (rd10 mouse). (**c**) Inhibition of slow oscillations and burst activity in the same retina as in B after high frequency electrical stimulation. (**d**) Recurrence of pathologic activity 5 min after termination of HF stimulation. Panels (**a–d**) are showing representative recordings from one electrode of a 64 channel Multielectrode Array (Multichannel Systems, Reutlingen, Germany) obtained from an ex-vivo retina preparation of the rd10 mouse

retinal surface using standard biphasic pulses may also induce the activation of RGCs inhibiting interneurons possibly Amacrine cells or Bipolar cells making a "nearly physiologic" stimulation of the retina even more difficult. Inhibition of RGCs by "misrouted" electrical stimulation will result in an unfavourable outcome in the clinical situation. Therefore we found it necessary to record and analyze the type of intrinsic activity in the retina adjacent to the stimulating electrodes before setting the parameters for stimulation in this area. This should be done ideally with the same bi-directional implant. Preliminary experiments were performed to overcome the limitations of the above mentioned altered intrinsic activity of the degenerated retina using modified stimulation protocols. The experiments proved that the concept of a bi-directional implant providing useful information on the local intrinsic activity of retinal neurons to modify the stimulus properties at a certain electrode is helpful to considerably improve the outcome of retinal prosthesis approaches (Fig. 12.5).

Future Directions

The VLARS Modification

Another problem of currently available retinal stimulators is the limited size of the stimulators. The aim to restore vision for blind patients with RP is not only to restore a very small central field but also to restore a larger field making orientation and mobility more likely to improve. Therefore, based on the EPIRET device platform we fabricated retinal stimulators covering 37° of the retina providing a much larger visual field compared to the currently approved implants. The stimulator form is designed to minimize implantation trauma on one hand but to achieve a larger retinal coverage. We performed surgical feasibility tests and also functional tests. The results obtained so far confirmed the usefulness of this modification but further experiments are necessary to demonstrate the superiority of this concept compared to currently available small stimulators [21].

The Intraretinal Prosthesis

In advanced cases of retinal degeneration retinal neurons leave their usual position in the retinal layers; e.g. retinal ganglion cells move more to the outer retina. Therefore it could be an ideal approach to insert 3D multielectrode arrays into the retina to provide the closest contact between electrodes and retinal neurons as possible. Such 3D multielectrode arrays have already been fabricated for recordings from the brain in neurophysiologic research. They have been applied to record local field potentials and action potentials from within the retina. Further electronic devices have been developed to optimize the problem of dealing with stimulation artifacts [22]. It is intended to further miniaturize such devices to make them suitable for the application within the thin retina. First prototypes have been designed and fabricated and very preliminary results in terms of recording and stimulation in ex-vivo retina preparations are obtained but more research is necessary before consistent data can be reported.

Acknowledgements Results were obtained with support by the following grants: DFG PAK 469/1, DFG WA 1472/6-1, BMBF 01IN501B, 01IN501F9, 01IN501K7, 01KP0004, 01KP0006, 01KP0402, 01KP0404, 01KP0405, 01PK0001, Jackstädt Foundation, and Hans Lamers Foundation.

The BIMEA research group: Peter Walter, Wilfried Mokwa, Rainer Kokozinski, Anton Grabmaier, Frank Müller, Andreas Offenhäusser, Sandra Johnen, Joachim Weis, and Florent Haiss.

References

1. Humayun MS, Dorn JD, Ahuja AK, Caspi A, Filley E, Dagnelie G, et al. Preliminary 6 month results from the Argus II epiretinal prosthesis feasibility study. Conf Proc IEEE Eng Med Biol Soc. 2008;2009:4566–8.

2. Humayun MS, Dorn JD, da Cruz L, Dagnelie G, Sahel J-A, Stanga PE, et al. Interim results from the international trial of second sight's visual prosthesis. Ophthalmology. 2011;119(4):779–88.
3. Ho AC. Long-term results from an epiretinal prosthesis to restore sight to the blind. Ophthalmology. 2015;5:1–8.
4. Stingl K, Bartz-Schmidt KU, Besch D, Braun A, Bruckmann A, Gekeler F, et al. Artificial vision with wirelessly powered subretinal electronic implant alpha-IMS. Proc Biol Sci. 2012;280(1757):20130077.
5. Stingl K, Bartz-Schmidt KU, Gekeler F, Kusnyerik A, Sachs H, Zrenner E. Functional outcome in subretinal electronic implants depends on foveal eccentricity. Invest Ophthalmol Vis Sci. 2012;54(12):7658–65.
6. Stingl K, Bartz-Schmidt KU, Besch D, Chee CK, Cottriall CL, Gekeler F, et al. Subretinal visual implant alpha IMS – clinical trial interim report. Vision Res. 2015;111:149–60.
7. Fujikado T, Kamei M, Sakaguchi H, Kanda H, Morimoto T, Ikuno Y, et al. Clinical trial of chronic implantation of suprachoroidal-transretinal stimulation system for retinal prosthesis. Sensor Mater. 2012;24(4):181–7.
8. Fujikado T, Morimoto T, Kanda H, Kusaka S, Nakauchi K, Ozawa M, et al. Evaluation of phosphenes elicited by extraocular stimulation in normals and by suprachoroidal-transretinal stimulation in patients with retinitis pigmentosa. Graefes Arch Clin Exp Ophthalmol. 2006;245(10):1411–9.
9. Fujikado T, Kamei M, Sakaguchi H, Kanda H, Morimoto T, Ikuno Y, et al. Testing of semichronically implanted retinal prosthesis by suprachoroidal-transretinal stimulation in patients with retinitis pigmentosa. Invest Ophthalmol Vis Sci. 2010;52(7):4726–33.
10. Ayton LN, Blamey PJ, Guymer RH, Luu CD, Nayagam DAX, Sinclair NC, et al. First-in-human trial of a novel suprachoroidal retinal prosthesis. Mori K, editor. PLoS One. Public Library of Science. 2014;9(12):7.
11. Mokwa W, Goertz M, Koch C, Krisch I, Trieu HK, Walter P. Intraocular epiretinal prosthesis to restore vision in blind humans. Conf Proc IEEE Eng Med Biol Soc. 2007;2008:5790–3.
12. Marzouk AM, Stanitzki A, Kokozinski R. Towards pulse-density modulated functional electrical stimulation of neural cells with passive membranes. VDE; 2012. p. 1–4.
13. Roessler G, Laube T, Brockmann C, Kirschkamp T, Mazinani B, Goertz M, et al. Implantation and explantation of a wireless epiretinal retina implant device: observations during the EPIRET3 prospective clinical trial. Invest Ophthalmol Vis Sci. 2008;50(6):3003–8.
14. Klauke S, Goertz M, Rein S, Hoehl D, Thomas U, Eckhorn R, et al. Stimulation with a wireless intraocular epiretinal implant elicits visual percepts in blind humans. Invest Ophthalmol Vis Sci. 2010;52(1):449–55.
15. Menzel-Severing J, Laube T, Brockmann C, Bornfeld N, Mokwa W, Mazinani B, et al. Implantation and explantation of an active epiretinal visual prosthesis: 2-year follow-up data from the EPIRET3 prospective clinical trial. Eye (Lond). 2011;26(4):501–9.
16. Walter P, Szurman P, Vobig M, Berk H, Lüdtke-Handjery HC, Richter H, et al. Successful long-term implantation of electrically inactive epiretinal microelectrode arrays in rabbits. Retina. 1998;19(6):546–52.
17. Menzel-Severing J, Sellhaus B, Laube T, Brockmann C, Bornfeld N, Walter P, et al. Surgical results and microscopic analysis of the tissue reaction following implantation and explantation of an intraocular implant for epiretinal stimulation in minipigs. Ophthalmic Res. 2010;46(4):192–8.
18. Walter P, Heimann K. Evoked cortical potentials after electrical stimulation of the inner retina in rabbits. Graefes Arch Clin Exp Ophthalmol. 1999;238(4):315–8.
19. Walter P, Kisvárday ZF, Görtz M, Alteheld N, Rössler G, Stieglitz T, et al. Cortical activation via an implanted wireless retinal prosthesis. Invest Ophthalmol Vis Sci. 2004;46(5):1780–5.

20. Eckhorn R, Wilms M, Schanze T, Eger M, Hesse L, Eysel UT, et al. Visual resolution with retinal implants estimated from recordings in cat visual cortex. Vision Res. 2005;46(17):2675–90.
21. Waschkowski F, Hesse S, Rieck AC, Lohmann T, Brockmann C, Laube T, et al. Development of very large electrode arrays for epiretinal stimulation (VLARS). Biomed Eng Online BioMed Central Ltd. 2014;13(1):11.
22. Schloesser M, Cota O, Heil R, Brusius J, Offenhausser A, Waasen SV, et al. Embedded device for simultaneous recording and stimulation for retina implant research. Sensors, 2013 IEEE, IEEE; 2013, p. 1–4.

Part III
Orbital and Intracranial Approaches

Chapter 13
Penetrative Optic Nerve-Based Visual Prosthesis Research

Menghui Li, Yan Yan, Kaijie Wu, Yiliang Lu, Jingjing Sun, Yao Chen, Xinyu Chai, Steven Katz, Pengjia Cao, Zengguang Ma, Pengcheng Sun, Qiushi Ren, and Liming Li

Abstract A number of research groups around the world have been dedicated to restoring some functional vision for blind patients through visual prostheses. The C-sight project (Chinese Project for Sight) proposed a visual prosthesis with penetrative stimulating electrode array implanted into the ON as a neural interface to couple the encoded electrical stimuli for vision recovery, since then a decade of effort has been devoted to the development of the first-generation prototype. In this article, the outcomes of this approach and its status quo were briefly summarized and introduced from different perspectives. Besides hardware system and surgical methods description, the cortical response characteristics in response to penetrating ON stimulation in *in vivo* animal experiments were extensively introduced. Firstly, as a widely used methodology of evaluating the effect of a certain electrical stimulus, the basic spatiotemporal properties of the electrically evoked cortical potentials (EEPs) elicited by penetrating ON stimulation were investigated. Secondly, the exact implantation sites of ON electrode array were considered and evaluated taking account of realizing fine visuotopic correspondence between ON electrical stimulation sites and the visual field. Thirdly, the optimal stimulus parameters were explored, as well as the relationship between response properties of electrical vs. visual stimulation. Furthermore, several potential future directions of this approach were also briefly discussed.

M. Li, PhD • Q. Ren, PhD (✉)
Department of Biomedical Engineering, College of Engineering, Peking University, Beijing, People's Republic of China
e-mail: renqsh@coe.pku.edu.cn

Y. Yan, PhD • K. Wu, PhD • Y. Lu, PhD • J. Sun, PhD • Y. Chen, PhD • X. Chai, PhD • P. Cao, PhD • Z. Ma, PhD • P. Sun, PhD • L. Li, PhD (✉)
School of Biomedical Engineering, Shanghai Jiao Tong University, Shanghai, People's Republic of China
e-mail: lilm@sjtu.edu.cn

S. Katz, MD
Department of Ophthalmology & Visual Science, Havener Eye Institute, Ohio State University, Columbus, OH, USA

V.P. Gabel (ed.), *Artificial Vision*, DOI 10.1007/978-3-319-41876-6_13

Keywords Visual prosthesis • Optic nerve • Electrical stimulation • Penetrative electrode array • Electrically evoked potentials

Key Points

- Biomedical engineering methods of electrically stimulating a certain site on the visual pathway to restore some functional vision for blind patients have been proved feasible by several scientific groups in the world
- The C-sight project (Chinese Project for Sight) proposed an ON approach with a penetrating multi-electrode array implanted into the ON as a neural interface to couple the encoded electrical stimuli
- The feasibility of penetrative ON electrical stimulation has been preliminarily proved by our *in vivo* electrophysiological experiments in animals.
- Some advantages of penetrative ON visual prosthesis, such as lower stimulating threshold and comparatively high spatial resolution have also been demonstrated.

Principal Idea

For human beings, 70–80 % of the external information is obtained via the visual system that once is impaired or lost, most likely due to a certain incurable disease, psychological suffering as well as difficulty in conducting normal activities would be inevitably incurred. In order to restore some functional vision for blind patients, the biomedical engineering method of electrically stimulating a certain site on the visual pathway by implanting an electronic device was introduced, largely driven by the advancement of biological microelectromechanical and biomaterials technology [1]. Such an attempt was first made by electrical stimulation of the visual cortex in 1968 [2]. To date a number of various technical schemes, mostly based on retina stimulation, have been proposed and are currently at different stages of basic research or clinical trials [2–15]. Optic nerve (ON) based visual prosthesis was first proposed by Veraart et al in 1998 [16, 17]. They successfully implanted a cuff surface electrode array around the ON of a blind subject and demonstrated that electrical stimulation of the ON can also elicit useful phosphenes [16–18].

As the first multidisciplinary research project on visual prosthesis in China, the C-sight project (Chinese Project for Sight) proposed an ON approach with penetrating electrodes. Briefly, the external optical information captured by a CCD camera and then processed by an image processor is transferred wirelessly to an internal micro-stimulator, which generates current pulses to stimulate the ON by a penetrating multi-electrode array implanted into the ON. In this approach, the penetrating multi-electrode array acts as a neural interface to couple the encoded electrical stimuli to the ON fibers, i.e. axons of the retinal ganglion cells (RGCs) for vision recovery. The ON based C-Sight visual prosthesis has several potential advantages. Firstly, compared with a cuff surface electrode array, penetrating electrodes have lower stimulation thresholds and higher spatial resolution [19, 20]. Secondly, the elicited phosphenes might cover large areas of the visual field and could maintain relatively satisfactory visuotopical correspondence with the ON stimulation sites close to the eyeball, due to the way the ON fibers are organized as they leave the ON head [21–23]. Thirdly, the implantation requires no trans-scleral tunnel, therefore avoiding the risk of rupture. Lastly, the implantation site is close to the globe which is thus intraorbitally accessible, without disturbing the already diseased retinal tissue. Since 2005, the C-sight group has been dedicated to investigating basic scientific issues on ON stimulation and developing a whole package of related technologies of designing and manufacturing a hermetic device that can be penetratively implanted to the ON and elicit functional vision by electrically stimulating the ON fibers of the blind patients.

The feasibility of this stimulation methodology and basic stimulation strategies must be carefully studied and evaluated prior to any human implantation. To this end, the C-sight group conducted a plethora of animal electrophysiological experiments as one of the essential parts of the fundamental visual prosthesis research, which is reviewed in this section together with the hardware description.

Indication for Certain Forms of Blindness

Untreatable blindness can be induced by severe retinal pathologies such as retinitis pigmentosa (RP) and age-related macular degeneration (AMD). Our device is designed mainly to restore functional vision lost due to these two major ophthalmological diseases. Both of them are characterized by a massive and irreversible loss of photoreceptor cells, as well as survival of most other retinal neurons, such that a substantial fraction of the retinal ganglion cells (RGC) can still form an relatively functional visual pathway to the visual cortex. Since the ON is composed of more than 1 million RGC fibers, the ON may be one of the ideal sites for stimulating array implantation to circumvent the damaged photoreceptors and avoid disturbing the diseased retina.

Technical Description

The hardware system of the C-sight visual prosthetic device was briefly depicted in Fig. 13.1. The external part includes a micro-camera for capturing the external optical information, a video processor for image processing, a stimulation encoder for data encoding as well as an RF amplifier and an RF emitting coil for RF transmission. The surrounding images are first captured by a micro-camera mounted on the glasses. Then, the key features of images are extracted from the original scenes by advanced image processing algorithms and encoded into trains of digital signals with specific spatiotemporal stimulation patterns. The encoded signals of

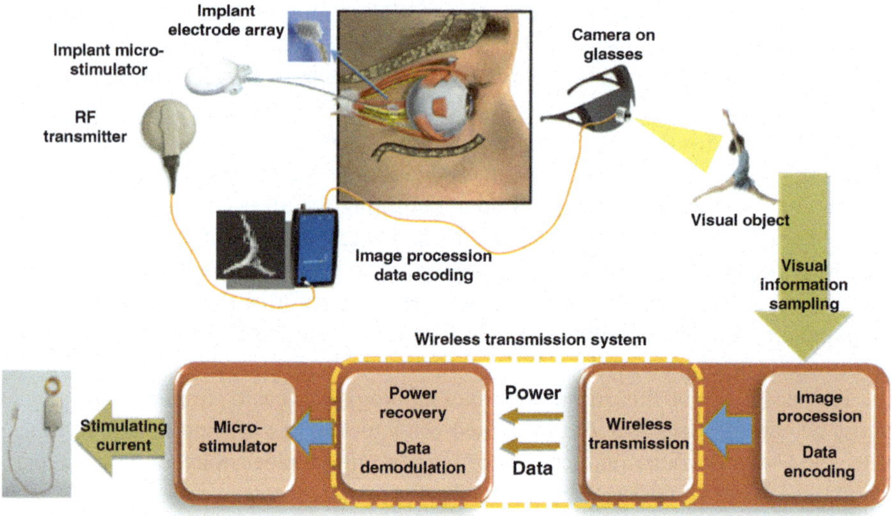

Fig. 13.1 A diagram of the first-generation C-Sight visual prosthetic device

electrical pulses are forwarded by RF transmission. The implant part comprises an RF receiving coil, a multi-channel stimulator, electrode connecting wires and a micro electrode array for implantation. The internal coil transfers the received radio power and data to the implant micro-stimulator. After power recovery and data demodulation, the multi-channel stimulator generates and transmits the micro-current pulses to the multichannel microelectrode array implanted into the ON. The electrode array was made of platinum (70 %)-iridium (30 %) wire-electrodes. At the current stage, there were total 18 electrodes arranged in four lines, consisting of one electrode used for common ground with low impedance below 1 kΩ, one electrode for reference, and the others for stimulating channels with impedance around 10 kΩ. The length of electrodes was ranged from 0.65 to 0.85 mm with 0.05 mm increment for each line. The distance between every two adjacent electrodes was about 0.4 mm. The electrode array was bundled by ceramic substrate and then embedded into the self-crimping silicon strip which can make the fixture convenient.

Surgical Methods

Apart from the fundamental researches necessary for prosthesis development, a simple low-risk surgical procedure that can protect both the globe and ON from secondary disturbance or impairment and at the same time achieve satisfactory ON exposure is also desirable for ON electrode implantation. Surgical approaches were explored in both animal experiments and human cadavers. In rabbits, through an orbital process of the frontal bone without removal of the bony orbit and resection

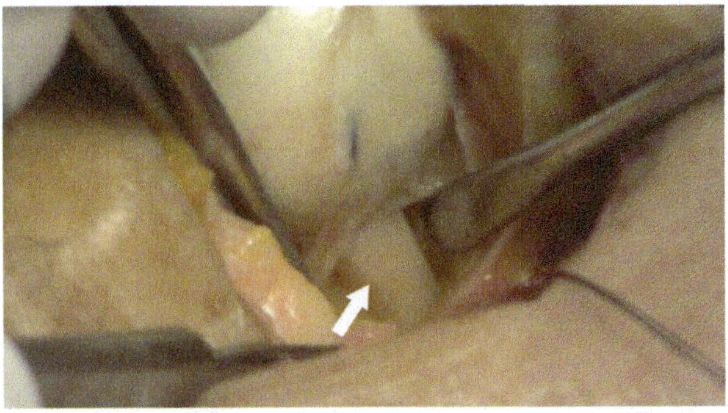

Fig. 13.2 Exposure of the ON (*white arrow*) via lateral orbitotomy on human cadaver

of the rectus muscles the ON could be exposed thoroughly and clearly [24]. And the ON of the cat can be exposed by an craniotomy over the frontal sinus just above the eyeball [33]. Due to the anatomic differences, the approaches in rabbits and cats are not suitable for the human, thus a more feasible surgery solution to achieve optimal access to intraorbital space and the ON via lateral orbitotomy has been explored. Surgery on human cadaver shows that this approach allows desirable exposure of the ON for stimulating electrode array implantation (Fig. 13.2).

Experimental Results

Besides establishing the hardware system of the C-sight visual prosthetic device, the cortical response characteristics in response to penetrating ON stimulation were extensively explored in animal models using electrophysiological methods. Firstly, as a widely used methodology of evaluating the effect of a certain electrical stimulus, the basic spatiotemporal properties of the electrically evoked potentials (EEPs) elicited by penetrating ON stimulation were investigated [25, 26]. Secondly, the exact implantation sites of ON electrode array were considered and evaluated taking account of realizing fine visuotopic correspondence of ON electrical stimulation. Thirdly, the optimal stimulus parameters were explored. And finally the relationship between response properties of electrical vs. visual stimulation was investigated.

Spatiotemporal Properties of the EEPs

To design optimal stimulation strategies for an ON visual prosthesis, it is necessary to investigate basic spatiotemporal properties of the cortical responses elicited by penetrative ON stimulation. The ON of the rabbit was stimulated and the visual cortex contralateral to the operated eye was used for EEP recording using an

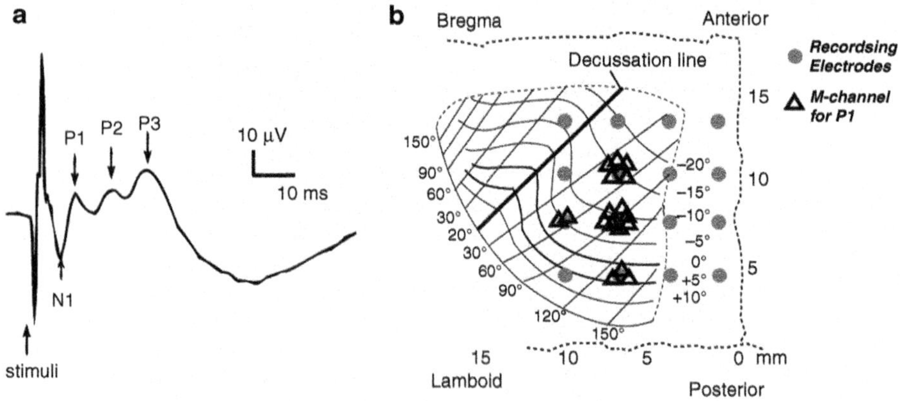

Fig. 13.3 (**a**) Waveform of multipeaked EEPs, including N1, P1, P2, and P3 components. EEPs were elicited by a pair of ON-stimulating electrodes separated by 1 mm. (**b**) Spatial distribution of the M-channel locations (*open triangles*) of the P1 component of the EEPs superimposed on a visual field map modified from [30]. Data were obtained using a current strength of 100 μA with a pulse duration of 0.5 ms. *Gray dots*: positions of recording electrode array. The data were from 17 stimulating electrode pairs in seven rabbits. The figure represents a view of the skull/cortex from above

epidually placed 4×4 electrode array. Biphasic charge-balanced rectangular stimuli with cathode-first pulse were used to stimulate the ON.

The experimental results showed that there were mainly four components (N1, P1, P2, P3, see Fig. 13.3a) in EEPs, with great variations not only in their implicit times, time courses but also in the stimulation thresholds (the minimum currents needed to elicit them) [19]. It has been reported that there are parallel processing pathways within the mammalian visual system that differ in cell morphology and conduction velocity and transfer distinct visual information [27, 28]. The variations in properties of different EEP components suggest electrically stimulating the ON may activate multiple types of the ON fibers, and it may be possible to activate distinct ON fibers selectively with a certain stimulation strategy to transfer distinct types of visual information.

The P1 was found to be the most reliable component among the multi-components of EEPs, [19] and the cortical location of the recording channel with the highest P1 amplitude (M-channel) was also exhibiting a good spatial correspondence to the ON stimulation sites (Fig. 13.3b). [29, 30]

Spatial discrimination of the ON stimulation is a crucial issue for a visual prosthesis to restore functional vision. We examined shifts in the location of the M-channel of P1 in response to monopolar ON stimulation from adjacent electrodes. Our experimental results showed that with two penetrating electrodes spaced 0.15 mm and implanted perpendicularly to the ON axis, the spatial profiles of elicited P1 responses could be distinguished from each other very well, which suggests a good spatial discrimination ability of penetrative ON stimulation [19, 21].

Visuotopic Mapping for Electrical Stimulation by ON Electrode Array

The ON is composed of RGC axons that tend to scatter to some extent as they leave the retina and pass through the ON head [21–23], which may result in poor visuotopic correspondence between the ON electrical stimulation and visual field for an ON visual prosthesis and hence poor pattern recognition. To address this issue, we conducted *in vivo* cat experiments to investigate the retinotopic organization of ON stimulation and its spatial resolution by studying the retinotopic correspondence between localized penetrative ON stimulation and the EEPs responses [31].

The results show that electrical stimulation with penetrating ON electrodes just located behind the globe could produce cortical responses in visuotopographically corresponding areas of the visual cortex (Fig. 13.4), implying a relatively good visuotopic organization within the ON close to the ON head as reported by Fitzgibbon et al. [21]. In addition, stimulating the temporal side of the ON elicited cortical responses corresponding to the central visual field and the visual field position shifted from the lower to central visual field as the electrode penetrated through the depth of the ON, which are consistent with a previous anatomical study on cats [22]. By measuring the cortical responsive region to ON electrical stimulation by a single electrode and the responsive shift elicited by two adjacent stimulating electrodes, we estimated that a spatial resolution of ~2–3° could be obtained by this approach, which may be slightly less than that by epi- and sub-retinal stimulation [6, 32].

This study shows that implanting electrodes penetratively behind the globe at multiple site or depths can potentially create visuotopic electrical stimulation with a relatively fine spatial resolution. Improvement on spatial resolution could be expected by using electrodes with smaller multi-stimulation points at different ON locations as well as current steering strategy [33].

Effects of Stimulus Pulse Shape and Frequency on Response Properties of EEPs

Pulse shape and pulse frequency are two of the most critical parameters for electrical stimulation. Charge-balanced biphasic pulses were adopted for its advantage in reducing tissue and electrode damage, facilitating channel interactions and increasing spatial resolution [34, 35].

Analysis of the EEPs shows that charge-balanced biphasic pulses with various shapes have different stimulation threshold. Compared with other stimuli, a stronger cortical response with a larger spatial spread could be produced by a stimulus with high-amplitude short-duration (HASD) cathodic phase when the total charge of the stimulus was fixed. In addition, the EEP amplitudes were significantly increased if an inter-phase gap was added to the stimulus between the its two

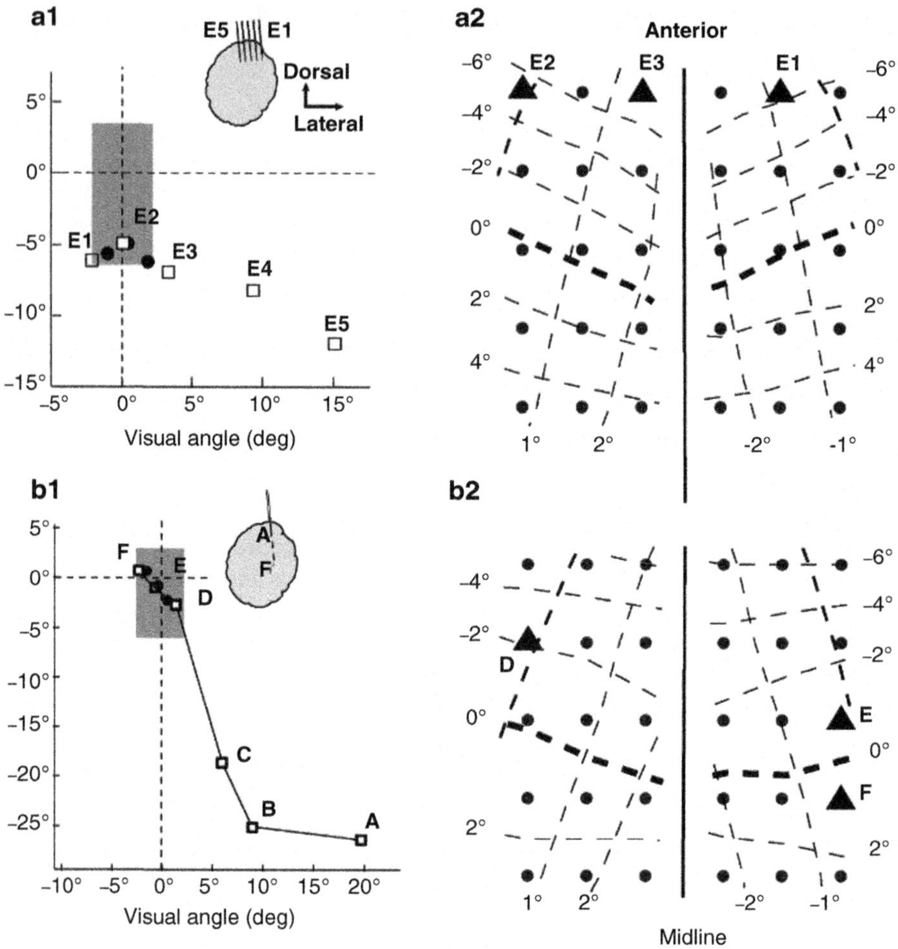

Fig. 13.4 Visuotopic organization by an array of 5 electrodes and one single electrode at different depths within the ON. (**a1**) The visual field positions of five ON stimulating electrodes (*E1–E5*; temporal to nasal; inter-electrode distance of 150 μm) determined by sparse noise stimuli (*open squares*). (**a2**) ON electrical stimulation through electrodes *E1*, *E2* and *E3* elicited M-channels at different cortical positions (*solid triangles*) within the visuotopic map. (**b1**) Visual field positions of six ON stimulating sites 150 μm apart in depth (*A–F*; *open squares*). (**b2**) Cortical M-channel locations following ON electrical stimulation by sites *D, E & F* in (**b1**). The shaded area in (**a1**) and (**b1**) is the recordable region of the visual cortex covered by the 5×6 epidural array

phases, and a saturation was seen when the gap was lengthened to ~0.2 ms. Gradually increasing the stimulating frequency resulted in monotonically decreased EEP amplitudes. In conclusion, an cathodic-first biphasic stimulus waveform with an inter-phase gap of ~0.2 ms might be optimal for ON stimulation, with possible advantages of less tissue damage, minimal electrode etching, and lower power consumption [34].

Relationship of Electrically and Visually Evoked Cortical Response

The ultimate goal of a visual prostheses is to mimic the natural visual input with electrical stimulation, it is thus crucial to find out the intrinsic relationship of the visually and electrically evoked cortical responses.

We designed experiments to explore this issue on a cat ON stimulation model. Platinum-iridium electrodes (100 Ω, PI20030, Micro Probe Inc., USA) were inserted into the cat ON 1–2 mm behind the eyeball. The visuotopic position of the ON electrode was first determined by a sparse noise method [31], and flash-light spot stimulation with varied size and brightness were applied at the same visual field location of the ON electrode. A cathodic-first biphasic rectangle stimulus was used with a phase duration of 0.5 ms at 1 Hz. The stimulating current was varied from below threshold (Thr) to 5 times of Thr (5 Thr). The electrically and visually evoked cortical responses were recorded using a 5×6 epidural silver-ball electrode array, with 15 electrodes on each cortical hemisphere. The amplitudes of multi-channel cortical responses were plotted and further fitted by a Gaussian curve. The Half-Width of Half-Maximum (HWHM) value of the fitted curve was used to represent the spatial spread of the cortical responses.

The spatial spread of the cortical VEPs increased as the radius of light spot was enlarged from 0.5 to 10° visual angle with fixed brightness, or as the light brightness was increased from 10 to 60 cd/cm^2 with a fixed radius of light spot. The current threshold to evoke stable EEPs was 3.6 ± 1.5 μA (mean ± SD), which corresponded to a charge threshold of 1.8 ± 0.8 nC or a charge density threshold of 293.2 ± 122.1 μC/cm with our penetrating ON electrode (n = 13 cats). When the stimulating current was raised from 1 to 5 Thr, the spatial spread of EEPs also enlarged gradually.

The spatial spread of electrically evoked responses using a current of 1–5 Thr was compared with that of the visually evoked responses using light spots of 0.6–5° visual angle with a luminance of 60 cd/cm^2 at the same retinotopic location. The results showed that the spatial spread of the cortical responses using 1 Thr current ON stimulation was equivalent to that of flash-light visual stimulation using a light-spot with a radius of 1.25 ± 0.49° visual angle, and a 5 Thr electrical ON stimulation corresponded to 6.85 ± 0.94° spot flash-light stimulation (n = 9 from 4 cats). The possible phosphene sizes evoked by ON electrical stimulation with different current intensities were evaluated and exhibited in Fig. 13.5(b), though further confirmation is required by clinical trials in the future.

Future Direction

The C-sight visual prosthesis group has been focusing its efforts on investigating basic scientific issues on ON visual prosthesis and developing a whole package of related technologies to design and manufacture a hermetic device that can be

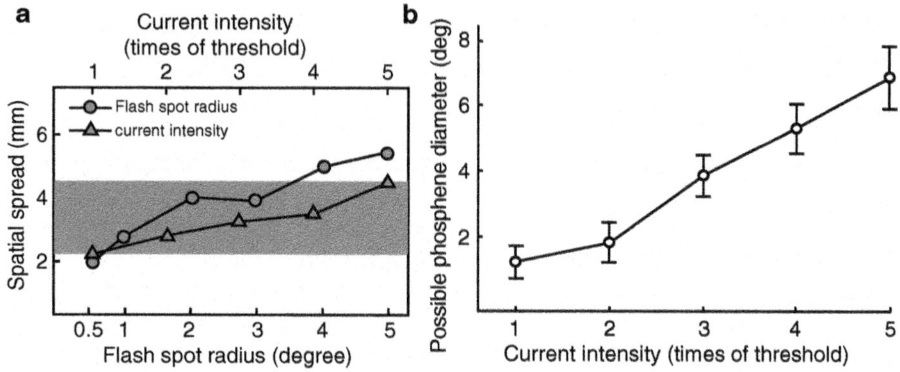

Fig. 13.5 Comparisons between electrically and visually evoked cortical response and possible phosphene size by ON stimulation with various current intensities. (**a**) An example showing the comparison of cortical spread to ON electrical stimulation and visual stimulation at the same visual field positions. (**b**) Estimated ON stimulation-induced phosphene sizing ($n=9$ in 4 cats). The spatial spread on the cortex was converted to visual angle using the cortical magnification factors in cat [36]

implanted to the ON in a penetrative way and elicit usable phosphenes by electrically stimulating the ON fibers of the blind patients. The first generation of the C-sight visual prosthetic device has been successfully developed.

So far, the feasibility of penetrative ON electrical stimulation has been preliminarily proved by our *in vivo* electrophysiological experiments in animals. In addition, the basic stimulation parameters and possible application of field shaping technology to this approach have been explored as well. Some advantages of penetrative ON visual prosthesis, such as lower stimulating threshold and improved spatial resolution compared to the cuffed one, have also been demonstrated. Further validation of this technological approach would be achieved by our undergoing behavioral experiments on implanted primates. New technologies such as ON-based "virtual channel" stimulating strategy are also under research to further improve the performance of the prototype [33, 37].

With the rapid advancement of relevant techniques and maturity of manufacturing procedures, the C-sight project is now progressing toward pilot clinical studies. Before taking this significant step, however, numerous additional preparations have to be completed, amongst which setting the inclusion and exclusion criteria for volunteer recruitment based on weighing the risks/potential benefits for patients has already been initiated.

The results of our electrophysiological experiments on animals carried out by the C-sight group have showed that our first-generation prototype based on penetrative ON stimulation is a promising approach. Some additional work remains to be done before conducting pilot clinical trials.

Acknowledgments This work was supported by the National Basic Research Program of China (Nos. 2011CB707502/3), and the National Natural Science Foundation of China (Nos. 61171174/60971102/61472247/91120304/61273368).

References

1. Zrenner E. Will retinal implants restore vision? Science. 2002;295(5557):1022–5.
2. Brindley GS, Lewin WS. The sensations produced by electrical stimulation of the visual cortex. J Physiol. 1968;196(2):479–93.
3. Rizzo 3rd JF, Wyatt J, Loewenstein J, Kelly S, Shire D. Perceptual efficacy of electrical stimulation of human retina with a microelectrode array during short-term surgical trials. Invest Ophthalmol Vis Sci. 2003;44(12):5362–9.
4. Eckmiller R. Learning retina implants with epiretinal contacts. Ophthalmic Res. 1997; 29(5):281–9.
5. Humayun MS, et al. Visual perception in a blind subject with a chronic microelectronic retinal prosthesis. Vision Res. 2003;43(24):2573–81.
6. Wilms M, Eger M, Schanze T, Eckhorn R. Visual resolution with epi-retinal electrical stimulation estimated from activation profiles in cat visual cortex. Vis Neurosci. 2003;20(5):543–55.
7. Zrenner E, et al. The development of subretinal microphotodiodes for replacement of degenerated photoreceptors. Ophthalmic Res. 1997;29(5):269–80.
8. Chow AY, Chow VY, Packo KH, Pollack JS, Peyman GA, Schuchard R. The artificial silicon retina microchip for the treatment of vision loss from retinitis pigmentosa. Arch Ophthalmol. 2004;122(4):460–9.
9. Palanker D, Vankov A, Huie P, Baccus S. Design of a high-resolution optoelectronic retinal prosthesis. J Neural Eng. 2005;2(1):S105–20.
10. Pardue MT, Ball SL, Phillips MJ, Faulkner AE, Walker TA, Chow AY, Peachey NS. Status of the feline retina 5 years after subretinal implantation. J Rehabil Res Dev. 2006;43(6):723–32.
11. Tsai D, Morley JW, Suaning GJ, Lovell NH. Direct activation and temporal response properties of rabbit retinal ganglion cells following subretinal stimulation. J Neurophysiol. 2009;102(5):2982–93.
12. Dobelle WH, Mladejovsky MG. Phosphenes produced by electrical stimulation of human occipital cortex, and their application to the development of a prosthesis for the blind. J Physiol. 1974;243(2):553–76.
13. Troyk P, et al. A model for intracortical visual prosthesis research. Artif Organs. 2003; 27(11):1005–15.
14. Schmidt EM, Bak MJ, Hambrecht FT, Kufta CV, O'Rourke DK, Vallabhanath P. Feasibility of a visual prosthesis for the blind based on intracortical microstimulation of the visual cortex. Brain. 1996;119(Pt 2):507–22.
15. Normann RA, Maynard EM, Rousche PJ, Warren DJ. A neural interface for a cortical vision prosthesis. Vision Res. 1999;39(15):2577–87.
16. Veraart C, Raftopoulos C, Mortimer JT, Delbeke J, Pins D, Michaux G, Vanlierde A, Parrini S, Wanet-Defalque MC. Visual sensations produced by optic nerve stimulation using an implanted self-sizing spiral cuff electrode. Brain Res. 1998;813(1):181–6.
17. Veraart C, Wanet-Defalque MC, Gerard B, Vanlierde A, Delbeke J. Pattern recognition with the optic nerve visual prosthesis. Artif Organs. 2003;27(11):996–1004.
18. Brelen ME, Duret F, Gerard B, Delbeke J, Veraart C. Creating a meaningful visual perception in blind volunteers by optic nerve stimulation. J Neural Eng. 2005;2(1):S22–8.
19. Sun J, Lu Y, Cao P, Li X, Cai C, Chai X, Ren Q, Li L. Spatiotemporal properties of multipeaked electrically evoked potentials elicited by penetrative optic nerve stimulation in rabbits. Invest Ophthalmol Vis Sci. 2011;52(1):146–54.
20. Rosahl SK, Mark G, Herzog M, Pantazis C, Gharabaghi F, Matthies C, Brinker T, Samii M. Far-field responses to stimulation of the cochlear nucleus by microsurgically placed penetrating and surface electrodes in the cat. J Neurosurg. 2001;95(5):845–52.
21. Fitzgibbon T, Taylor SF. Retinotopy of the human retinal nerve fibre layer and optic nerve head. J Comp Neurol. 1996;375(2):238–51.
22. Naito J. Course of retinogeniculate projection fibers in the cat optic nerve. J Comp Neurol. 1986;251(3):376–87.

23. Horton JC, Greenwood MM, Hubel DH. Non-retinotopic arrangement of fibres in cat optic nerve. Nature. 1979;282(5740):720–2.
24. Li X, Cai C, Li L, Chai X, Ren Q. Low-hemorrhage-risk surgical approach to expose the optic nerve in rabbits without bony removal and rectus resection. Vet Ophthalmol. 2009;12(4): 227–33.
25. Sun J, Chen Y, Chai X, Ren Q, Li L. Penetrating electrode stimulation of the rabbit optic nerve: parameters and effects on evoked cortical potentials. Graefes Arch Clin Exp Ophthalmol. 2013;251(11):2545–54.
26. Cai C, Li L, Li X, Chai X, Sun J, Lu Y, Sui X, Chen P, Ren Q. Response properties of electrically evoked potential elicited by multi-channel penetrative optic nerve stimulation in rabbits. Doc Ophthalmol. 2009;118(3):191–204.
27. Schiller PH, Malpeli JG. Functional specificity of lateral geniculate nucleus laminae of the rhesus monkey. J Neurophysiol. 1978;41(3):788–97.
28. Cleland BG, Levick WR, Morstyn R, Wagner HG. Lateral geniculate relay of slowly conducting retinal afferents to cat visual cortex. J Physiol. 1976;255(1):299–320.
29. Vaney DI, Hughes A. The rabbit optic nerve: fibre diameter spectrum, fibre count, and comparison with a retinal ganglion cell count. J Comp Neurol. 1976;170(2):241–51.
30. Thompson JM, Woolsey CN, Talbot SA. Visual areas I and II of cerebral cortex of rabbit. J Neurophysiol. 1950;13(4):277–88.
31. Lu Y, Yan Y, Chai X, Ren Q, Chen Y, Li L. Electrical stimulation with a penetrating optic nerve electrode array elicits visuotopic cortical responses in cats. J Neural Eng. 2013;10(3):036022.
32. Eckhorn R, et al. Visual resolution with retinal implants estimated from recordings in cat visual cortex. Vision Res. 2006;46(17):2675–90.
33. Li M, Yan Y, Wang Q, Zhao H, Chai X, Sui X, Ren Q, Li L. A simulation of current focusing and steering with penetrating optic nerve electrodes. J Neural Eng. 2013;10(6):066007.
34. van Wieringen A, Macherey O, Carlyon RP, Deeks JM, Wouters J. Alternative pulse shapes in electrical hearing. Hear Res. 2008;242(1–2):154–63.
35. Macherey O, van Wieringen A, Carlyon RP, Deeks JM, Wouters J. Asymmetric pulses in cochlear implants: effects of pulse shape, polarity, and rate. J Assoc Res Otolaryngol. 2006; 7(3):253–66.
36. Tusa RJ, Palmer LA, Rosenquist AC. The retinotopic organization of area 17 (striate cortex) in the cat. J Comp Neurol. 1978;177(2):213–35.
37. Khalili Moghaddam G, Lovell NH, Wilke RG, Suaning GJ, Dokos S. Performance optimization of current focusing and virtual electrode strategies in retinal implants. Comput Methods Programs Biomed. 2014;117(2):334–42.

Chapter 14
Thalamic Visual Prosthesis Project

Margee J. Kyada, Nathaniel J. Killian, and John S. Pezaris

Abstract The lateral geniculate nucleus of the thalamus (LGN) is a well-studied structure in the early visual pathway that links the retina to the primary visual cortex. As a deep structure, it has been long overlooked by the visual prosthesis field due to surgical inaccessibility. The unrelated field of deep brain stimulation has developed safe and effective means for clinical implantation of stimulating electrodes in structures that are near the LGN, removing the primary barrier for consideration of the thalamus as a stimulation target for artificial vision. In this chapter we review current progress toward creation of a thalamic visual prosthesis, describing initial animal experiments as proof-of-concept with single microwire electrodes, computer simulations of electrode placement and the resulting pattern of phosphenes in the visual field, experiments with sighted human volunteers to assess effective acuity of artificial vision using virtual reality simulations, and finally results from training animals in an artificial vision simulation in preparation for implantation of stimulating electrodes.

Keywords Artificial vision • LGN • Microstimulation • Phosphene • Visual function • Blindness

Abbreviations

CT	Computerized Tomography (X-ray)
DBS	Deep Brain Stimulation
LGN	Lateral Geniculate Nucleus
logMAR	logarithm of the minimum angle of resolution
MNREAD	Minnesota Reading Test of Visual Acuity
MRI	Magnetic Resonance Imaging
V1	Primary Visual Cortex

M.J. Kyada
Department of Behavioral Neuroscience, Northeastern University, Boston, MA, USA

N.J. Killian • J.S. Pezaris (✉)
Department of Neurosurgery, Massachusetts General Hospital, Harvard Medical School, Boston, MA, USA
e-mail: john@pezaris.com; pezaris.john@mgh.harvard.edu

V.P. Gabel (ed.), *Artificial Vision*, DOI 10.1007/978-3-319-41876-6_14

Key Points

- The field of Deep Brain Stimulation has made placement of stimulating electrodes in midbrain structures routine, creating the possibility of easily implanting stimulating electrodes in LGN.
- In monkeys, stimulation through microwires in LGN evokes phosphenes that are readily incorporated into a simple behavioral task.
- In normally sighted humans, a virtual reality simulation of thalamic artificial vision showed that about 500 phosphenes total will provide reasonably useful vision, both with a letter recognition task, and a reading task. More phosphenes provide better performance.
- The same virtual reality simulation showed that monkeys perform at levels comparable to humans in a letter recognition task in the easiest conditions, but somewhat worse in harder conditions, and only after significant training.
- Current work involves development of a prototype device with 64-contact electrodes implanted bilaterally (128 contacts total) in monkeys.

Introduction

Millions of people worldwide are at risk for complete vision loss [1]. There has been substantial recent progress made in the field of artificial vision, with the regulatory approval of retinal implants to treat retinitis pigmentosa [2]. Significant progress has been made by other groups working on retinal or cortical approaches [3–7], along with those pursuing optic nerve [8] and thalamic implants [9–15]. In this chapter, we review our progress toward a thalamic visual prosthesis.

The success of the cochlear implant to restoring hearing [16] has inspired work in restoration of other sensory processes through electrical stimulation including the majority of visual prosthesis projects that utilize electrical stimulation to evoke visual percepts, or phosphenes, in the early visual pathway. Electrode designs vary according to the characteristics of the targeted structure: arrays of contacts are typically used in the retina to stimulate bipolar or retinal ganglion cells [2, 6, 17], cuff or penetrating electrodes in the optic nerve [8], microwire tuft electrodes in the lateral geniculate nucleus of the thalamus [11–13], and surface or penetrating electrodes in the visual cortex [3, 4, 6].

Early Visual System Organization

The early visual system is organized as a sequence of specialized stages. The retina receives images from the optics of the eye and transforms them to neural signals. The optic nerve conveys these signals to the lateral geniculate nucleus in the thalamus (LGN), an intermediary relay station [18, 19]. From the LGN, visual information is passed to the primary visual cortex where conscious perception begins [20].

The LGN is unique among the visual structures in that it has the only macroscopic segregation of the major visual channels with koniocellular, magnocellular, and parvocellular cells segregated into layers [21]. These different classes of neurons encode different aspects of visual information with similar response characteristics to the retinal neurons from which they receive their first visual input [22]. The LGN then projects to the input layer of the primary visual cortex, where the fundamental response characteristics are shaped by precisely combined activity from multiple LGN cells [23, 24]. The LGN also receives substantial non-retinal input, including from the cortex, which is thought to mediate attention (discussed below).

A hallmark of the visual system is non-uniform acuity or resolution across the visual field, with higher levels of acuity toward the center and lower toward the periphery. This central over-representation begins at the retina where the density of photoreceptors and retinal ganglion cells at the fovea can be an order of magnitude higher than at the periphery [25]. The centrally-weighted profile is carried through the rest of the early visual pathway, but the compressed cellular density is not, resulting in an apparent magnification of central vision areas in structures after the retina, starting at LGN [7, 26, 27]. For example, the central 3° of the visual field occupy 60 % of the LGN volume [12, 28].

Approaches to Artificial Vision

Multiple approaches to artificial vision are possible from the rich architecture of the early visual pathway as reviewed by Pezaris and Eskandar [13]: the retina, the optic nerve, the optic tract, the LGN, the optic radiation and V1 (Fig. 14.1).

The first stage in the visual system, the retina, is a common approach for visual prostheses. It provides substantial benefits over other approaches, especially a less invasive implantation surgery, and the potential for a coverage of the entire visual field with a unilateral implantation. The retina is, however, a delicate tissue and the eye presents limited space for implantation, making the bioengineering goals challenging to achieve. Results from retinal work have demonstrated the difficulty inherent in providing high-resolution vision [6, 29, 30]. Perhaps the most significant restriction is the requirement for a population of healthy retinal ganglion cells for stimulation, which counter-indicates retinal implants for blindness caused by trauma to the eyes or diseases such as glaucoma.

The optic nerve has been investigated with both cuff-style [31] electrodes and penetrating microelectrodes [32, 33]. While cuff-style electrodes at present offer low-resolution performance, an approach using penetrating microelectrodes could provide higher acuity through higher contact count.

The optic tract (the projection between the chiasm and the LGN) and radiation (the projection between the LGN and primary visual cortex) could also be targeted

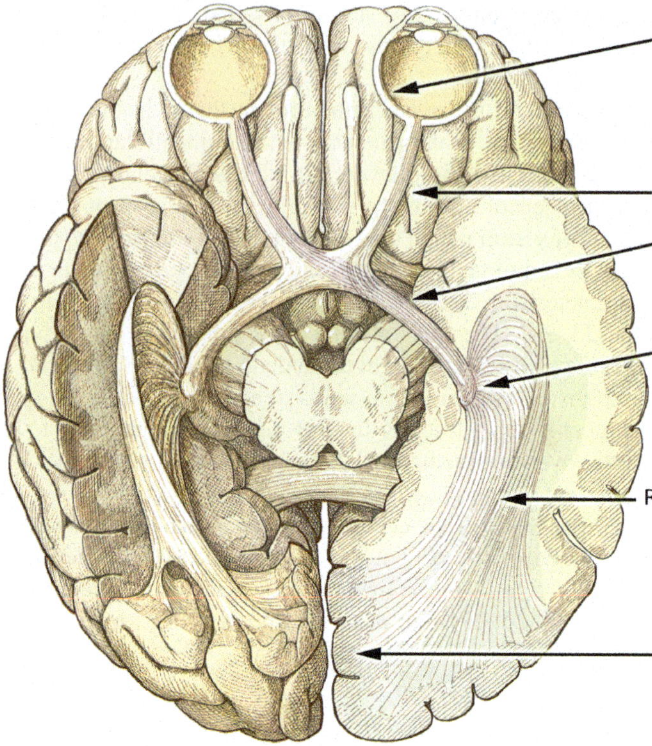

Fig. 14.1 Ventral view of the human brain. The early visual system is depicted in this ventral view of the human brain. Light enters through the optics of the eye and is focused on the retina where photons are converted to neural action potentials by the retinal circuitry. Signals pass from the retina along the optic nerve, chiasm, and tract to the lateral geniculate nucleus of the thalamus (LGN). Whereas each retina represents the entire visual scene, each LGN represents only the contralateral visual hemifield but from both eyes, after the fiber shuffling in the chiasm. From the LGN, signals pass along the optic radiation to the input layers of the primary visual cortex. Each of the labeled stages presents a potential stimulation site for artificial vision, with various advantages and disadvantages to each; electrical stimulation at any stage relies upon a remaining population of healthy cells to be activated (Reprinted from Pezaris and Eskandar [13]. With permission from American Association of Neurological Surgeons)

for phosphene generation, but they have few advantages over the LGN, and, at least for the radiation, a more challenging physical structure for electrode design.

Cortical implants have the longest history of investigation, including the first artificial vision experiments [3, 4, 34–36]. Our deep understanding of primary visual cortex [37] suggests that a cortical visual prosthesis is a realistic goal. Physically, the cortex is the largest among potential targets, allowing for a large number of electrode contacts [38, 39] and therefore potentially high-resolution artificial vision. This advantage is tempered by cortical folding that makes some parts of the visual field more difficult to access than others, and the position of the central-most visual region within the interhemispheric fissure [10].

Thalamic prostheses have been shown to be a viable approach [11]. While previous stages of the visual system allow for a less invasive implant, the techniques from the unrelated field of deep brain stimulation (DBS) have made surgical access to midbrain regions routine [40–42] and discussed below. The LGN offers a compact representation of the entire visual field, allowing for complete coverage with bilateral implants [11]. Magnification of the central field simplifies creation of a high-resolution implant [12]. Finally, electrical stimulation at the LGN that mimics input from the optic nerve allows the visual system to use the normal corticothalamic feedback system [9].

Indication for Certain Forms of Illnesses

The thalamic approach supports a wide range of indications. Any agent that results in blindness due to a cessation of neural output from the eye can potentially be treated with a thalamic visual prosthesis. These conditions include glaucoma, macular degeneration, and retinitis pigmentosa. Important additional indications include medically necessary enucleation and trauma to the globe or optic nerve. Existing drug-based or non-cranial surgical therapies such as lens replacement would be preferable in blindness caused by infection, cataract, and corneal scarring.

Attention

Because attention is a vital part of visual system processing, visual prostheses should support attentional effects to optimize utility to the patient. The classical view of LGN being a simple relay station is slowly changing to one where it has a more complex role [43] following observations of activity being modulated during visual attention [21, 43–45]. Spatial attention, as one example of attention, has been shown to affect LGN activation in both humans and macaques [43, 46, 47]. As the LGN receives projections from the cortex, the brain stem, and the thalamic reticular nucleus in addition to the retina, the LGN is architecturally poised for a central role [43, 48]. While we expect a thalamic prosthesis to support the natural integration of modulatory, non-retinal input to LGN, it might be difficult to establish the same level of functionality with a cortical device.

Technical Description

The thalamic visual prosthesis as a device has a similar overall design as other approaches using electrical stimulation (Fig. 14.2). A *scene camera,* mounted in an external frame worn like a set of glasses, serves as a stand-in for the retina. Its

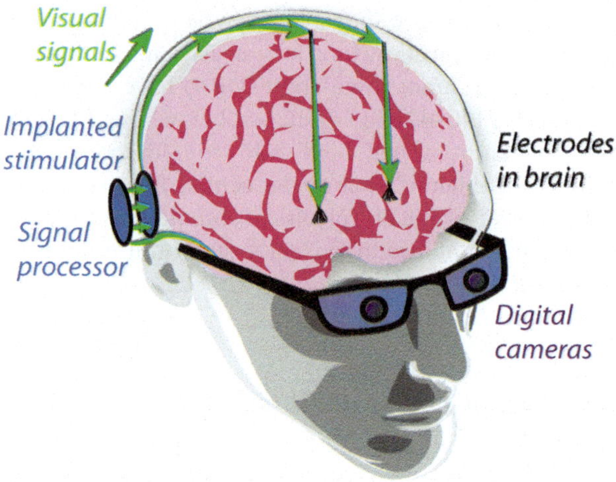

Fig. 14.2 Schematic view of the thalamic visual prosthesis. The overall design of the thalamic visual prosthesis follows a theme that is common among many projects. A video camera (here, shown as two cameras, one for each eye) sends signals to an externally worn signal processor that continually extracts information from the video stream and converts it to a neural code. The encoded signals are transmitted wirelessly to a permanently implanted simulator that drives brush-style electrodes that are bilaterally placed in LGN

signals are transformed by an externally worn processor into a form appropriate for stimulation of neural tissue. The transformed signals are sent over a secure wireless connection to a permanently implanted stimulator that drives a set of brush-style microwire electrodes. Each individual electrode contact generates a single pixel-like percept called *a phosphene*. However, unlike pixels in a computer display, the arrays of phosphenes generated by visual prostheses are neither uniformly spaced, nor abutting, but instead tend to be discrete, separated visual elements on an unstimulated background [13].

Because the precise placement of individual microwires in a brush-style depth electrode is not presently possible, our project is taking an approach that accommodates uncertainty in location. There are, however, general characteristics of brush-style implants that result from the combination of electrode mechanical characteristics and LGN functional characteristics. The visual scene is smoothly mapped onto the retina by the optics of the eye, establishing an orderly progression that can be recognized at nearly every later stage of visual processing. The largest adjustment of the map reflects the non-uniformity of visual acuity, or equivalently, cellular density on the retina. Photoreceptor and retinal ganglion cell density is highest in the foveal area, tapering off substantially toward the periphery. A conceptually one-to-one functional relationship exists from retinal ganglion cells to thalamic cells, but unlike the retina, the LGN has an even anatomical cellular density, resulting in an apparent magnification of representation as mentioned above. This change in representational density is reflected in the pattern of phosphenes generated by a regular placement of stimulating electrodes. In the retina, regular electrode placement results in phosphene patterns that appear close to a regular grid in visual space, but the same sort of regular placement creates a phosphene pattern that is strongly center-weighted in the thalamus and visual cortex [13]. As a result, thalamic implants are anticipated to be somewhat more natural in use than regular arrays implanted retinally (Pezaris Laboratory, 2009).

Transformation of the video stream into stimulation trains requires knowledge of the exact location of each phosphene in the visual field. At present, we rely upon the well-understood anatomical mapping of the retinotopic field onto the LGN, although a higher-accuracy map would ultimately improve utility. Various methods have been described for refining phosphene locations [49], but these become somewhat tedious and unattractive for electrode counts in the hundreds-to-thousands, and the ultimate answer remains elusive. Nevertheless, given a description of the phosphene pattern in visual space, each video frame from the scene camera is translated into a set of independent per-electrode stimulation trains based on a straightforward veridical function that adjusts stimulation intensity according to brightness. Details of the encoding function also remain open until we have more informative feedback from human experiments, and are likely to change.

Our current design calls for 128 stimulating electrodes in bilateral groups of 64. While there is an understanding that having more phosphenes is universally preferable as it translates to higher resolution, there is a threshold effect in the range of a few hundred to a thousand points for tasks of daily living [14, 15]. At present, our electrode count is limited only by technical reasons as the volume of human LGN can accommodate thousands of microwires [12]. Future generations of our bench-based system will increase the phosphene count, incorporate a wireless connection between the external processor and the stimulator, and include a permanently implanted stimulator.

Surgical Methods

The thalamic approach has been made possible because of advances in the unrelated field of deep brain stimulation. DBS was initially developed for treatment of motor disorders such as Parkinsonian tremor [41, 42] and has become a well-developed clinical technique that is safe and effective [50]. Electrode implantation is considered minimally invasive [51, 52] as only small holes are required in the skull, and excellent placement accuracy is routine [53]. The implanted components for DBS therapy are highly similar to those required for a visual prosthesis – bilateral stimulating electrodes and permanently implanted stimulators – and the typical targets for DBS of the subthalamic nucleus and globus pallidus are only one centimeter or so away from the LGN. The description that follows is a speculative adaptation of the standard DBS implantation method to use with a visual prosthesis.

A titanium reference frame is temporarily attached to the skull and MRI and CT scans of the head with the frame in place are taken immediately prior to implantation surgery. After surgical planning, a small burr-hole is cut in the skull and an insertion mechanism temporarily affixed using the reference frame to ensure accuracy. Traditional microelectrodes are introduced and advanced toward the target area while neural electrical activity is monitored for the expected functional characteristics of overlying structures. Once the putative location of LGN is found, stimulation is applied through the microelectrode to validate phosphene position within the visual field. Two or three additional penetrations are made to orient the neurosurgeon within LGN. Prosthesis electrodes are then introduced to the finalized location and their operation verified. Electrodes are cemented in place at the skull, the leads routed subcutaneously to a stimulator placed in the subclavical space, and the reference frame removed. This process is logically repeated for both hemispheres, although it typically happens in coordinated stages. The entire surgical procedure typically takes 1–2 h.

Measurement of individual electrode stimulation thresholds and phosphene characteristics must be undertaken as the first part of post-implant therapy. We anticipate that repeated sessions with specialized staff will be required to adjust stimulation settings and encoding parameters for each patient to optimize benefit and utility.

Experimental Results

The line of inquiry into a thalamic visual prosthesis was established with an experiment demonstrating proof of concept by Pezaris and Reid [11] in a monkey model. Stimulation through microwires placed in LGN were shown to evoke phosphenes that were immediately incorporated into a behavioral task as alternatives to small points of light presented on a computer screen. Phosphene location could be controlled through careful placement of stimulating electrodes, and corresponded to the location of the response fields of cells recorded prior to stimulation. This work included a brief secondary experiment with two electrodes that demonstrated independent control of two non-simultaneous phosphenes.

Shortly thereafter, Pezaris and Reid [12] investigated basic engineering questions into different electrode designs and their expected phosphene patterns along with the physical limitations of implanting a large number of microwires. They modeled implantation of regular 3D arrays of electrodes into monkey LGN, for which an accurate functional atlas exists [54], and described the center-weighted patterns of phosphenes that resulted. In particular, a microwire spacing of 600 microns resulted in approximately 300 phosphenes per visual hemifield in the monkey. Although an accurate functional atlas does not yet exist for the human LGN, the area is about twice as large in volume than in monkey [12], such that electrodes at 800 micron spacing could support nearly 400 phosphenes within the central-most 10° of visual space with a bilateral implant.

To understand the utility of such center-weighted patterns that reflect the underlying representational density across the visual field, experiments were then performed to measure the effective acuity that example patterns would provide [14]. Normal, sighted human subjects used a virtual reality simulation of thalamic artificial vision to perform a two-alternative forced choice letter recognition task that was based on standard acuity charts used in clinical assessment of basic visual function. Approximately 100 phosphenes in central vision were found to be sufficient for 20/470 vision (logMAR 1.37) and approximately 400 phosphenes for 20/240 vision (logMAR 1.08). It was suggested that for each pattern, the effective acuity could be determined by measuring the size of the circle that circumscribed the central-most 20 phosphenes. Although the most important aspect of this work was to guide selection of channel count in the first prototype device, the level of improvement in subject performance over the short, 2-h experimental time hints at the critical role that rehabilitative post-implant training will have.

Verification of the usability of phosphenes in a real-world application was then pursued with a more advanced virtual reality system that normal, sighted subjects used to perform the MNREAD test of visual acuity [15]. This test requires subjects to read three-line simple sentences at varying font sizes, measuring reading speed and accuracy which are expected to worsen as font size decreases. Not surprisingly, it was found that the combination of high phosphene count patterns with large font sizes produced the fastest and most accurate reading, and that lowering either phosphene count or font size resulted in reduced performance. Translation of reading performance into measurements of visual acuity were consistent with those from the letter recognition task described above, but with substantially reduced subject burden, suggesting the reading task will form an important tool for future non-invasive assessment of prosthesis designs.

The laboratory is currently developing a bench-based prototype device with 128 electrodes that are placed bilaterally (half in each LGN) to cover both left and right portions of central vision. In preparation for testing, monkeys have been trained on the same letter recognition task as described above in a third virtual reality simulation of artificial vision (Killian et al., 2016). While monkeys do not understand the letters with the same depth of meaning as humans, they are adept at recognizing arbitrary visual objects (reviewed in [55]), and with substantial training have been able to perform at levels comparable to our human results. This training has been undertaken as a prerequisite to testing with the bench-based system driving implanted electrodes with the same task presented through electrically-driven phosphenes to demonstrate a full circuit visual prosthesis.

Future Direction

The Thalamic Prosthesis Project will continue to advance toward the goal of human implantation. Results from both animal and sighted human subjects have demonstrated the utility of a multi-pronged approach, obtaining answers to critical scientific and engineering questions with the most appropriate model system.

In the near future, we anticipate demonstration of a 128-electrode prosthesis in an animal model. Assessing the effectiveness of this bench-based device will guide transformation of our results into an implantable prototype to be tested in a second suite of animal subjects with the follow-on aim of initial tests in human volunteers.

The remaining significant challenges include scientific, engineering, and medical issues that all must be addressed. Scientific questions about the appearance of phosphenes (color, size) and their controllability are most easily answered in human subjects. Engineering questions remain about translation of video streams into neural stimulation, as well as adaptation of existing stimulator technologies to use as visual prostheses, and addressing device biocompatibility and lifetime issues. Medical issues include developing a means for improving the accuracy of standard anatomical maps of deep brain structures in blind individuals so as to refine target identification during implantation, and creating a more thorough understanding the role of post-implant rehabilitation therapy in long-term implant performance.

In particular, the uncertainty of which encoding method to translate the video stream to neural stimulation carries questions about how stimulation is best patterned across many electrodes. Potential challenges include generation of unintended phosphenes with multiple simultaneously activated electrodes [56] and decreasing effectiveness of stimulation [57]. These may be potentially solved by careful selection of stimulation parameters [58, 59]. While we expect such questions to be addressed initially in animal models, a more expedient approach would include human volunteers.

Long-Term Adaptation

One of the large open questions relates to plasticity and long-term adaptation in the visual system of prosthesis recipients. The success that cochlear implants have achieved is due to the acceptance and usage of the device, and the concomitant long-term learning effects that span many years [60].

Just as cochlear implant use leads to long-term perceptual modification [6, 60], artificial visual percepts may also change in perceived location and size in visual space over time [61]. For children with the advantage of developmental plasticity, such adaptation may prove quite fruitful and provide justification for early intervention with a visual prosthesis for the congenitally blind. In adults, where plasticity is thought to be more limited [62], cortical reorganization is likely to follow thalamic plasticity associated with electrical stimulation [26, 63]. While we have evidence that humans quickly adapt to new visual modalities [15], we speculate that the corticothalamic feedback loop may provide a critical mechanism to modulating thalamic phosphenes, adapting the perceptual structures to make seeing easier with artificial vision.

An Ultimate Goal

Ultimately, we must continue to strive to create a device that provides a substantial improvement in the quality of life for the affected patient population without undue side-effects or operational burden. Sight, to those with natural vision, is effortless, and that should be the goal for researchers in artificial vision.

References

1. World Health Organization (WHO). Visual impairment and blindness. Fact Sheet N°282. Updated August 2014.
2. Brant Fernandes RA, Diniz B, Ribeiro R, Humayun M. Artificial vision through neuronal stimulation. Neurosci Lett. 2012;519(2):122–8.
3. Brindley GS, Lewin WS. The sensations produced by electrical stimulation of the visual cortex. J Physiol. 1968;196(2):479–93.
4. Dobelle WH, Mladejvosky MG. Phosphenes produced by electrical stimulation of human occipital cortex and their application to the development of a prosthesis for the blind. J Physiol. 1974;243(2):553–576.1.
5. Weale RA. Senile ocular changes, cell death, and vision. In: Sekuler R, Kline D, Dismukes K, editors. Aging and human visual function. New York: Alan R Liss; 1982. p. 161–71.
6. Humayun MS, Weiland JD, Fujii GY, Greenberg R, Williamson R, Little JM, et al. Visual perception in a blind subject with a chronic microelectronic retinal prosthesis. Vision Res. 2003;43:2573–81.
7. Dow BM, Snyder AZ, Vautin RG, Bauer R. Magnification factor and receptive field size in foveal striate cortex of the monkey. Exp Brain Res. 1981;44(2):213–28.
8. Kanda H, Morimoto T, Fujikado T, Tano Y, Fukuda Y, Sawai H. Electrophysiological studies of the feasibility of suprachoroidal- transretinal stimulation for artificial vision in normal and RCS rats. Invest Ophthalmol Vis Sci. 2004;45(2):560–6.
9. Panetsos F, Sanchez-Jimenez A, Diaz-de Cerio E, Diaz-Guemes I, Sanchez FM. Consistent phosphenes generated by electrical microstimulation of the visual thalamus. An experimental approach for thalamic visual neuroprosthesis. Front Neurosci. 2011;5:84.
10. Panetsos F, Diaz-de Cerio E, Sanchez-Jimenez A, Herrera-Rincon C. Thalamic visual neuroprostheses: comparison of visual percepts generated by natural stimulation of the eye and electrical stimulation of the thalamus. IEEE/EMBS Conference on Neural Engineering, 2009.
11. Pezaris JS, Reid RC. Demonstration of artificial visual percepts generated through thalamic microstimulation. Proc Natl Acad Sci U S A. 2007;104(18):7670–5.
12. Pezaris JS, Reid RC. Simulations of electrode placement for a thalamic visual prosthesis. IEEE Trans Biomed Eng. 2009;56(1):172–8.
13. Pezaris JS, Eskandar EN. Getting signals into the brain: visual prosthetics through thalamic microstimulation. Neurosurg Focus. 2009;27(1):E6.
14. Bourkiza B, Vurro M, Jeffries A, Pezaris JS. Visual acuity of simulated thalamic visual prostheses in normally sighted humans. PLoS One. 2013;8(9):e73592.
15. Vurro M, Crowell AM, Pezaris JS. Simulation of thalamic prosthetic vision: reading accuracy, speed, and acuity in sighted humans. Front Human Neurosci. 2014;8:816.
16. Papsin BC, Gordon KA. Cochlear implants for children with severe-to-profound hearing loss. N Engl J Med. 2007;357:2380–7. doi:10.1056/NEJMct0706268.
17. Chow AY, Chow VY, Packo KH, Pollack JS, Peyman GA, Schuchard R. The artificial silicon retina microchip for the treatment of vision loss from retinitis pigmentosa. Arch Ophthalmol. 2004;122(4):460–9.
18. Spear SD, Moore RJ, Kim CB, Xue JT, Tumosa N. Effects of aging on the primate visual system: spatial and temporal processing by lateral geniculate neurons in young adult and old rhesus monkeys. J Neurophysiol. 1994;72(1):402–20.
19. Sherman SM, Guillery RW. Exploring the thalamus and its role in cortical function. Cambridge: MIT Press; 2005.
20. Schmid MC, Mrowka SW, Turchi J, Saunders RC, Wilke M, Peters AJ, Ye FQ, Leopold DA. Blindsight depends on the lateral geniculate nucleus. Nature. 2010;466:373–7.
21. Denison RN, Vu AT, Yacoub E, Feinberg DA, Silver MA. Functional mapping of the magnocellular and parvocellular subdivisions of human LGN. Neuroimage. 2014;102(Pt 2):358–69.
22. Nakauchi K, Fujikado T, Kanda H, Morimoto T, Choi JS, Ikuno Y, Sakaguchi H, Kamei M, Ohji M, Yagi T, Nishimura S, Sawai H, Fukuda Y, Tano Y. Transretinal electrical stimulation by

an intrascleral multichannel electrode array in rabbit eyes. Graefes Arch Clin Exp Ophthalmol. 2005;243(2):169–74. Epub 2004 Dec 7.
23. Kara P, Pezaris JS, Yurgenson S, Reid RC. The spatial receptive field of thalamic inputs to single cortical simple cells revealed by the interaction of visual and electrical stimulation. Proc Natl Acad Sci U S A. 2002;99(25):16261–6.
24. Reid RC, Alonso JM. Specificity of monosynaptic connections from thalamus to visual cortex. Nature. 1995;378:281–4.
25. Orban G. Neuronal operations in the visual cortex. New York: Springer; 1984.
26. Born BT, Trott AR, Hartmann TS. Cortical magnification plus cortical plasticity equals vision? Vis Res. 2015;111(B):161–9.
27. Malpeli JR, Baker FH. The representation of the visual field in the lateral geniculate nucleus of Macaca mulatta. J Comp Neurol. 1975;161(4):569–94.
28. Schneider KA, Richter MC, Kastner S. Retinotopic organization and functional subdivisions of the human lateral geniculate nucleus: a high-resolution functional magnetic resonance imaging study. J Neurosci. 2004;24(41):8975–85.
29. Reppas JB, Usrey WM, Reid RC. Saccadic eye movements modulate visual responses in the lateral geniculate nucleus. Neuron. 2002;35:961–74.
30. Dagnelie G, Barnett D, Humayun MS, Thompson RW. Paragraph text reading using a pixelized prosthetic vision simulator: parameter dependence and task learning in free-viewing conditions. Invest Ophthalmol Vis Sci. 2006;47(3):1241–50.
31. Veraart C, Raftopoulos C, Mortimer JT, Delbeke J, Pins D, Michaux G, Vanlierde A, Parrini S, Wanet-Defalque M-C. Visual sensations produced by optic nerve stimulation using an implanted self-sizing spiral cuff electrode. Brain Res. 1998;813(1).
32. Li L, Sun M, Cao P, Cai C, Chai X, Li X, et al. A visual prosthesis based on optic nerve stimulation: in vivo electrphysiological study in rabbits. In: Peng Y, Weng X, editors. APCMBE 2008, IFMBE Proceedings 19. New York: Springer; 2008. p. 54–7.
33. Sakaguchi H, Fuikikado T, Kanda H, Osanai M, Fang X, Nakauchi K, et al. Electrical stimulation with a needle-type electrode inserted into the optic nerve in rabbit eyes. Jpn J Opthalmol. 2004;48:552–7.
34. Bradley DC, Troyk PR, Berg JA, Bak M, Cogan S, Erickson R, et al. Visuotopic mapping through a multichannel stimulating implant in primate V1. J Neurophysiol. 2005;93: 1659–70.
35. Dobelle WH. Artificial vision for the blind by connecting a television camera to the visual cortex. ASAIO J. 2000;46:3–9.
36. Tehovnik EJ, Slocum WM. Phosphene induction by microstimulation of macaque V1. Brain Res Rev. 2007;53:337–43.
37. Hubel DH, Wiesel TN. Brain and visual perception: the story of a 25-year collaboration. Oxford: Oxford University Press; 2004.
38. Sommerhalder J, Rappaz B, de Haller R, Fornos AP, Safran AB, Pelizzone M. Simulation of artificial vision: II. Eccentric reading of full-page text and the learning of this task. Vis Res. 2004;44:1693–706.
39. Sommerhalder J, Oueghlani E, Bagnoud M, Leonards U, Safran AB, Pelizzone M. Simulation of artificial vision: I. Eccentric reading of isolated words, and perceptual learning. Vis Res. 2003;43:269–83.
40. Seddighi A, Seddighi AS, Zali AR, Afaghi V, Afaghi A, Ashrafi F. Therapeutic effects of thalamic electrical stimulation in Parkinson's disease. Global J Heath Sci. 2011;3(2):102–8.
41. Kumar R, Lozano AM, Kim YJ, Hutchison WD, Sime E, Halket E, Lang AE. Double-blind evaluation of subthalamic nucleus deep brain stimulation in advanced Parkinson's disease. Neurology. 1998;51(3):850–5.
42. Limousin P, Pollak P, Benazzouz A, Hoffman D, Broussolle E, Perret JE, Benabid A-L. Bilateral subthalamic nucleus stimulation for severe Parkinson's disease. Mov Dis. 1995;10(5):672–4.
43. O'Connor DH, Fukui MM, Pinsk MA, Kastner S. Attention modulates responses in the human lateral geniculate nucleus. Nat Neurosci. 2002;5(11):1203–9.

44. Schneider KA. Subcortical mechanisms of feature-based attention. J Neurosci. 2011;31(23):8643–53.
45. Schneider KA, Kastner S. Effects of sustained spatial attention in the human lateral geniculate nucleus and superior colliculus. J Neurosci. 2009;29(6):1784–95. doi:10.1523/JNEUROSCI. 4452-08.2009.
46. McAlonan K, Cavanaugh J, Wurtz RH. Guarding the gateway to cortex with attention in visual thalamus. Nature. 2008;456(7220):391–4. doi:10.1038/nature07382. Epub 2008 Oct 5.
47. Casagrande VA, Sáry G, Royal D, Ruiz O. On the impact of attention and motor planning on the lateral geniculate nucleus. Prog Brain Res. 2005;149:11–29.
48. Kastner S, Schneider KA, Wunderlich K. Beyond a relay nucleus: neuroimaging views on the human LGN. Prog Brain Res. 2006;155:125–43.
49. Stronks HC, Dagnelie G. Phosphene mapping techniques for visual prostheses. In: Dagnelie G, editor. Visual prosthetics. New York: Springer; 2011. p. 367–83.
50. Okun MS. Deep-brain simulation for Parkinson's disease. N Engl J Med. 2012;367:1529–38.
51. Yamamoto T, Katayama Y, Hirayama T. Minimally invasive neurosurgery for involuntary movement and intractable pain: from destructive surgery to electrical stimulation therapy. Funct Neurosurg. 1997;36:23–8.
52. Molinger AY, Benabid A-L, Rezai AR. Brain stimulation: current applications and future prospects. Thalamus Relat Syst. 2001;1:255–67.
53. Burchiel KJ, McCartney S, Lee A, Raslan AM. Accuracy of deep brain stimulation electrode placement using intraoperative computed comography without microelectrode recording. J Neurosurg. 2013;119(2):301–6.
54. Erwin E, Baker FH, Busen WF, Malpeli JG. Relationship between laminar topology and retinotopy in the rhesus lateral geniculate nucleus: results from a functional atlas. J Comp Neurol. 1999;407:92–102.
55. Logothetis NK, Sheinberg DL. Visual object recognition. Ann Rev Neurosci. 1996;19: 577–62.
56. Dobelle WH, Mladejovsky MG, Girvin JP. Artificial vision for the blind: electrical stimulation of visual cortex offers hope for a functional prosthesis. Science. 1974;183(4123):440–4.
57. Heming EA, Choo R, Davies JN, Kiss ZHT. Designing a thalamic somatosensory neural prosthesis: consistency and persistence of percepts evoked by electrical stimulation. IEEE Trans Neural Syst Rehab Eng. 2011;19(5):477–82.
58. Lee SW, Eddington DK, Fried SI. Responses to pulsatile subretinal electric stimulation: effects of amplitude and duration. J Neurophysiol. 2013;109(7):1954–68.
59. Dowden BR, Frankel MA, Wilder AM, Hiatt SD, Ledbetter NM, Warren DA, Clark GA, Normann RA. Coordinated, multi-joint, fatigue-resistant feline stance produced with intrafascicular hind limb nerve stimulation. J Neural Eng. 2012;9(2):026019.
60. Beadle EA, McKinley DJ, Nikolopoulos TP, Brough J, O'Donoghue GM, Archbold SM. Long-term functional outcomes and academic-occupational status in implanted children. After 10 to 14 years of cochlear implant use. Otol Neurotol. 2005;26(6):1152–60.
61. Marc RE, Jones BW. Retinal remodeling in inherited photoreceptor degenerations. Mol Neurobiol. 2003;28(2):139–47
62. Buonomano DV, Merzenich MM. Cortical plasticity: from synapses to maps. Annu Rev Neurosci. 1998;21:149–86.
63. Moore BD, Kiley CW, Sun C, Usrey WM. Rapid plasticity of visual responses in the adult lateral geniculate nucleus. Neuron. 2011;71(5):812–9.

Chapter 15
CORTIVIS Approach for an Intracortical Visual Prostheses

Eduardo Fernández and Richard A. Normann

Abstract Cortical prostheses are a subgroup of visual neuroprostheses capable of evoking visual percepts in profoundly blind people through direct electrical stimulation of the occipital cortex. This approach may be the only treatment available for blindness caused by glaucoma, end-stage retinitis pigmentosa, optic atrophy, trauma to the retinas and/or optic nerves or by diseases of the central visual pathways such as brain injuries or stroke. However the selection of a specific person for a cortical implant is not straightforward and currently there are not strict standardized criteria for accepting or rejecting a candidate. We are now facing the challenge of creating such an intracortical visual neuroprosthesis designed to interface with the occipital visual cortex as a means through which a limited but useful visual sense could be restored to these blind patients.

Keywords Visual prosthesis • Artificial vision • Electrode arrays • Surgical technique • Phosphenes • Electrical stimulation • Human striate cortex • Plasticity

Key Points

- The intracortical approach may be the only treatment available for pathologies affecting the entire retina, optic nerve, thalamus or the brain.
- While the full restoration of vision seems to be unlikely in the near future, a cortical device can create meaningful visual percepts, resulting in a substantial improvement in the quality of life of blind and visually impaired persons.
- The surgical approach for the implantation of intracortical microelectrodes is straightforward and follows standard neurosurgical procedures.
- A modulation and better understanding of adaptive brain changes following vision loss is crucial for restoring a useful vision.

E. Fernández, MD, PhD (✉)
Department of Neural Engineering, Miguel Hernández University, CIBER BBN, Elche, Alicante, Spain
e-mail: e.fernandez@umh.es

R.A. Normann, PhD
Department of Bioengineering, University of Utah, Salt Lake City, UT, USA

V.P. Gabel (ed.), *Artificial Vision*, DOI 10.1007/978-3-319-41876-6_15

Principal Idea

Loss of vision affects millions of people worldwide and poses extraordinary challenges to individuals in our society that relies heavily on sight. Although in recent years the techniques of molecular genetics have led to a rapid identification of a great number of genes involved in visual diseases (see https://sph.uth.edu/Retnet/sum-dis.htm for an update of genes and loci causing retinal diseases), and there are significant advancements in the development of different approaches for artificial vision, at present there is no effective treatment for many patients who are visually handicapped as a result of degeneration or damage to the inner layers of the retina, the optic nerve or the visual pathways. Therefore, there are compelling reasons to pursue the development of a cortical visual prosthesis capable of restoring some useful sight in these profoundly blind patients.

As blindness results from an interruption in the normal flow of signals along the visual pathways, a visual prosthesis has to excite the neurons of the pathway at some point after the damage site [1]. The only requirement is that the device should contact with still functioning neural elements. Since retinal diseases frequently reduce visual acuity and result in non-curable blindness, several groups worldwide are working on the development of various prostheses designed to interact with the remaining healthy retina, optic nerve and LGN. However the output neurons of the eye, the ganglion cells, often degenerate in many retinal blindnesses [2], and therefore a retinal, optic nerve or even a LGN prosthesis are not helpful for blindness caused by glaucoma or optic atrophy nor for diseases of the visual pathways. Because this extensive degeneration usually respects the neurons in the higher visual regions of the brain, this suggests the enormous potential of a cortical prosthesis designed to stimulate these cortical neurons directly [3–6]. Thus if these higher visual centers could be stimulated with visual information in a format somewhat similar to the way they were stimulated before the onset of blindness, a blind individual may be able to use this stimulation to extract information about the physical world around him/her [1, 4, 5, 7].

The Case for a Cortical Visual Neuroprosthesis

The concept of a cortical visual prosthesis began with studies of the functional architecture of the cerebral cortex and has a long history in biomedical engineering. An important source of information in this field is provided by the analysis of the visual perceptions elicited by cortical stimulation during surgical operations. Löwenstein and Borchardt reported in 1918 the case of a patient that was able to see flickering in the opposite half of their visual field after stimulation of the occipital pole, and few years later a German neurosurgeon, Foerster, was the first to expose the human occipital pole under local anesthesia and to electrically stimulate it [8]. He noted that electrical stimulation induced the perception of points of light, called phosphenes that were usually described as 'stars in the sky', 'clouds' and 'pinwheels' with locations that were dependent on where the stimulation probe was placed. These findings together with the earlier studies of Wilder Penfield and co-workers during the course of neurosurgical interventions for the treatment of epilepsy [9] established the physiological basis for present efforts to develop a visual prosthesis for the blind.

Figure 15.1 illustrates the basic idea. If we stimulated a single electrode positioned in the visual cortex, the patient can perceive a single phosphene. With two electrodes simultaneously, it is possible to induce the perception of a horizontal or vertical line (Fig. 15.1a); with three electrodes arranged as a triangle it is possible to perceive a triangle (Fig. 15.1b) and so on. If even a crude representation of visual space can be delivered to electrodes implanted in the visual cortex, the blind subject should eventually be able to use it to create an image (Fig. 15.1c). Thus the learning

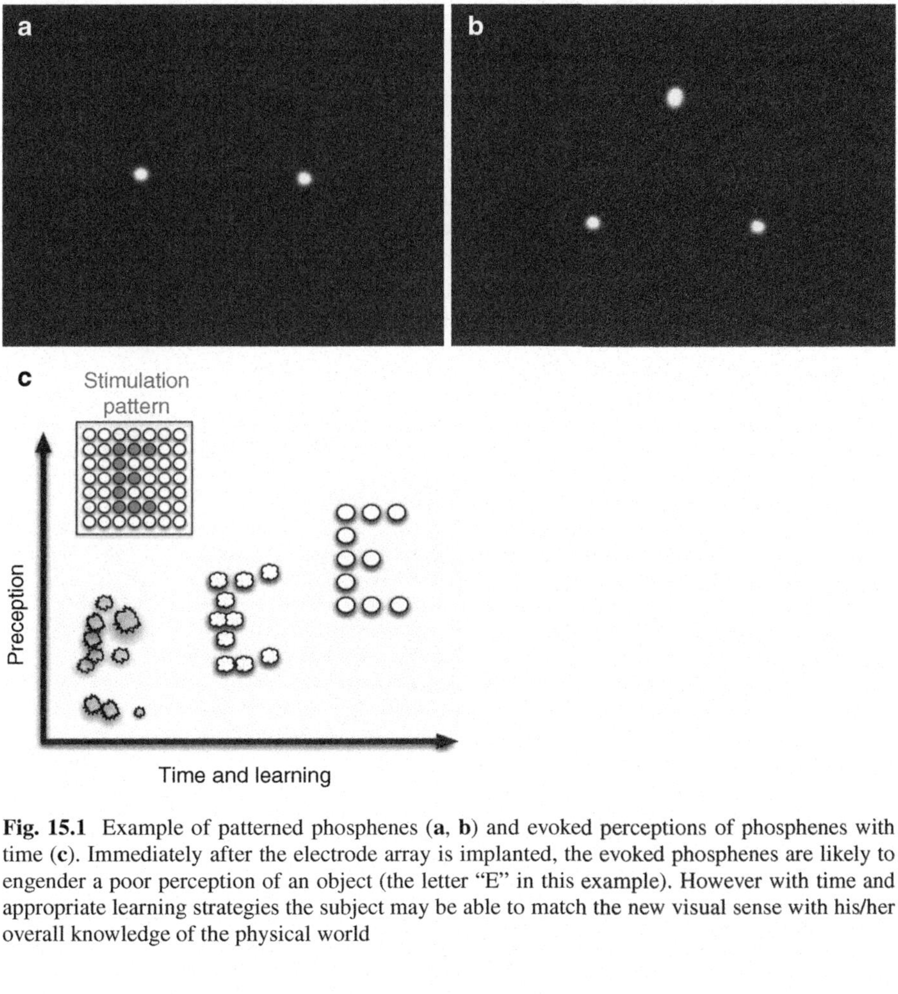

Fig. 15.1 Example of patterned phosphenes (**a**, **b**) and evoked perceptions of phosphenes with time (**c**). Immediately after the electrode array is implanted, the evoked phosphenes are likely to engender a poor perception of an object (the letter "E" in this example). However with time and appropriate learning strategies the subject may be able to match the new visual sense with his/her overall knowledge of the physical world

and adaptation that occurs in the visual cortex will allow perceiving an image that comports with his or her sense of the surrounding physical world.

In this framework experiments by the group of Giles Brindley in England, William Dobelle at the University of Utah and others, showed that stimulation of multiple electrodes simultaneously allowed blind volunteers to recognize simple patterns, including letters and Braille characters [10–12]. Unfortunately, these early efforts did not culminate in the restoration of a useful visual sense. Problems with this early work were associated mainly with the large surface electrodes that were used to evoke phosphenes. Thus, relatively high electrical currents were required to evoke phosphenes and when multiple electrodes were stimulated, these large currents could interact in a non-linear fashion, evoking phosphenes with unpredictable spatial properties. Furthermore they also found that a visual prosthesis based on relatively large surface electrodes implanted subdurally would have limited usefulness because of occasional elicitation of pain due to meningeal or scalp stimulation, and the risk of inducing epileptic seizures.

A promising approach, which can activate populations of neurons with greater spatial specificity and lower levels of stimulation than is possible with larger electrodes on the surface of the brain, is the use of intracortical microelectrodes [13]. This cortical approach requires the use of intracortical penetrating electrodes, with sizes of the same order of magnitude as the neurons intended to be stimulated, and located preferably in layer 4 of the occipital cortex, since this stratum receives the main central connection from the LGN and optic nerve (Fig. 15.2b). In this context, one microelectrode array that has been used extensively in acute and chronic recording experiments is the Utah Electrode Array (UEA). This array has been designed to compromise as little cortical volume as possible and has 100 narrow silicon shanks protruding 1.0–1.5 mm from a flat rectangular base that rests on the surface

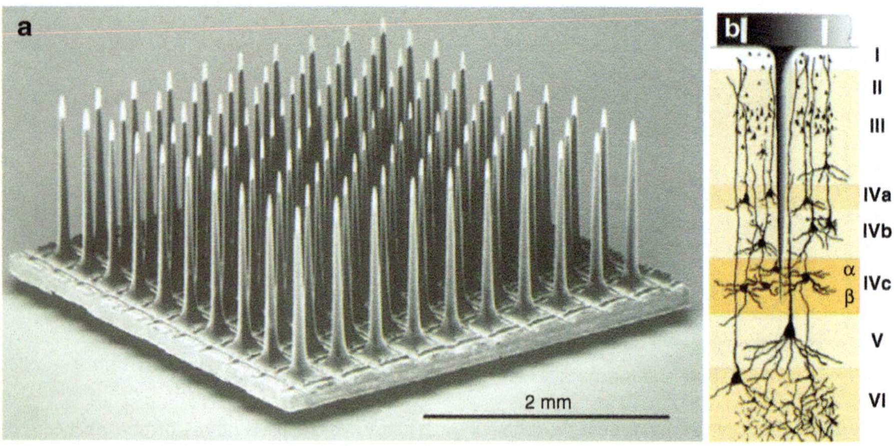

Fig. 15.2 (**a**) Scanning electron micrograph of a 10-by-10-electrode array designed to be inserted into the primary visual cortex. (**b**) Drawing of the visual cortex with one implanted intracortical microelectrode. Note the electrode tips are located in layer IVc

of the cortex (see Fig. 15.2a). The base of each microelectrode is surrounded by a moat of glass that insulates each electrode from neighboring electrodes, and the entire structure, with the exception of the electrode tips, is insulated from the neural tissues. Stimulation sites are located on the shank tips that have been metalized with activated iridium oxide. In present day embodiments, each electrode is connected to a scalp mounted connector with a 25 micron diameter insulated wire. The UEA has been used in BrainGate clinical trials [14–16], in research with epilepsy patients [5, 17] and is the only intracortical microelectrode array that has been FDA approved for long-term human studies.

Technical Description

Figure 15.3 illustrates the basic components of a cortical visual neuroprosthesis. One or two cameras provide image acquisition, which is then processed by a bioinspired retina-like encoder in order to transform the visual world into electrical signals [18]. This first stage performs a multichannel spatio-temporal filtering to extract and enhance the most relevant features of the scene and also re-encodes this information into a neuromorphic stream of electrode addresses (Fig. 15.3a). The second

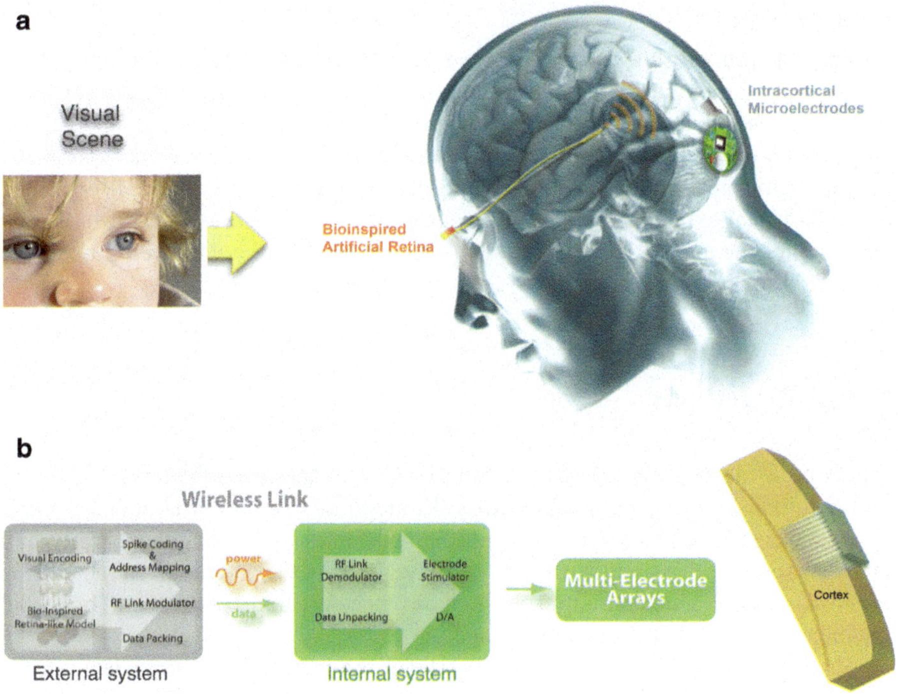

Fig. 15.3 Basic components of an intracortical visual neuroprosthesis (see text for more details)

stage serializes the information and transmits it through a radio-frequency link (RF) to the implanted device (Fig. 15.3b). This RF block provides a wireless transfer of power and data to the internal system. The implanted electronics package must decode the signals, identify the target electrodes and control the voltage shape (D/A converter) and amplitude of the waveform to be applied to the appropriate electrodes located near the target neurons [19, 20].

While the full restoration of vision seems to be unfeasible, it is expected that a cortical device can create truly meaningful visual percepts that can be translated into functional gains such as the recognition, localization and grasping of objects or skillful navigation in familiar an unfamiliar environments resulting in a substantial improvement in the standard of living of blind and visually impaired persons. Such assistive devices have already allowed thousands of deaf patients to hear sounds and acquire language abilities and the same hope exists in the field of visual rehabilitation.

Indications

The intracortical approach is expected to provide a potential solution to pathologies affecting the entire retina, optic nerve, thalamus or the brain. This approach it is the only treatment available for blindness caused by glaucoma or optic atrophy as well as for diseases of the central visual pathways such as brain injuries or stroke [4, 5, 7, 21–23].

The selection of a specific person for a cortical visual implant is not straightforward and currently there are no strict standardized criteria for accepting or rejecting a candidate nor for the best rehabilitation procedure for every type of blindness [24]. In general it is considered crucial that the subject should have no residual vision and had no significant benefit from a conventional visual aid. Furthermore it is needed previous visual experience. In this context, it has been presumed that if blindness occurs after the age of 10 years of age, visual pathways should develop normally and thus remain excitable.

Surgical Methods

Intracortical electrodes must penetrate into the brain and reach the level of the normal neuronal input to the visual cortex. In humans, this region is about 1.5 mm below the cortical surface, but we should also take into account that there are several layers of tissue separating the surface of the scalp from the cortex. From the outside in, these structures are: skin, muscles that cover the cranium, periosteum, bone and the meninges (dura mater, arachnoid and pia mater).

The surgical method for the implantation of the intracortical microelectrodes is straightforward and follows the standard neurosurgical procedures. Briefly, after the scalp is prepped with an antiseptic, a small skin incision is made. Then the skin and muscles are lifted off from the bone and folded back. Next, one small burr hole or a minicraniotomy of approximately 1.5 cm is made in the skull. This is a minimally invasive procedure that allows an easy access to the brain and is a standard procedure widely used in neurosurgery. After opening the dura with surgical scissors the neurosurgeon cuts the pia arachnoid and exposes the surface of the brain where the electrode array is inserted (Fig. 15.4). A high-resolution MRI is of paramount importance to avoid big blood vessels and help to find the best location of the electrode array.

Although each electrode in the array has a very sharp tip, it is a formidable task to implant a large number of electrodes into the cortex. Each needle has been made as slender as possible yet retain sufficient strength to withstand the implantation procedure. However even though the individual microelectrodes of the UEA are extremely sharp, early attempts to implant an array of 10 × 10 electrodes into the visual cortex in different animal models only deformed the cortical surface and resulted in incomplete implantation. Thus, while one or a few needles can be readily inserted, trying to insert a large number of electrodes only dimples the cortical surface. This problem is solved using a high velocity, impact insertion technique [25, 26]. This procedure allows the complete and safe insertion of the array in a manner that minimizes dimpling and compression of the subjacent structures. After implantation, the very large surface area of the 100 microelectrodes acts to integrate the array with the cortical tissues thereby providing a stable interface.

The latest step is to close the craniotomy. A Gore-Tex surgical membrane is laid over the array to inhibit adhesions [27] and the dura is closed with sutures. A second layer of Gore-Tex is laid over the dura and then the bone flap is replaced back in its original position and secured to the skull with titanium plates and screws. Finally the muscles and skin are sutured back together and a turban-like or soft adhesive dressing is placed over the incision for some days. The whole procedure takes approximately 1–1.5 h.

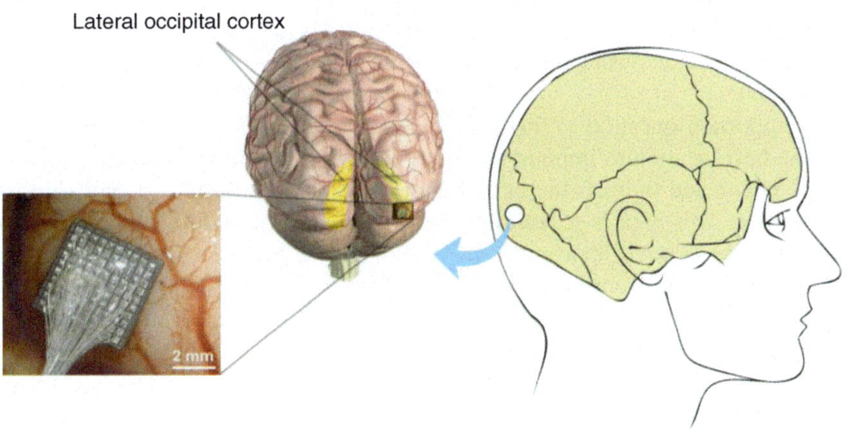

Fig. 15.4 Overview of the Implantation procedure of the electrode array near the occipital pole. *Scale bar* 2 mm

Experimental Results

Physiological and behavioral experiments in different animal species have shown that the UEA can be safely used for stimulation and recording of populations of neurons in visual cortex [5, 7, 28, 29]. Furthermore the amount of electrical current that must be injected into the tissues to excite the neurons is in the 1–10 microamp range. This is clearly two to three orders of magnitude smaller than the currents required to evoke phosphenes in previous attempts of developing a cortical visual prosthesis using surface electrodes [10–12]. At the same time, the data from non-human primates indicate that the monkeys perceive the cortical microstimulation as another visual stimulus and respond according to their training [5, 28]. The results of these experiments demonstrate that much selective stimulation can be achieved by implanting penetrating microelectrodes within the visual cortex, and altogether, establish the foundations for experiments in human volunteers.

With approved clinical protocols by the University of Utah (USA) and by the Hospital General Universitario of Alicante (Spain), we undertook preliminary investigations to establish the safety of the implantation procedures and to adapt the insertion technique to human requirements. These experiments were performed in 12 persons suffering from epilepsy or brain tumors that had to undergo a surgical resection of a brain region.

Our experimental results demonstrate that the implantation can be done without major complications and that high-quality recordings from human neurons can be consistently obtained in both acute (intraoperative) and chronic (epilepsy monitoring unit) settings. No adverse effects associated with these implantations have been reported. Furthermore we have also performed preliminary experiments to study the visual perceptions elicited by electrical stimulation at different locations of the human occipital cortex. The most common perceptions consisted of elementary visual images described as flashing, colored or uncolored lights and stars. No other symptoms such as seizures, nausea, or neurological deficits occurred during or after stimulation. The size of the perceived phosphenes ranged from a "pinpoint" to almost the whole visual field, depending on the location and stimulation parameters.

An important question in this field, which is not yet fully answered, is related with the best location to implant the microelectrodes. 90 % of projections from the eye are channeled through the lateral geniculate nucleus (LGN) to primary visual cortex (V1). This area is located on the medial surface of the occipital lobe and because of the layered appearance in Nissl stains, it is called the striate cortex. It includes the calcarine cortex and extends around the occipital pole. Since the striate cortex is involved in the initial cortical processing of all visual information, it has been proposed as the best site for implantation. However this area is difficult to reach (it is in the medial surface of the occipital lobe) and contains the calcarine artery, a branch of the posterior cerebral artery, which supplies the region. Therefore, we have been studying other suitable sites of implantation in order to avoid potential complications. Our preliminary results show that the electrical stimulation of the lateral occipital cortex (see Fig. 15.4) induces visual perceptions with consistent retinotopic organization and suggest that electrodes implanted near the occipital pole or in extrastriate areas could be able to elicit patterned perceptions and provide a limited but useful sense in blind subjects [30]. Furthermore, we have to take into account the learning processes and the neural plasticity of the visual cortex, which should allow an ever-improving correlation between the physical world and the evoked phosphenes. Nevertheless more data on the most effective means of stimulating the visual cortex using intracortical multielectrode arrays is still needed.

Future Directions

Like auditory brainstem implants in the profoundly deaf and recent work with "deep brain" stimulation in those afflicted by severe Parkinson's disease, cortical visual prostheses for the blind are now on the verge of entering a phase of human experimentation. Due to the complexity of the visual system and because verbal feedback is crucial, most core questions will be centered on the nature of the visual percepts that are elicited by electrical stimulation.

While many attributes characterize a visual scene (for example, color, form, motion and field of view), current strategies in visual prosthesis development are aimed to address only the most basic component, that is, spatial detail. In this context, it has been presumed that the quality of visual percepts is likely to improve, as remaining technical challenges are resolved. For example, more complex perceptions could be generated by simply increasing the number of stimulating electrodes, thereby increasing the potential resolution of images being produced [31, 32]. However, given that the complex relationship between patterns of electrical stimulation and target visual percepts remains largely unknown, this view appears to be an oversimplification. Thus, an increase in stimulus resolution may initially be perceptually meaningless rather than helpful [33]. At the same time, current psychophysical evidence suggest that the human visual system is able to identify and extract complex information (such as identifying human faces) from relatively poor quality images by relaying upon multiple salient visual features and cues [34]. This suggests that the assumption that visual perception will improve by concentrating on efforts geared toward increasing image resolution alone (as opposed to other visual attributes such as for example the temporal encoding related to motion perception) may be incorrect.

We should also be aware that the stimulation patterns used to evoke visual perception can vary with a number of parameters such as pulse duration, duty cycle, amplitude, number of pulses in a train, etc. Furthermore these parameters vary for every channel and might take very different values for each implanted patient. Even for a given subject, these values could change due to electrode encapsulation or neuroplastic changes. Thus many issues remain to be answered in these human experiments before useful vision can be provided for blind patients. In addition, we should take into account how the visual brain adapts to the loss of vision. This would particularly involve effective patient selection and a "custom-tailoring" of the cortical visual prosthetic devices for the needs of each patient.

A key issue that has often been utterly underrated in this context is the role of neural plasticity. Thus, we should take into consideration not only standardized methods and employ current clinical and technological expertise, but also consider newly emerging developmental and neurophysiological evidence. For example, there is considerable evidence that adaptive and compensatory changes occur within the brain following the loss of sight [35–38]. These studies have suggested that in some blind patients the occipital parts of the brain that sighted subjects utilize to process visual information are transformed and can be utilized to process tactile and auditory stimuli. This adaptive process in the brain probably allows blind subjects to extract greater information from touch and hearing, thus improving their quality of life and enhancing the integration of the blind in the social and working environment of a sighted society. The modulation and better understanding of these neuroplastic changes is crucial for restoring a limited but useful functional vision to those with profound blindness.

References

1. Normann RA, et al. Cortical implants for the blind. IEEE Spectrum. 1996;1996:54–9.
2. Marc RE, et al. Extreme retinal remodeling triggered by light damage: implications for age related macular degeneration. Mol Vis. 2008;14:782–806.
3. Troyk P, et al. A model for intracortical visual prosthesis research. Artif Organs. 2003;27(11):1005–15.
4. Fernandez E, et al. Development of a cortical visual neuroprosthesis for the blind: the relevance of neuroplasticity. J Neural Eng. 2005;2(4):R1–12.
5. Normann RA, et al. Toward the development of a cortically based visual neuroprosthesis. J Neural Eng. 2009;6(3):035001.
6. Tehovnik EJ, Slocum WM. Electrical induction of vision. Neurosci Biobehav Rev. 2013;37(5):803–18.
7. Fernandez E, et al. Acute human brain responses to intracortical microelectrode arrays: challenges and future prospects. Front Neuroeng. 2014;7:24.
8. Foerster O. Beitrage zur pathophysiologie der sehbahn und der spehsphare. J Psychol Neurol. 1929;39:435–63.
9. Penfield W, Rasmussen T. The cerebral cortex of man. New York: Macmillan; 1950.
10. Brindley GS, Lewin WS. The sensations produced by electrical stimulation of the visual cortex. J Physiol (Lond). 1968;196:479–93.
11. Dobelle WH, et al. 'Braille' reading by a blind volunteer by visual cortex stimulation. Nature. 1976;259:111–2.
12. Dobelle WH. Artificial vision for the blind by connecting a television camera to the visual cortex. Asaio J. 2000;46(1):3–9.
13. Schmidt EM, et al. Feasibility of a visual prosthesis for the blind based on intracortical microstimulation of the visual cortex. Brain. 1996;119(Pt 2):507–22.
14. Perge JA, et al. Intra-day signal instabilities affect decoding performance in an intracortical neural interface system. J Neural Eng. 2013;10(3):036004.
15. Homer ML, et al. Sensors and decoding for intracortical brain computer interfaces. Annu Rev Biomed Eng. 2013;15:383–405.

16. Hochberg LR, et al. Neuronal ensemble control of prosthetic devices by a human with tetraplegia. Nature. 2006;442(7099):164–71.
17. Truccolo W, et al. Single-neuron dynamics in human focal epilepsy. Nat Neurosci. 2011;14(5):635–41.
18. Morillas CA, et al. A design framework to model retinas. Biosystems. 2007;87(2–3):156–63.
19. Romero S, et al. Reconfigurable retina like preprocessing platform for cortical visual neuroprosthesis. In: Akay M, editor. Handbook of neural engineering. Hoboken: Wiley-IEEE Press; 2007. p. 267–79.
20. Rush AD, Troyk PR. A power and data link for a wireless-implanted neural recording system. IEEE Trans Biomed Eng. 2012;59(11):3255–62.
21. Bradley DC, et al. Visuotopic mapping through a multichannel stimulating implant in primate V1. J Neurophysiol. 2005;93(3):1659–70.
22. Kane S, et al. Electrical performance of penetrating microelectrodes chronically implanted in cat cortex. IEEE Trans Biomed Eng. 2013;60:2153–60. doi:10.1109/TBME.2013.2248152.
23. Lewis PM, et al. Restoration of vision in blind individuals using bionic devices: a review with a focus on cortical visual prostheses. Brain Res. 2015;1595:51–73.
24. Merabet LB, et al. 'Who is the ideal candidate?': decisions and issues relating to visual neuroprosthesis development, patient testing and neuroplasticity. J Neural Eng. 2007;4(1):S130–5.
25. Rousche PJ, Normann RA. A method for pneumatically inserting an array of penetrating electrodes into cortical tissue. Ann Biomed Eng. 1992;20:413–22.
26. House PA, et al. Acute microelectrode array implantation into human neocortex: preliminary technique and histological considerations. Neurosurg Focus. 2006;20(5):E4.
27. Maynard EM, Fernandez E, Normann RA. A technique to prevent dural adhesions to chronically implanted microelectrode arrays. J Neurosci Methods. 2000;97(2):93–101.
28. Davis TS, et al. Spatial and temporal characteristics of V1 microstimulation during chronic implantation of a microelectrode array in a behaving macaque. J Neural Eng. 2012;9(6):065003.
29. Stacey WC, et al. Potential for unreliable interpretation of EEG recorded with microelectrodes. Epilepsia. 2013;54(8):1391–401.
30. Fernandez E, et al. Perceptions elicited by electrical stimulation of human visual cortex. Invest Opthalmol Vis Sci. 2015;56: ARVO E-Abstract 777.
31. Dagnelie G, et al. Paragraph text reading using a pixelized prosthetic vision simulator: parameter dependence and task learning in free-viewing conditions. Invest Ophthalmol Vis Sci. 2006;47(3):1241–50.
32. Thompson Jr RW, et al. Facial recognition using simulated prosthetic pixelized vision. Invest Ophthalmol Vis Sci. 2003;44(11):5035–42.
33. Veraart C, et al. Pattern recognition with the optic nerve visual prosthesis. Artif Organs. 2003;27(11):996–1004.
34. Sinha P. Recognizing complex patterns. Nat Neurosci. 2002;5(Suppl):1093–7.
35. Pascual-Leone A, et al. The plastic human brain cortex. Annu Rev Neurosci. 2005;28: 377–401.
36. Merabet LB, Pascual-Leone A. Neural reorganization following sensory loss: the opportunity of change. Nat Rev Neurosci. 2010;11(1):44–52.
37. Fernandez E, Merabet LB. Cortical plasticity and reorganization in severe vision loss. In: Dagnelie G, editor. Visual prosthetics, New York. Springer; 2011.
38. Merabet LB. Building the bionic eye: an emerging reality and opportunity. Prog Brain Res. 2011;192:3–15.

Chapter 16
The Intracortical Visual Prosthesis Project

Philip R. Troyk

Abstract The possibility of engineering, testing, and deploying a cybernetic interface to the visual areas of the human brain has inspired scientists, biomedical engineers, clinicians, and science fiction writers. Implemented as a cortical visual prosthesis, visual perception might be provided to individuals with blindness. Based upon pioneering work in the late 1960's, and the development of significant technology throughout the remainder of the twentieth century, the Intracortical Visual Prosthesis (ICVP) is being planned for clinical trial. Autonomous, wireless, 16-channel stimulator modules will be used to tile the dorsolateral surface of the human occipital lobe. Each module will contain 16 intracortical electrodes that penetrate the cortical surface and provide simulation currents to visual processing areas of the brain. Through the use of spatial and temporal integration, the expectation is that the brain will convert the artificial visual information into useful visual perceptions. While it is not expected that the ICVP will produce normal vision, prior work strongly suggests that the artificial visual perception may notably enhance the user's ability to recognize objects and navigate, and improve overall quality of life.

Keywords Visual prosthesis • Intracortical electrodes • Wireless implantable devices • Cortical visual prosthesis • Intracortical Visual Prosthesis (ICVP) • Psychophysics • Wireless Floating Microelectrode Array (WFMA)

Key Points

- Forming an artificial interface to the visual cortex was the first method attempted for a visual prosthesis. Although retinal prostheses have seen more recent successes, the cortical approach would be applicable to a larger user population.
- The intracortical approach uses microelectrodes that penetrate the cortex with tip sizes of unit micron size, rather than unit millimeter-sized electrodes placed over the pia. The pool of neurons recruited by the

P.R. Troyk, PhD
Department of Biomedical Engineering, Illinois Institute of Technology, Chicago, IL, USA
e-mail: troyk@iit.edu

V.P. Gabel (ed.), *Artificial Vision*, DOI 10.1007/978-3-319-41876-6_16

closely-spaced microelectrodes is substantially smaller than that recruited by surface electrodes, so the spatial resolution is higher.

- The Wireless Floating Microelectrode Array (WFMA) is powered by, and communicated through, a transcutaneous inductive link which eliminates both transcutaneous connectors and implanted cables that would be tethered to the array. Thus the 16-channel WFMA stimulator "floats" on the surface of the brain.
- Unlike retinal prostheses, cortical prostheses require mapping of the spatial visual percepts (phosphenes). Multimodal mapping techniques can minimize mapping errors.
- How the ICVP system might be used for visually-guided tasks is presently unknown. Because the system interfaces directly with the visual cortex, use of higher-order percepts may enable the formation of a "percept-based language" for communication of artificial visual information directly to the brain.

The Cortical Approach

Ideas for using electrical stimulation to communicate artificially-acquired visual information, i.e. from a technological imaging device, to the human visual system in order to compensate for visual deficit or disease date from the first half of the twentieth century. Conceptually, an artificial electrical connection to the visual system can be made in several physical locations including: retinal, choroid, optic nerve, lateral geniculate nucleus, and visual cortex. Although in the past 10 years the retinal approach has seen the most clinical success, a large majority of people with blindness are not candidates for retinal prostheses due to the pathology of their visual deficits which affects a combination of the retina and optic nerve functionality. Prior to the availability of modern ophthalmic surgical methods which now permit retinal, and other orbit-located artificial stimulation devices, to be connected to the eye, the brain was a more obvious target for interfacing a visual prosthesis. The basic premise of a cortical visual prosthesis is that by providing coordinated spatial-temporal electrical stimulation directly to the cortical visual system, one can manipulate the eloquent visual neural machinery of the brain, bypassing the retina, optic nerve, and thalamus, and creating a useful visual perception. Therefore, interest in developing a clinically-deployable cortical visual prosthesis remains high.

The understanding that artificial stimulation of the visual cortex could cause visual perceptions was known in the 1920's and subsequently researched by Penfield [31, 32], and others, through the 1950's. As early as 1955, a patent by Shaw [36] described a device to restore visual perception via electrical stimulation of the brain. Using technology of the time, it was proposed to connect the output of a photocell to percutaneous electrodes that were implanted into the occipital lobe. This concept was independently tested through experiments by Button and Putnam [8], in which three volunteers were implanted with four wires that penetrated cranial burr holes and were inserted into the occipital lobe. An electrical modulator circuit changed the electrical stimulus frequency and amplitude, applied to the electrodes, in accordance with the photocell output. During a testing time of several weeks, the subjects used the system to scan the area around them by moving their photocell with their hands. Functionally, they were able to locate illuminated objects in near proximity, including incandescent lamps and birthday cake candles. Unfortunately, at that time little was known about safe stimulation limits or how to appropriately drive implanted electrodes, and the resulting visual perception often filled the subjects' entire visual field, thus limiting the practical use to merely determining light from dark. However, this crude device did include all of the essential elements that were later implemented within a cortical prosthesis: a light-to-electric transducer, a means for changing electrical stimulation based upon the light transduction, and implanted cortical electrodes.

Following the Hubel and Wiesel [23] discovery of the functional structure of visual cortex, it became seriously considered that by using coherent patterns of cortical electrical stimulation, inducing useful artificial visual perceptions might be possible. In bold experiments, Brindley and Lewin [5], were the first to investigate chronic cortical stimulation directed towards the goal of a visual prosthesis. A 52-year old woman was implanted with a complex electronic stimulation system that consisted of 80 platinum electrode discs, placed on the surface of the occipital pole, and 80 trancutaneously-powered electrical stimulators, one for each electrode and measuring about the size of a U.S. Quarter, implanted subcutaneously within the right cortical hemisphere. Approximately 32 independent phosphenes, of various sizes and shapes, were obtained, and their electrical thresholds of perception were measured. Attempts were made to combine the phosphenes into crude letters and shape outlines. However, this early cortical visual prosthesis did not prove to be of any practical use to the subject. A second subject received a similar implanted system in 1972 [4, 6, 7, 34]. For these 80 implanted electrodes, and stimulators, 79 of them produced phosphenes, similar to those experienced in the first subject, and they were meticulously mapped over 3 years, post-implant. These pioneering experiments demonstrated: the feasibility of implanting a multitude of electrodes and associated electronics, the continued functionality of the visual cortex following years of blindness, and the long-term stability of phosphenes. However, little knowledge was gained about how cortically-induced phosphenes might be integrated to produce meaningful sensory perceptions.

The purposeful stimulation of the visual cortex via large (1–2 mm) surface electrodes placed upon the pia-arachnoid surface along the midline of the occipital pole, was further investigated by Dobelle [13–15, 33] and others, culminating in a series of implantations within 16 blind recipients by Dobelle in 2000–2005. The earlier Dobelle work tested the ability of the implanted subjects to use the artificial perceptions to "read visual Braille" [15]. However, reading rates were considerably less that what could be obtained by tactile Braille. Unfortunately the later work was not published, it remains shrouded in uncertainty about aspects of the subjects' recruitment and participation, reports in the popular press have described notable inducing of seizures from the cortical surface stimulation, and the knowledge about the visual function obtained from these surface-based cortical systems remain anecdotal.

Intracortical Visual Prostheses

Following the work of Brindley, in 1969 the NIH formed the neural prosthesis program, and later (1986) the intramural intracortical visual prosthesis program, with the goal of developing and implanting a cortical visual prosthesis that used intracortical, rather than surface, stimulation of the visual cortex. The premise was that small needle-like electrodes that penetrated striate cortex, with exposed tips areas (20–30 sq microns) about the size of cortical neurons, would be able to produce better-controlled and more distinct phosphenes, than had been obtained from the larger surface electrodes. Perceptual integration of tens, or hundreds, of these intracortical phosphenes would result in the desired visual perception. To accomplish this aggressive goal required development of enabling technology that allowed for safe implantation of large numbers of intracortical electrodes, and during the next 20 years (1976–1996) numerous extramural technology-development contracts were funded by the NIH. Based upon studies by Bartlett and Doty [2] in Macaques, as well as acute intracortical microstimulation studies in sighted patients undergoing occipital craniotomy [1], a short-term implantation of intracortical microelectrodes, using percutaneous wires, was done in a human volunteer who had been blind for 22 years secondary to glaucoma [35]. The goals of this study were to determine if intracortical electrodes could produce punctate phosphenes following many years of blindness. Although later suffering from technological complications, 34 of the 38 microelectrodes initially produced distinct phosphenes with threshold currents in the range of 1.9–25μA, orders of magnitude lower than the currents necessary for the earlier work using surface electrodes. Intracortical microelectrodes spaced 500 μm apart generated separate phosphenes, but microelectrodes spaced 250 μm typically did not. Importantly, this two-point resolution was about five times better than had previously been achieved with electrodes on the cortical surface. These encouraging results motivated further work to develop the technology, surgical methods, and functional implementation of an intracortical system.

The ICVP Project

The NIH intramural program ended in 1996, and was reconstituted in 2000 as the Intracortical Visual Prosthesis Project (ICVP) at the Illinois Institute of Technology. Following work in Macaques [3, 38], the ICVP concept was matured into that shown in Fig. 16.1. As first reported in [39–41], to replace the numerous implanted packages connected to electrodes by wires used in earlier work, the Wireless Floating Microelectrode Array (WFMA) was developed for the ICVP. Shown in

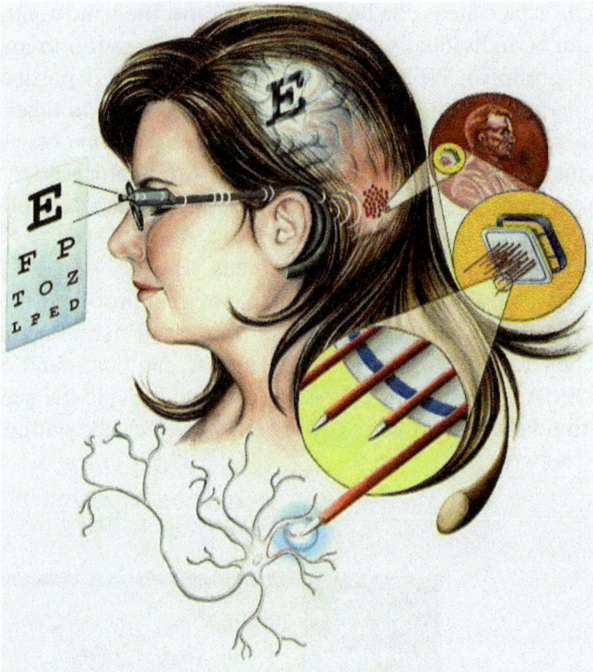

Fig. 16.1 Artist's concept drawing of the ICVP. A collection of miniature wireless stimulator modules (WFMA) implanted on the occipital lobe communicate artificial image information directly to the visual cortex. Electrode size is shown relative to a human hair (Courtesy of Illinois Institute of Technology)

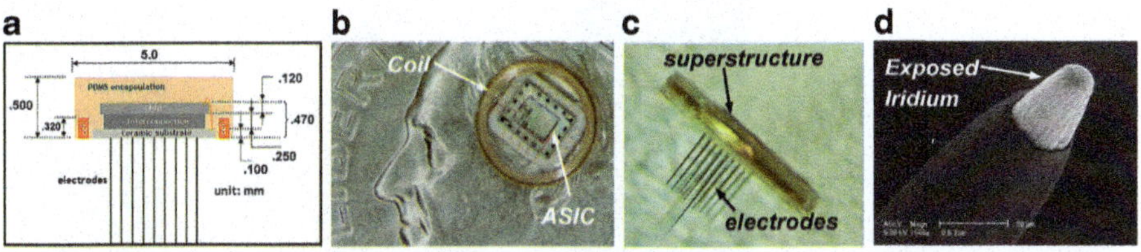

Fig. 16.2 Details of the WFMA stimulator module. (**a**) Sectional drawing of WFMA – for clarity not all drawing dimensions to scale. (**b**) Top view of WFMA on US Dime. (**c**) Side view of WFMA showing electrodes. (**d**) SEM photograph of typical electrode black is Parylene insulation, bright is iridium metal (Courtesy of Illinois Institute of Technology)

Fig. 16.2, the WFMA is physically comprised of a ceramic substrate platform that maintains the lateral position of eighteen (16 + reference + counter) Parylene-insulated iridium microelectrodes, and provides electrical interconnection between a superstructure that contains an electronic application-specific-integrated circuit (ASIC) and microcoil, to form a fully-integrated autonomous wireless stimulator module. The electrode tips are individually exposed by laser ablation of the Parlyene and the exposed surface areas can be individually specified and controlled; the electrode lengths can be individually controlled during fabrication to implement specified lengths. A group of WFMAs comprise the implanted portion of the ICVP System, each module controlling 16 electrodes. In contrast to other cortical-based neural interfaces, that use either percutaneous connectors or pacemaker-style implanted modules, the WFMA is an autonomous stimulator device that penetrates the pia-arachnoid membrane, floats within the subdural space and eliminates cable-induced tethering forces upon the brain.

Each WFMA device receives power and data wirelessly over a transcutaneous inductive link activated by an extracorporal telemetry controller (TC). As shown in Fig. 16.3, the ICVP recipient would wear a head-band that contains the TC, and connects to a belt-worn signal processor. The TC can command each electrode, within each WFMA, in a random-access fashion and provide the needed intracortical electrical stimulation – similar to calling up each electrode within an "implanted mobile-phone" network.

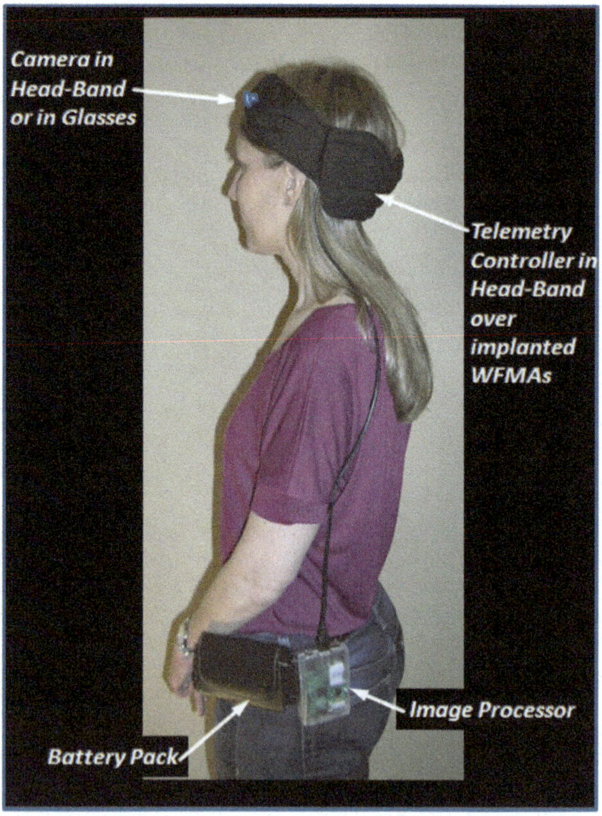

Fig. 16.3 Physical configuration of the portable ICVP system. The telemetry controller within the headband powers the implanted WFMAs and receives commands from the belt-worn signal processor. A camera within the headband, or in spectacles, provides the video image that gets communicated to the cortical visual system (Courtesy of Illinois Institute of Technology)

Surgical Methods

Clinical testing of the ICVP system has been planned, and of critical importance is the location and extent of WFMA implantation. These choices involve a balance between minimizing surgical risk and maximizing likelihood of visual function. There is long-standing and detailed information regarding the layout and variability of human visual cortical areas, the visual field representations in these areas, and the characteristics of phosphenes elicited in these areas. Methodologies used to collect this information range from post-mortem anatomical [19, 37] and in-vivo lesion (trauma and epilepsy; [21, 22]) studies, recording and stimulation with indwelling electrodes in sighted epilepsy patients [14, 24, 26] and blind individuals [5, 8, 35], more recently functional MRI [12, 27–29, 42], and transcranial magnetic stimulation [16]. The most relevant considerations are:

1. Without certain knowledge about providing visual function, minimizing the surgical risk suggests avoiding the placement of WFMAs in the calcarine fissure, on the medial wall, or near the torcula, and thus limits the available anatomical area to the occipito-dorso-lateral surface and posterior inferior gyrus.
2. Inter-individual variability of the size of cortical areas (by ~50 %) and occipitally-exposed V1 (0–10 mm, median 4 mm) will most likely force placement of some WFMA units in higher visual areas; WFMA placement is likely to range beyond V2 and V3 and thus cover multiple visual field representations.
3. While simple round phosphenes will typically be elicited in V1-V3, those in higher areas may have more complex shapes; it is possible that these higher-order percepts cannot be easily integrated into V1-V3-based image perceptions.
4. Based on available fMRI evidence, phosphenes from occipito-dorso-lateral implants may extend to ~25°, while the study reported by Schmidt et al. [35] reported phosphenes up to 45° eccentricity. One advantage of the anatomical choice of the occipito-dorso-lateral surface, for implanting the WFMAs, is that a larger phosphene eccentricity range may be obtained than if implantation was restricted to the minimal surgical risk regions of V1, albeit with an increase in the variability in the phosphene perception. However, having these electrodes in extrastriate cortex may allow, as some researchers have speculated, for the use of higher-order percepts. Figure 16.4 shows the cortical area most likely to be used for the proposed WFMA modules, and the expected resulting phosphene distribution in relative size and location.

For the early ICVP recipients, surgical implantation (using a high-speed inserter tool) of the WFMA modules will be restricted to one hemisphere. For the first implanted subject, a small number (about nine WFMA modules – 144 electrodes) will be implanted over the right lateral occipital region near the midline in a 3×3 pattern. Under aseptic technique, a 3 cm paramedian incision will expose the skull. Following the craniotomy, the dura will be opened with flaps based on the midline and inferior sinuses to allow access to the occipital tip and lateral cortex. As the

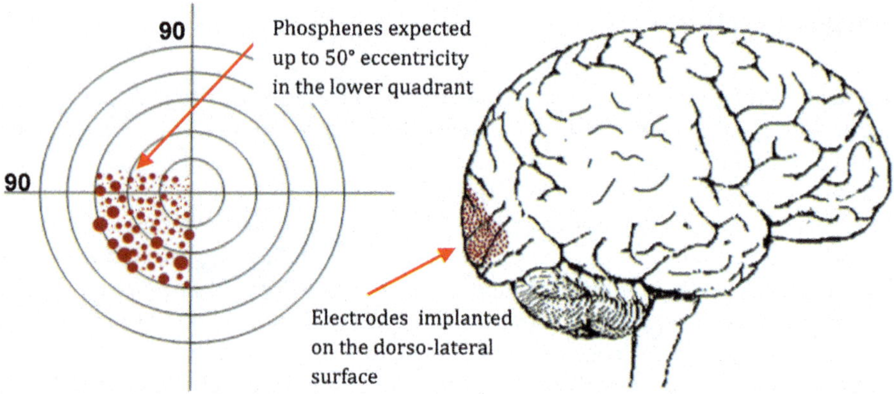

Fig. 16.4 Visual map (*left*) with various-sized phosphenes distributed up to 50° eccentricities, for electrodes implanted on the lateral surface area within a radius of 3 cm from the occipital pole, based on findings of [24, 35]; fMRI studies limit the likely eccentricities to ~25° (Courtesy of Illinois Institute of Technology)

WFMAs will be inserted, care will be taken to avoid superficial blood vessels. The dura will be closed in a water-tight fashion, the bone will be reconstructed with craniofacial plating, and the skin will be closed in layers using a water-tight technique. Following evaluation of the stability of the neural interface in the first subject, subsequent volunteers will be implanted with larger numbers of WFMAs; anticipating the available cortical area, implantation of up to 600 electrodes will be possible.

Clinical Pilot Study

Since a clinical trial of the ICVP system has yet to be implemented, a description of the anticipated components of the trial follows:

1. **Dynamic Characteristics of All Electrodes/Phosphenes:** For each electrode it will be necessary to determine its threshold (lowest current eliciting a visual percept), ceiling (lower of the current limits allowed by safe stimulation and perceptual comfort), and approximate number of just noticeable brightness difference steps: an indication of the maximum number of grey levels each electrode can convey. The effects of varying stimulation parameters including pulse amplitude, pulse width, burst length, burst frequency, and burst repetition rate will be measured.
2. **Phosphene Mapping:** Unlike retinal prostheses, for which the location of phosphenes in visual space can be estimated based upon the relative pattern and location of the electrodes on the retina, cortical prostheses require functional mapping in order to determine the spatial location of each phosphene, produced

by single or groups of electrodes, within visual space. This is due to the uncertainties in the form and intertwining of the cortical retinotopic maps that will be accessed by the intracortical electrodes. Established mapping strategies have been developed so as to construct a phosphene map for all functional electrodes, using touchscreen and eye movement procedures [9] for all electrodes, and the pair direction procedure for clustered phosphenes [25]. In the touchscreen procedure, fixation is maintained while the subject moves the index finger of the ipsilateral hand across a touchscreen to the perceived phosphene location. In the eye movement method the phosphene is shown briefly while fixation is maintained, and a saccade is then made to the remembered phosphene location. In the pair direction procedure, a pair of phosphenes is shown in quick sequence, and the subject traces on the touchscreen the perceived relative direction from the 1st to the 2nd phosphene. A least squares fitting method is used to unify the resulting maps.

3. **Ability to Convey Basic Visual Percepts:** The phosphene maps will be used to identify clusters that will allow presentation of solid objects and outlines (simple geometric shapes, Landolt C, Lea symbols), and explore basic visual properties of phosphene-based images, addressing questions such as:

    (a) If an outline is presented, are the phosphenes seen as isolated dots, or is there (partial) continuity?
    (b) Do adjacent phosphenes from distant electrodes show less "filling in" than those from adjacent electrodes?
    (c) Will there be any filling in of the center when a (small) object is presented as an outline?
    (d) Can filling in be improved by stimulating phosphenes inside a contour, even using distant electrodes?
    (e) Is there a perceptual difference between computer-generated objects/outlines and those generated from a camera image, and does this depend on the presence of eye/head/camera movements?
    (f) Does the perception of object movement generated by a head-mounted camera differ from that caused by object movement not elicited by the ICVP wearer?

Once the basic phosphene properties are established, and associated with a reliable map, image processing algorithms will be used to transform arbitrary images into cortical stimulation patterns, and the ICVP recipient will be trained in simple shape recognition and other elementary visual tasks. To assess the functional utility of the ICVP system multiple measuring instruments will be used:

1. Impact of Vision Impairment – Very Low Vision [18], a 32 item questionnaire with a Likert difficulty scale (0-not at all to 5-impossible) designed and validated for individuals with very low vision
2. Melbourne IADL-VLV assessment [17], with 11 instrumental activities of daily living for individuals with very low vision, to which observation-based performance scores are assigned

The VLV instruments named above were designed for individuals who have at least rudimentary form vision, and thus may not be sensitive to the visual perception levels mediated by the ICVP. Two emerging instruments, developed to specifically address ultra-low vision (ULV, limited to seeing hand movements, light projection, and bare light perception) are likely to yield useful quantitative measures of ICVP-mediated visual perception:

3. The PLoVR ULV questionnaire [10] consists of 150 items, but an adaptive version that yields a calibrated visual ability score after administration of 10–20 items is now available [11].
4. The PLoVR ADL assessment consists of 17 activities that can be administered at different difficulty levels and is currently being calibrated; an adaptive version of this set is under development.

Use of ICVP for Performing Functional Visual Tasks

In normal vision, the brain often "fills in details" (plasticity) for identifying familiar objects, and continued use of the ICVP may produce a similar progression in visual function, leading to increasingly successful visual discrimination and reduced reaction times. This assumes, however, that phosphenes elicited in different cortical areas can be combined into single compound percepts, but this is by no means guaranteed. For example, phosphenes in V1 may respond very differently to the spatio-temporal information gained from scanning than those in higher areas, and this may affect the perceptual coherence of the image, and thus the subject's performance. Outside of V1 some electrodes may not elicit punctate phosphenes, or may not initially evoke any conscious response [26, 30]. However, even for stimulating electrodes which do not evoke phosphenes, after many trials subjects can learn to perceive them [20]. In the best-case scenario, the ICVP recipients will learn to ignore these differences and progressively achieve integrated perception, even though this may differ from vision as they used to know it. In the worst-case scenario phosphenes elicited in higher visual areas will need to be excluded from the image processing, reducing the ability to present detail (e.g., visual acuity). It may be possible to exploit the properties of higher-order phosphenes and use specific aspects of their appearance to convey certain properties present in the scene. Colored phosphenes may be utilized to signal the presence of large swaths of that color in the scene; unusually shaped phosphenes might be used as abstract signs or codes to signal the presence of a person or the #7 city bus in the camera image; provided the implanted subject can distinguish them reliably from other phosphenes, each of these phosphenes could be given its own meaning through an intelligent image processing app, many of which are routinely available in smartphones. Use of the ICVP system, which can access higher visual centers, may permit, or require, the development of a new symbolic visual prosthetic "language" through which new visual scene recognition will be realized.

References

1. Bak M, Girvin JP, Hambrecht FT, Kufta CV, Loeb GE, Schmidt EM. Visual sensations produced by intracortical microstimulation of the human occipital cortex. Med Biol Eng Comput. 1990;28:257–9.
2. Bartlett JR, Doty RW. An exploration of the ability of macaques to detect microstimulation of the striate cortex. Acta Neurobiologiae Expermentalis (Warzawa). 1980;40:713–28.
3. Bradley DC, Troyk PR, Berg JA, Bak M, Cogan S, Erickson R, et al. Visuotopic mapping through a multichannel stimulating implant in primate V1. J Neurophysiol. 2005;93(3): 1659–70.
4. Brindley GS. Sensory effects of electrical stimulation of the visual and paravisual cortex in man. In: Jung R, editor. Handbook of sensory physiology, vol. VII/3. Berlin: Springer; 1973. p. 583–94.
5. Brindley GS, Lewin WS. The sensations produced by electrical stimulation of the visual cortex. J Physiol (Lond). 1968;196:479–93.
6. Brindley GS, Rushton DN. Observations on the representation of the visual field on the human occipital cortex. In: Hambrecht FT, Reswick JB, editors. Functional electrical stimulation: applications in neural prostheses. New York: Marcel Dekker; 1977. p. 261–76.
7. Brindley GS, Donaldson PEK, Falconer M, Rushton DN. The extent of the region of occipital cortex that when stimulated gives phosphenes fixed in the visual field. J Physiol (Lond). 1972;225:57P–8.
8. Button J, Putnam T. Visual responses to cortical stimulation in the blind. J Iowa Med Soc. 1962;LII(1):17–21.
9. Dagnelie G, Yin VT, Hess D, Yang L. Phosphene mapping strategies for cortical visual prosthesis recipients. J Vis. 2003;3(9):222.
10. Dagnelie G, Jeter PE, Adeyemo K, Rozanski C, Nkodo AF, Massof RW. Psychometric properties of the PLoVR ultra-low vision (ULV) questionnaire. Invest Ophthalmol Vis Sci. 2014;55(13):2150.
11. Dagnelie G, Barry MP, Adeyemo O, Jeter PE, Massof RW. Twenty questions: an adaptive version of the PLoVR ultra-low vision (ULV) questionnaire. Invest Ophthalmol Vis Sci. 2015;56(7):497.
12. DeYoe EA, Carman GJ, Bandettini P, Glickman S, Wieser J, Cox R, Miller D, Neitz J. Mapping striate and extrastriate visual areas in human cerebral cortex. Proc Natl Acad Sci. 1996; 93(6):2382–6.
13. Dobelle WH, Mladejovsky MG. Phosphenes produced by electrical stimulation of human occipital cortex, and their application to the development of a prosthesis for the blind. J Physiol (Lond). 1974;243:553–76.
14. Dobelle WH, Mladejovsky MG, Girvin JP. Artificial vision for the blind: electrical stimulation of visual cortex offers hope for a functional prosthesis. Science. 1974;183:440–4.
15. Dobelle WH, Mladejovsky MG, Evans JR, Roberts TS, Girvin JP. 'Braille' reading by a blind volunteer by visual cortex stimulation. Nature. 1976;259:111–2.
16. Fernandez E, Alfaro A, Tormos JM, Climent R, Martınez M, Vilanova H, Pascual-Leone A. Mapping of the human visual cortex using image-guided transcranial magnetic stimulation. Brain Res Protoc. 2002;10(2):115–24.
17. Finger RP, McSweeney SC, Deverell L, O'Hare F, Bentley SA, Luu CD, Ayton LN. Developing an instrumental activities of daily living tool as part of the low vision assessment of daily activities protocol developing the IADL-VLV. Invest Ophthalmol Vis Sci. 2014;55(12): 8458–66.
18. Finger RP, Tellis B, Crewe J, Keeffe JE, Ayton LN, Guymer RH. Developing the Impact of Vision Impairment–Very Low Vision (IVI-VLV) questionnaire as part of the LoVADA protocol developing the IVI-VLV. Invest Ophthalmol Vis Sci. 2014;55(10):6150–8.
19. Flores LP. Occipital lobe morphological anatomy: anatomical and surgical aspects. Arq Neuropsiquiatr. 2002;60(3A):566–71.

20. Histed MH, Ni AM, Maunsell JH. Insights into cortical mechanisms of behavior from microstimulation experiments. Prog Neurobiol. 2013;103:115–30.
21. Holmes G. Disturbances of vision by cerebral lesions. Br J Ophthalmol. 1918;2(7):353.
22. Horton JC, Hoyt WF. The representation of the visual field in human striate cortex: a revision of the classic Holmes map. Arch Ophthalmol. 1991;109(6):816–24.
23. Hubel DH, Wiesel TN. Receptive fields, binocular interaction and functional architecture in the cat's visual cortex. J Physiol. 1962;160(1):106–54.2.
24. Kaido T, Hoshida T, Taoka T, Sakaki T. Retinotopy with coordinates of lateral occipital cortex in humans. J Neurosurg. 2004;101(1):114–8.
25. Kaskhedikar GP, Yang L, Boucher T, Troyk P, Dagnelie G. Development of mapping methods with simulated phosphenes for implementation in intracortical visual prosthesis recipients. Invest Ophthalmol Vis Sci. 2015;56(7):4315.
26. Lee HW, Hong SB, Seo DW, Tae WS, Hong SC. Mapping of functional organization in human visual cortex electrical cortical stimulation. Neurology. 2000;54(4):849–54.
27. Levy I, Hasson U, Avidan G, Hendler T, Malach R. Center–periphery organization of human object areas. Nat Neurosci. 2001;4(5):533–9.
28. McFadzean R, Brosnahan D, Hadley D, Mutlukan E. Representation of the visual field in the occipital striate cortex. Br J Ophthalmol. 1994;78(3):185–90.
29. McFadzean RM, Hadley DM, Condon BC. The representation of the visual field in the occipital striate cortex. Neuro-Ophthalmol. 2002;27(1–3):55–78.
30. Ni AM, Maunsell JH. Microstimulation reveals limits in detecting different signals from a local cortical region. Curr Biol. 2010;20(9):824–8.
31. Penfield W, Jasper H. Epilepsy and the functional anatomy of the human brain. London: Churchill; 1954, p.116–26, 404–6.
32. Penfield W, Rasmussen T. The cerebral cortex in man. New York: Macmillan; 1950.
33. Pollen DA. Some perceptual effects of electrical stimulation of the visual cortex in man. In: Tower DB, editor. The nervous system, vol. 2: the clinical neurosciences. New York: Raven; 1975. p. 519–28.
34. Rushton DN, Brindley GS. Short- and long-term stability of cortical electrical phosphenes. In: Rose FC, editor. Physiological aspects of clinical neurology. Oxford: Blackwell; 1977. p. 123–53.
35. Schmidt EM, Bak MJ, Hambrecht FT, Kufta CV, O'Rourke DK, Vallabhanath P. Feasibility of a visual prosthesis for the blind based on intracortical microstimulation of the visual cortex. Brain. 1996;119(Pt 2):507–22.
36. Shaw D. Method and means for aiding the blind. U.S. Patent no. 2,721,316; 1955.
37. Stensaas SS, Eddington DK, Dobelle WH. The topography and variability of the primary visual cortex in man. J Neurosurg. 1974;40:747–55.
38. Troyk PR, DeMichele GA. Inductively-coupled power and data link for neural prostheses using a class-E oscillator and FSK modulation. In Engineering in medicine and biology society, 2003. Proceedings of the 25th annual international conference of the IEEE. 2003a. vol. 4, p. 3376–9. IEEE.
39. Troyk P, Bak M, Berg J, Bradley D, Cogan S, Erickson R, Kufta C, McCreery D, Schmidt E, Towle V. A model for intracortical visual prosthesis research. Artif Organs. 2003b;27: 1005–15.
40. Troyk PR, Bradley D, Bak M, Cogan S, Erickson R, Hu Z, Towle V. Intracortical visual prosthesis research-approach and progress. In Engineering in Medicine and Biology Society, 2005. IEEE-EMBS 2005. 27th Annual International Conference of the IEEE. 2006a. p. 7376–9.
41. Troyk PR, Detlefsen DEA, DeMichele GAD. A multifunctional neural electrode stimulation ASIC using NeuroTalk TM interface. In Engineering in medicine and biology society, 2006. EMBS'06. 28th annual international conference of the IEEE. 2006b. p. 2994–7. IEEE.
42. Wandell BA, Brewer AA, Dougherty RF. Visual field map clusters in human cortex. Philos Trans R Soc Lond B Biol Sci. 2005;360(1456):693–707.

Chapter 17
Monash Vision Group's Gennaris Cortical Implant for Vision Restoration

Arthur James Lowery, Jeffrey V. Rosenfeld, Marcello G.P. Rosa, Emma Brunton, Ramesh Rajan, Collette Mann, Mark Armstrong, Anand Mohan, Horace Josh, Lindsay Kleeman, Wai Ho Li, and Jeanette Pritchard

Abstract The *Gennaris bionic vision system* is a wireless device that has been designed to directly stimulate the primary visual cortex to restore useful vision to people with bilateral, irreversible blindness. Here, we describe the end-to-end system and the design of each component. The rationale for design decisions is provided, including the benefits of cortical stimulation, the need for wireless power and data transmission and the format of the autonomous implant tiles and penetrating micro-electrode arrays. We discuss the broad population of people for which this device may provide benefit, with reference to specific indications of blindness.

Details of laboratory and preclinical tests that we have used to verify the electrical functionality of the device are described. A description of the surgical method that has been developed for implanting tiles in the visual cortex is provided, which

A.J. Lowery, BSc Dunelm, PhD (✉) • E. Brunton, PhD • C. Mann, PhD • A. Mohan, BE (FCD), ME, PhD
Department of Electrical and Computer Systems Engineering, Monash University, Clayton, VIC, Australia
e-mail: arthur.lowery@monash.edu

J.V. Rosenfeld, MD, MS, FRACS, FRCS, FACS
Monash Institute of Medical Engineering, Monash University, Clayton, VIC, Australia

M.G.P. Rosa, BSc, MSc, PhD
Department of Physiology, Monash Vision Group, Australian Research Council Centre of Excellence for Integrative Brain Function, Monash University, Clayton, VIC, Australia

R. Rajan, BSc(Hons), PhD
Department of Physiology, Neuroscience Program, Biomedicine Discovery Institute, Monash University, Clayton, VIC, Australia

M. Armstrong, DIP, ART, RMIT
Department of Design, Monash Art Design and Architecture, Caulfield, VIC, Australia

H. Josh, BEng (Hons), PhD • L. Kleeman, BE, BMath, PhD • W.H. Li, BE (HONS I), PhD
J. Pritchard, BSc (Hons), MPhil, PhD
Department of Electrical and Computer Systems Engineering, Monash University, Clayton, VIC, Australia

V.P. Gabel (ed.), *Artificial Vision*, DOI 10.1007/978-3-319-41876-6_17

will be used to demonstrate proof-of-concept of the system in first-in-human studies. Highlighted is the importance of post-surgical device calibration, psychophysics testing and training of recipients in using the system in both controlled and unsupervised environments. Signal processing algorithms that have been developed to enhance the user experience are described and details provided of how these have been tested to optimise their integration into the full system. Finally, we describe how the Gennaris technology can be applied to a broad spectrum of other technological and health-related challenges.

Keywords Cortical stimulation • Bionic vision • Wireless link • Implant tile • Hermetic • Penetrating electrodes • Annulus • Neurosurgery • Neural plasticity • Academic-industry partnership

Key Points

- Cortical stimulation for vision restoration has the potential to address a large number of cases of irreversible blindness, including those resulting from optic nerve damage.
- Wireless power and data transmission reduces risk of post-operative infection.
- Autonomous implant tiles allow for flexible electrode placement and hence we expect to optimise the functional outcome for each recipient of the device.

The Monash Vision Group's *Gennaris* cortical implant is designed to restore some vision to recipients who suffer from a wide variety of untreatable profound vision loss. It is based on a set of implantable tiles that have penetrating electrodes, to reach layer IV of the human visual cortex. It is known that precise stimulation of neuronal groups in the visual cortex generates visual percepts of light called phosphenes. Each tile has 43 electrodes, with the first generation of Gennaris able to support up to 11 tiles. The tiles receive power and data from a common wireless transmitter that is held at the back of the head on a custom designed glasses frame. Each tile is able to decode commands from a common data stream, to activate several electrodes at a time. The original image is received from a small camera mounted in the headgear. The image from the camera is processed to extract the most important information depending on the activity of the user. Gennaris is currently under the final stages of testing, with human trials planned for late 2017.

Introduction

The aim of the Monash Vision Group (MVG) system – called Gennaris – is to restore sufficient vision to the blind recipients so that they will be able to identify objects in front of them including the shapes of people and whether they are moving and to navigate the environment.

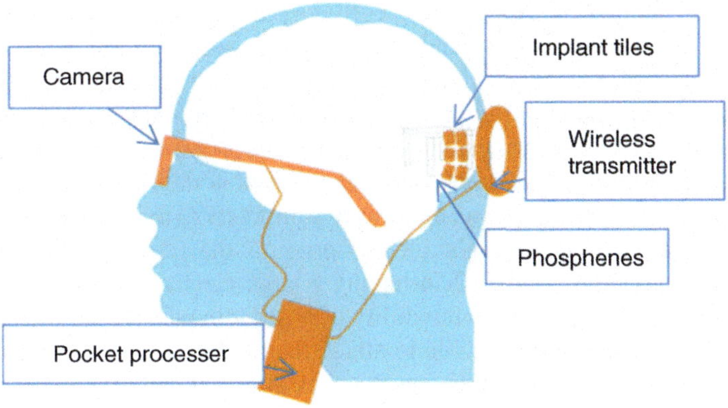

Fig. 17.1 Artistic impression of MVG's Gennaris bionic vision system showing the main components

MVG was established to provide an alternative approach to the development of a 'bionic vision prosthesis' in Australia, one based around cortical implants. Initial funding of A$10M, from 2010 to 2015, was granted by the Australian Research Council (ARC) under its Strategic Research Initiative in Bionic Vision Science and Technologies.

The multidisciplinary team was drawn together in mid-2009, by hand-picking individuals and partners that had the relevant skills and experience to design, develop, manufacture and test the devices. This team included Grey Innovation – an electronic products company, MiniFAB – a designer and manufacturer of medical devices, and clinicians at The Alfred Hospital – a leading trauma and general hospital in Melbourne. Within Monash University, skills were drawn from the faculties of Engineering, Science and Medicine; including researchers in electronics, robotic vision, neuroscience, bio-materials, physiology, industrial design and mathematics.

Principal Idea

The principal idea (Fig. 17.1) is to electrically stimulate the cell bodies and axons near the middle layers of human primary visual cortex (V1). Layer IV was chosen as the optimal target as this is where information from the visual thalamus is input to the cortex, and so the processing functions of V1 would not be lost. However, the targeting of a specific layer will necessarily be approximate, due to factors such as the variable curvature of the cortex, which introduces differences in relative thickness [3]. Also, previous studies by [7] had shown that the currents required to elicit a visual response (a phosphene) are much reduced when penetrating electrodes are used compared with cortical surface or subdural electrodes. Surface electrodes, as used by Dobelle in his wired stimulators [2], typically required more than 20× the stimulation current. Higher currents have the obvious disadvantage that the electronics system has to deliver these currents – impacting the design of the wireless power transmission system, and ultimately the lifetime of the battery – but also may cause epileptic seizures. Excessive heat may also be generated which may damage the neural tissue in the vicinity. A comprehensive review of approaches to cortical visual prostheses was published by [5].

A key design choice was to use a number of autonomous implant tiles to cover the visual cortex. This choice was made as it is impractical to image the smaller calibre blood vessels of the brain's surface prior to the craniotomy (see *Surgical Methods* section). Thus, rather than having a large electrode grid, several smaller tiles would be used to give some flexibility of positioning during surgery. It was also realised that it would be impossible to attach the tiles to a common wiring harness without this harness putting stress on the tiles after implantation. These tethering forces tend to progressively displace the tiles and therefore the electrodes. Thus, the tiles were designed to have their own individual wireless links to the external wireless transmitter, to provide them with power and data. A consequential design challenge has been the incorporation of a complete wireless receiver within such a tiny package – each tile package is only $9 \times 9 \times 2.5\text{-mm}^3$ – both from the point of view of the receiver coil being able to intersect enough of the transmitted power, but also because very small electronic components have to be used within the package (Fig. 17.2).

The wireless link also has to feed data to all of the tiles, and the individual tiles must be able to decode which commands are meant for them. Fortunately, or more accurately because of a huge and continuing investment by the electronics industry and the dedication of tens of thousands of engineers, electronics has shrunk in size to such a point that our Application-Specific Integrated Circuits (ASICs) have enough processing power to decode and correct the wireless messages that are sent

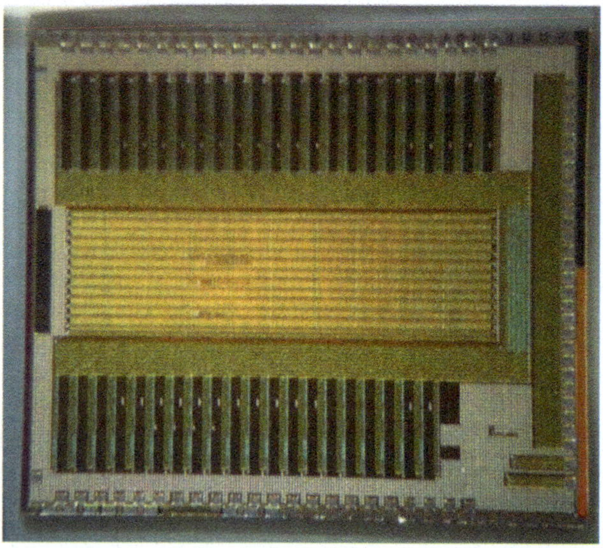

Fig. 17.2 As-fabricated mixed-signal ASIC photomicrograph

to them, and enough silicon area left over to provide independent drive currents to each electrode.

The data to activate the tiles is generated by an externally worn pocket-sized processor. This takes megapixel-sized images from a small video camera mounted in the headgear, and processes them down to a stimulation pattern of only a few-hundred pixels. The experience of our robotic-vision researchers was especially pertinent here, as robots have the same issues in analysing complex and cluttered images to extract the key information from them. In our case, work with groups of individuals who are blind, with the help of Vision Australia, identified situations such as meetings, where the key information includes how many people are paying attention. Thus, we developed algorithms to replace people's faces with emoticons. This field of research is known as Transformative Reality, in which a realistic image is transformed into a more useful image.

Indication for Certain Forms of Blindness

Gennaris effectively bypasses most of the visual system up until the primary visual cortex, or V1. Thus, it is expected to provide benefits to patients where, for example, retinal implants would not be suitable. Examples include severe retinal degeneration where the neural elements are lost such as end-stage glaucoma, optic nerve/chiasm disease or injury and patients who have lost their eyes through traumatic damage, or cancer (e.g. bilateral retinoblastoma). Thus, it is clear that a cortical approach will serve many causes of blindness, with the exception of cases where damage has occurred to the cortical visual systems. Another unresolved issue is whether people who have lost their vision at an early age, or who have congenital blindness, will have cortical circuits that could interpret the stimulation that we give them, or could possibly learn to use such stimulation usefully. This is a question for future research.

Technical Description

The system will be described by working backwards – that is, in the opposite direction to that which the signals flow. This is because the design is first constrained from the brain-end, rather than the camera end. An overview of the Gennaris system is described by [6].

Figure 17.3 shows a complete implant tile. It is a ceramic package with electrodes penetrating its underside (the side closest to the cortex). The electrodes are mostly insulated, apart from annular regions that are at the depth of layer IV of the human primary visual cortex. This 'annular' stimulating region design was chosen as it allows a better control of the electric fields around the electrode than stimulating from the electrode's tip, where the electric field would be highly dependent on

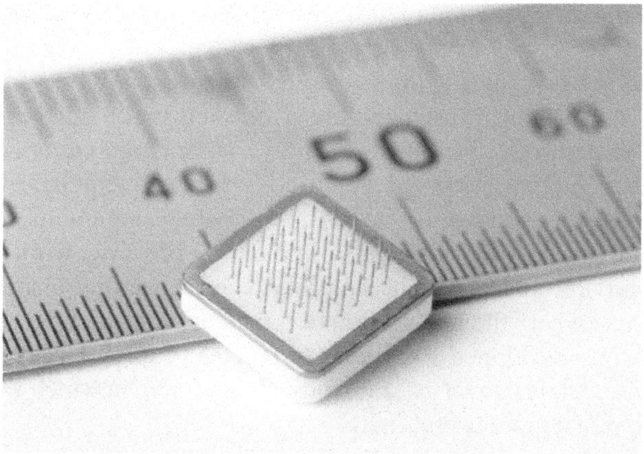

Fig. 17.3 An implant tile before Parylene coating

the exact radius of the tip. We also designed the electrodes assuming that there would be some tissue damage close to the electrode, so that the design objective was to have a sufficient electric field some distance from the electrode, rather than a field at the surface of the electrode. This leads to a mathematical optimisation, which suggests that a large uninsulated area is preferable to a smaller area. After testing we opted for an active surface area of around 40,000 μm^2 per electrode. The electrodes themselves are platinum-iridium (PtIr), which is a conventional and well-characterised material for human implants. As a result of the annular design, these electrodes are able to evoke stimulation responses while working at safe charge densities.

The wireless link is a conventional inductive link, in which inductors resonating with capacitors are used in the transmitter and receiver. The resonant coupling increases the coupling efficiency between the transmitter and receiver, though also reduces the available data bandwidth. Thus the data protocol has been made efficient by only sending 'activate' commands to the electrodes, rather than the actual waveforms. Flexibility to change the stimulation waveforms has been preserved by allowing the waveforms to be described during a programming phase of the tiles, which can be initiated at any time during the stimulation. A 500,000 transistor ASIC stores the simulation waveforms, and sends appropriate currents to each electrode when commanded to do so by the transmitter. The stimulation waveforms have a negative then a positive phase, with the intention of generating zero net charge after each stimulation. Any residual charge is removed during a 'grounding' phase.

Figure 17.4 shows a prototype of the headgear. This includes a camera at the front, and the transmitter coil at the rear. The position of the coil is adjustable, and can be locked into position post-surgery, to suit the positions of the implanted tiles. The headgear has been designed by Monash Art, Design and Architecture (MADA) to be comfortable over long periods, by careful selection of pressure points, the centre of gravity, choice of materials, adjustability, and minimisation of mass.

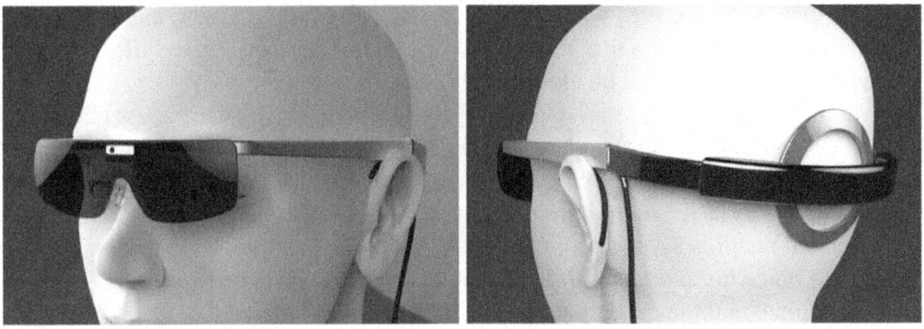

Fig.17.4 Headgear concept

Surgical Methods

The initial recipients of Gennaris will be medically and psychologically fit adults who have acquired blindness and who have total vision loss bilaterally. They will be required to undergo a detailed consent process to ensure they, and their supporters, have a realistic understanding of what to expect following the surgery. They will require medical screening tests and a brain magnetic resonance (MR) scan as part of the selection. They will need to have normal architecture of the visual cortex on the MR scan.

The surgical procedure itself will include a preoperative stereotactic localising MR scan so that the calcarine fissure and visual cortex can be accurately identified at surgery. For the first participants, the implantation of Gennaris device will be unilateral. We hypothesize that head movement, neural plasticity and visual cognitive systems will enable more complete visual constructs to be perceived from this unilateral input.

The operative procedure has been designed to enable a general neurosurgeon with some preliminary orientation and training to be able to perform the procedure. Each tile will be verified as being electrically functional before the sterilisation process prior to implantation. Perioperative antibiotics and anticonvulsants will be administered and then the patient placed under general anaesthesia, and placed prone on the operating table. The patient's head will be fixed in a frame and a small unilateral craniotomy will be performed in the occipital region to expose the occipital pole, adjacent cortex and the falx cerebri. Care will be taken to avoid any injury to the adjacent venous sinuses. The peri-calcarine cortex and occipital pole will be identified using the stereotactic guidance system.

The tiles will be placed in the primary visual cortex in an orientation that is approximately parallel to the external coil. This will ensure efficient and reliable wireless transmission. We do not intend to place tiles on the medial aspect of the hemisphere as they would be orthogonal to the wireless coil. Moreover, we will not place any tiles within the calcarine fissure, as this would unduly damage the adjacent cortex and the occipital lobe; our vision processing modelling in normally sighted subjects wearing a head-up display glasses suggests that stimulating this area is not necessary.

After insertion, the tiles will be covered with dural replacement and the cranial defect will be repaired so that there is no downward pressure on the tiles from the cranial flap. The scalp will be closed in the usual way.

We initially aim to place up to 6 tiles (giving a total of 258 electrodes) above and below the calcarine fissure at the occipital pole. Therefore, the tiles will be situated in the macular (central vision) area of the primary visual cortex. The tiles will be located in positions that avoid their electrodes passing through major blood vessels. If the visual result is satisfactory and as the technology improves in design we will be able to place more tiles in future recipients. The tiles can be removed if they are non-functional and the participant requests this.

Psychophysics and Patient Training

Once the patient has recovered from the operation and is mobile, the testing of the device and the rehabilitation phase commences. It is important to verify that the device is performing as we predicted; this will be achieved through extensive psychophysics testing with the participant.

The first phase of psychophysics assessment is phosphene mapping - measuring the spatial location and physical characteristics of phosphenes in relation to stimulating electrodes. An accurate map allows Gennaris to produce a more useful representation of the visual world. This mapping will vary between participants due to individual differences in brain anatomy and surgical variations in electrode placement. We expect that with several months of training, participants will be able to unconsciously identify shapes, movement and possibly large print letters.

Upon completion of the phosphene mapping, each participant will also need to learn how to use the device; that is, their brain needs to learn to adapt to this new form of visual input. Neural plasticity is thought to be necessary for the perception of these new images. This will likely take a number of months.

Integral to the testing and training phase is the use of image processing algorithms, that modify the camera data to represent the world in its simplest form and provide the most useful information to the participant. We have developed a library of algorithms that have been tested using the 'Hatpack'; a custom-built, portable, real-time and non-invasive head-worn device that presents a simulation of the world in bionic form to the user (Fig. 17.5). This has enabled us to optimise our image-processing algorithms for real-world situations that can present challenges to blind individuals. Details of the Hatpack device are described by [4].

Experimental Results

The safety and efficacy of the system have been verified in a number of ways. As with any electronic system, the development of electronic test systems is critical to the development of a product. The ASIC itself can perform a self-test, or 'boundary scan'

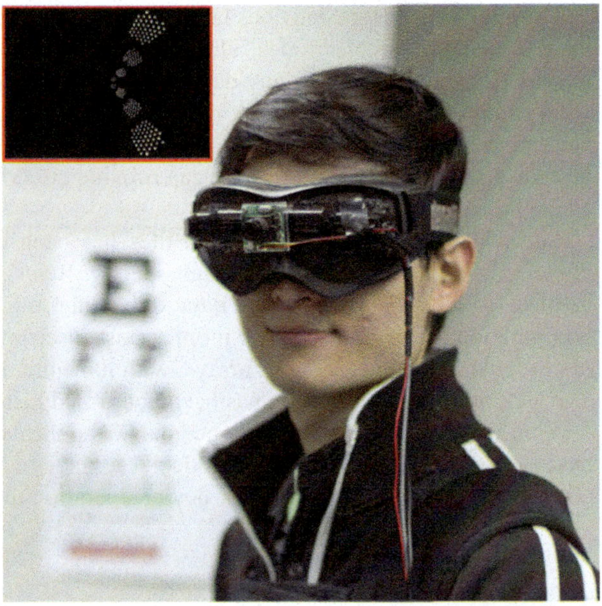

Fig. 17.5 Real-time head mounted simulator for Gennaris showing 8 implant tiles mapping into the user's visual field. Note the *top left insert* shows what the user sees with all electrodes activated

to verify the digital processing within it. When a batch of ASICs is manufactured, half of the chips are packaged in a manner that enables each analog output of the ASIC to be compliance tested. The remaining half are used in the tile manufacturing process. Firstly the ASICs are wire-bonded to a circuit board incorporating components for the wireless receiver. This complete assembly can then be tested before the final stages of packaging. After packaging, the tiles can be tested by illuminating them from a wireless transmitter, while monitoring the electrode currents. We have also placed the tiles in various stress tests, such as operation at elevated temperatures in a saline bath. The hermeticity of the tiles is also verifiable by using helium leak testing.

In addition to modelling studies of the electrodes, we have also conducted in-vivo studies in rats of real electrodes with the annulus design, comparing different materials, primarily PtIr with and without a coating of porous titanium nitride (TiN). This work is described by [1, 8]. Single electrodes or electrode arrays were implanted into the motor cortex of rats to determine the current required to evoke a motor response (whisking) and to measure the charge injection capacity (CIC) of the electrodes in the short-term experiments.

Long-term studies involved chronic implantation for up to 40 days, with electrodes stimulated for at least 4 h per day for up to 26 days with charge densities ranging from 1.3 to 71.4 $\mu C/cm^2/ph$. We collected electrochemical impedance spectroscopy and voltage transients daily before and after stimulation to monitor the condition of the electrodes and the surrounding tissue during the period of implantation; then at the end of the experiment brain tissue was collected and immunohistochemical staining performed for NeuN (a marker of neurons, to determine the number of live neurons) and GFAP (a marker of astrocytes, as a marker of the inflammatory response).

Despite using charge densities larger than what had previously been measured to be safe on the PtIr electrodes, electrochemical measures and scanning electron microscopy did not identify any damage to the electrodes that could be associated with stimulation. Further, histology demonstrated that healthy neurons were in close proximity to the electrodes and there was minimal astrogliosis. These studies provide a secure foundation that we can provide effective stimulation without damage to the cortex.

Surgical implantation of Gennaris tiles has been demonstrated using a sheep model. The technique is based on high-speed (>8 m/s) insertion using a pneumatic surgical tool, with preliminary data indicating minimal injury to the cortex. Examination of the brain up to 6 months post-insertion revealed a 50 micron zone of neuronal loss adjacent to the arrays, with the animal suffering no complications. The lack of long-term damage has been confirmed histologically.

Wireless transmission of power and data from the external coil to implanted tiles has also been achieved in a sheep model. The range of transmission is up to 30 mm, consistent with the requirement for device operation through the human skull.

Future Direction

The development of fully-implantable autonomous electronic stimulating tiles has encompassed many skills and has built up a large amount of knowledge on the design, manufacturing, testing and implantation techniques. Although the primary goal is to restore vision, it is easy to envisage how such technology could be used elsewhere in the body. Other regions of the cortex are an obvious choice: other regions of the cerebral cortex could be stimulated to replace particular senses, such as a proprioception, peripheral touch sensation and hearing.

An obvious development is for a recording tile to complement the stimulating tiles. This has some additional difficulty, as the signals being recorded are usually very small, so that the wireless power might disturb them. Ultimately, it may be possible to have reconfigurable electronics within the implants, allowing several applications to be serviced by a single device design.

Acknowledgement Special acknowledgement goes to Dr. Collette Mann, who sadly passed away before publication of this Book. As Monash Vision Group's Clinical Coordinator, Dr. Mann's contribution to this Chapter included the generation of human response data using our Hatpack bionic vision simulator, in addition to proof reading Chapter content.

References

1. Brunton EK, et al. In vivo comparison of the charge densities required to evoke motor responses using novel annular penetrating microelectrodes. Front Neuroeng. 2015; doi:10.3389/fneng.2015.00005.

2. Dobelle WH. Artificial vision for the blind by connecting a television camera to the visual cortex. ASAIO J. 2000;46:3–9.
3. Hilgetag CC, Barbas H. Role of mechanical factors in the morphology of the primate cerebral cortex. PLoS Comput Biol. 2006;2(3):e22.
4. Josh H, et al. 2012. Mobile, real-time simulator for a cortical visual prosthesis. Paper presented at BioDevices 2012 – Proceedings of the International Conference on Biomedical Electronics and Devices, Portugal. p. 37–46.
5. Lewis PM, et al. Restoration of vision in blind individuals using bionic devices: a review with a focus on cortical visual prostheses. Brain Res. 2015;1595:51–7.
6. Lowery AJ, et al. 2015. Restoration of vision using wireless cortical implants: the Monash Vision Group Project. Presented at the 37th Annual International Conference of the IEEE Engineering in Medicine and Biology Society, Milan, Paper WeBPoT14.8.
7. Schmidt EM, et al. Feasibility of a visual prosthesis for the blind based on intracortical micro-stimulation of the visual cortex. Brain. 1996;119(Pt 2):507–22.
8. Wang C, et al. Characteristics of electrode impedance and stimulation efficacy of a chronic cortical implant using novel annulus electrodes in rat motor cortex. J Neural Eng. 2013;10(4):046010.

Index

V.P. Gabel (ed.), *Artificial Vision*, DOI 10.1007/978-3-319-41876-6

The manufacturer's authorised representative in the EU is Springer Nature Customer Service Centre GmbH, Europaplatz 3, 69115 Heidelberg, Germany. If you have any concerns regarding our products, please contact ProductSafety@springernature.com

Printed and bound by CPI Group (UK) Ltd, Croydon, CR0 4YY
22/09/2026
02220946-0003